CHANGING CANCER PATTERNS
AND
TOPICS IN CANCER EPIDEMIOLOGY

Gann Monograph on Cancer Research

The "Gann Monograph on Cancer Research" series is promoted by the Japanese Cancer Association. This semiannual series of monographs was initiated in 1966 by the late Dr. Tomizo Yoshida (1903–1973) and is now published jointly by Japan Scientific Societies Press, Tokyo and Plenum Press, New York and London. Each volume consists of collected contributions on current topics in cancer problems and allied research fields. The planning for each volume is done by the Monograph Committee of the Japanese Cancer Association, with the final approval of the Board of Directors. It is hoped that the series will serve as an important source of information in the field of cancer research.

The publication of these monographs owes much to the financial support given by the late Professor Kazushige Higuchi, the Jikei University School of Medicine.

Japanese Cancer Association

JAPANESE CANCER ASSOCIATION

Gann Monograph on Cancer Research No.33

CHANGING CANCER PATTERNS AND TOPICS IN CANCER EPIDEMIOLOGY

IN MEMORY OF PROFESSOR MITSUO SEGI

Edited by
MINORU KURIHARA
KUNIO AOKI
ROBERT W. MILLER
CALUM S. MUIR

JAPAN SCIENTIFIC SOCIETIES PRESS, Tokyo
PLENUM PRESS, New York and London

April 1987

Published jointly by
JAPAN SCIENTIFIC SOCIETIES PRESS
2-10 Hongo, 6-chome, Bunkyo-ku, Tokyo 113, Japan
ISBN-13: 978-1-4684-1290-1   e-ISBN-13: 978-1-4684-1288-8
DOI: 10.1007/978-1-4684-1288-8

       and
PLENUM PRESS
233 Spring Street, New York, NY 10013, USA

Distributed in all areas outside Japan and Asia between Pakistan and Korea by PLENUM PRESS, New York and London.

PREFACE

Despite an enormous investment of effort throughout the world, cancer is still a major barrier to human longevity. Cancer deaths are estimated to be more than five million globally. Currently responsible for about 20% of all deaths in developed countries, the burden of cancer is steadily increasing in the developing world, following the control of malnutrition and infectious and parasitic diseases.

Deeply impressed by the report of the Symposium on Geographic Pathology and Demography of Cancer held at Oxford in 1950, and through his preliminary work on cancer mortality statistics in Japan, Professor M. Segi decided to devote his life to the fight against cancer by establishing worldwide comparative cancer statistics—one of the landmarks in cancer studies and in cancer prevention strategies.

He and his associates published six volumes of Cancer Mortality in 24 Countries with reliable mortality statistics covering 1950–1967, using the world population which he had derived as a standard. These publications rapidly became standard works of reference on the subject throughout the world.

Professor Segi was a pioneer of cancer epidemiology in Japan. He cleaved a path through the jungle of cancer using epidemiological methods. By promoting cancer studies, he overcame the poor understanding of malignant disease which existed after World War II, when cancer mortality rates were still low.

It is of great significance that the commemorative Monograph on Professor Segi appears as one of the Gann Monograph series supported by the Japanese Cancer Association, as cancer epidemiology currently plays an important role in the understanding and control of cancer in most parts of the world.

The title of the monograph "Changing Cancer Patterns and Topics in Cancer Epidemiology—in Memory of Professor Mitsuo Segi" characterizes Dr. Segi's continuous interest in not only static figures of cancer but also dynamic changes in trends which, as he repeatedly stated, reflect the influence of causal factors. This monograph consists of five parts, all of which are related to the research work Dr. Segi initiated in Japan: Changing cancer patterns, Cancer registration, Migrant studies, Topics in cancer epidemiology and International comparative studies.

The editors would like to express their sincere gratitude for the twenty-one papers contributed to this issue from various parts of the world. It was a great honor and pleasure to be able to include dedications to Dr. Segi from five distinguished scientists in the field of cancer research: Dr. Kaneyoshi Akazaki of Japan, Dr. Johannes Clemmesen of Denmark, Sir Richard Doll of the United Kingdom and Mr. William Haenszel and Dr. John Higginson of the United States of America, who were all on close terms with

Dr. Segi. We also express our deep appreciation to Dr. H. Sugano for suggesting this monograph and his encouragement during the prepublication stage.

We hope that this monograph will advance the study of cancer and will speed the day when this most tenacious enemy of mankind is overcome.

February 13, 1987

M. Kurihara
K. Aoki
R. W. Miller
C. S. Muir

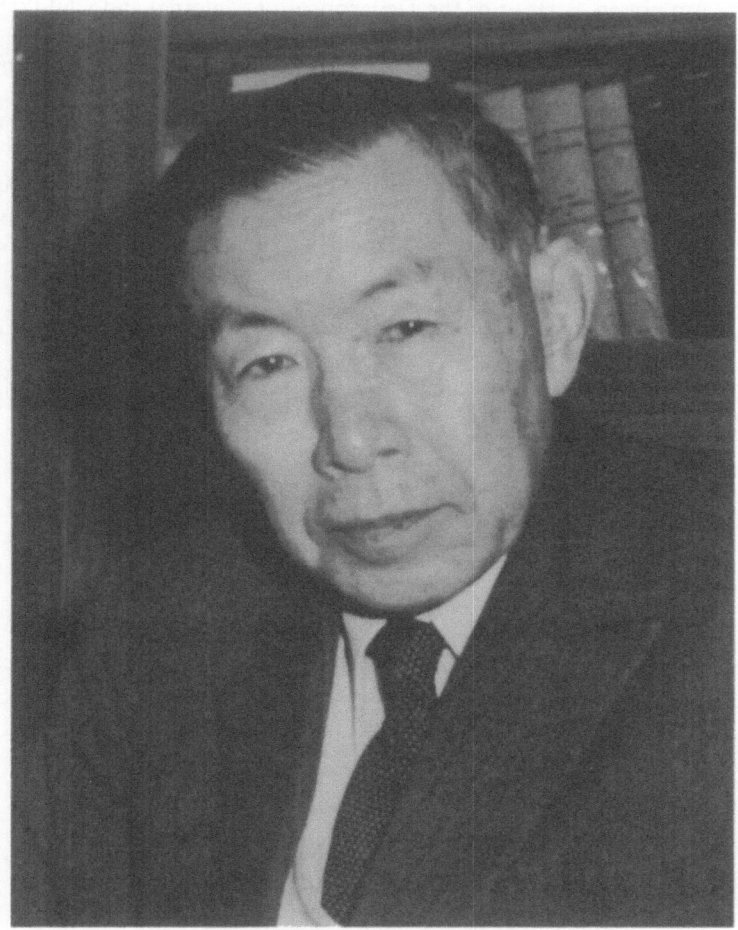

Mitsuo Segi, M.D. (1908–1982)

March 2, 1908   Born in Nagoya.

1932   Graduated from the Faculty of Medicine, Tokyo Imperial University. Entered Graduate School of the same University, majored in anatomy.

1936   Became a research member in the Department of Obstetrics and Gynecology, Tokyo Imperial University.

1937   Received doctor of philosophy.

1938   Went to Europe and America to study gynecology and maternal health administration.

1941   Appointed to a part-time staff of the Ministry of Health and Welfare.

1947   Appointed as Head of the Department of Maternal and Child's Health, Ministry of Health and Welfare.

1949   Moved to the Health and Welfare Statistics Division, Ministry of Health and Welfare.

1950   Appointed Professor of Tohoku University School of Medicine (Department of Public Health).

1971   Retired from Tohoku University. Appointed Professor Emeritus of Tohoku University. Became President of Mizuho (Junior) College, and consultant of the Aichi Cancer Center Research Institute.

1971   Received the Japan Cancer Society Award for his works on cancer epidemiology.

1974   Received the Health Culture Award (Hoken-bunka-sho) from the Ministry of Health and Welfare.

1975   Received the Chunichi Newspaper Culture Award (Chunichi-bunka-sho).

May 8, 1982   Died.

MEMORIES OF PROFESSOR MITSUO SEGI

More than three years have passed since the sudden demise of Professor Mitsuo Segi, whose contributions to cancer epidemiology are internationally renowned; yet our sense of loss is still great.

Because Professor Segi's elder brother, Dr. Mototatsu Segi, had been my classmate at the University of Tokyo, Faculty of Medicine, I heard of Professor Segi who was three years junior in the same faculty but had no opportunity to meet and get acquainted with him at that time.

Upon his graduation from the University of Tokyo in 1932, Professor Segi's first step in starting his career was to continue his study as a researcher in the Department of Anatomy where he was assigned to conduct research on the genesis of intestinal epithelial cells. Professor Michio Inoue was Chairman of the Department. During his study, Professor Segi discovered a large aggregation of basal-granulated cells on the intestinal villi of human fetuses. The discovery of this peculiar cell apparatus was reconfirmed and its biological significance was clarified by later researchers after 45 years in oblivion and is widely accepted as "Segi's cap" today. No doubt, his early study reveals the outstanding competence of Professor Segi as a histologist as well.

In 1935 Professor Segi moved to the Department of Gynecology and Obstetrics where he chose to study cervical cancer as his research work, because the research projects of the Department at that time were mainly focused on cervical cancer and sex hormones.

In 1938 Professor Segi was selected as an advanced student to go to Germany to study modern medicine, where his principal interest focused on cancer research, and on mother and child care. After his return to Japan Professor Segi was appointed Head of the Division of Mother and Child Care at the newly founded Ministry of Health and Welfare. There he devoted himself to solve the facing problem concerning mother and himself to solve the facing problem concerning mother and child care, established the new system for a maternity book in 1942 which enabled the individual pregnant women to possess her medical record of health. This system continues successfully even today under the name of the maternity passbook.

Meanwhile Professor Segi discontinued cancer research including epidemiological work. In 1950 he was appointed Professor of the newly established Department of Public Health at Tohoku University School of Medicine, and resumed his study of cancer epidemiology. With the collaboration of his staff, Professor Segi completed epidemiological analysis of age-adjusted cancer mortality for selected sites in 24 countries using the newly invented world standard population and published six volumes of monographs in serial form from 1950 to 1967. This was the very first extensive study on cancer epidemiology ever achieved in the world, and it brought him high worldwide appreciation for its usefulness. In fact, the monographs served many cancer researchers as a good and convenient reference book for worldwide epidemiological data on cancer. Thereafter, Professor Segi analyzed age-adjusted cancer mortality in 46 prefectures of Japan over 9 years and published the results obtained. The significance of this distinguished and informative work is also highly praised.

I had been in the position of Professor of Pathology at Niigata University School of Medicine until 1954 when I was offered a professorship at Tohoku University where Professor Segi had been appointed.

This encounter at Tohoku University initiated our fellowship which soon became a close one through our common works. Shortly after that Mr. William Haenszel, Chief of Biometry Branch of National Cancer Institute proposed to Professor Segi a cooperative study on cancer mortality of Japanese migrants to the United States. For this study, mutual collaboration of pathologists in the United States and Japan was required, and Dr. Grant N. Stemmermann, Director of Laboratories of Kuakini Hospital in Honolulu and I, together with my co-workers, joined in this U.S.-Japan cooperative cancer study. The participation in this study was tremendously significant for me and through this cooperation, I became greatly interested in cancer epidemiology.

In 1965 I left Tohoku University to accept the position of Director of Aichi Cancer Center Research Institute which was newly founded in Nagoya. A few years later Professor Segi, having retired from Tohoku University, also returned to Nagoya—his hometown, and established the Segi Institute of Cancer Epidemiology which was a private institution.

Here Professor Segi continued his epidemiologic study of cancer and was appointed advisor of the Aichi Cancer Center. It was fortunate for us that we could have his advice for the research activity of our Laboratory of Epidemiology.

Although Professor Segi had already felt his gradually progressive illness during these years, his strenuous study of cancer epidemiology was continued under the best medical care until, to our great sorrow, he suddenly succumbed to a heart attack on May 8, 1982.

This sad news was conveyed to the scientists in the field of cancer epidemiology throughout the world by Dr. C. S. Muir of International Agency for Research on Cancer in Lyon. Many cables and letters of condolence were sent from not only epidemiologists but also cancer researchers from many countries, who expressed their deepest sympathy and their admiration for Professor Segi, a most prominent figure in international studies of cancer epidemiology.

Publication of recent studies in cancer epidemiology in this Gann Monograph on Cancer Research of the Japanese Cancer Association in commemoration of the great work of Professor Segi is an extremely significant event.

Kaneyoshi AKAZAKI
Nagoya, Japan

I take great pleasure in paying my tribute to the memory of my late friend and colleague Professor Mitsuo Segi.

Already in 1950 at the Oxford Symposium on the Endemiology of Cancer, it was realized that significant contributions to Cancer Epidemiology could be expected from Japan in view of past national achievements in Cancer Research. Such expectation were, however more than fulfilled with the appearance of Segi's world-wide tables, the field where I met with his achievements. His system of publications formed a reliable and widely accessible basis for study of the international pattern of cancer mortality as a useful prelude to the development in cancer registration, serving as the indispensable starting ground for the more elaborate statistics to follow.

The quiet and unassuming authority of Mitsuo Segi and his silent friendly attitude made his appearance and personality equally unforgettable.

It is therefore highly satisfactory that tribute is paid to his memory at a time when his personality is still alive—in the recollection of his contemporaries.

Johannes CLEMMESEN
Copenhagen, Denmark

MITSUO SEGI

Mitsuo Segi was a personal friend whose death has left a gap that can never be filled. Quiet and unassuming, he might be overlooked on first acquaintance; but he had a tenacity of purpose, which ensured that anything he took up was carried through to a successful conclusion, and a warmth of feeling and sense of loyalty which made temporary colleagues turn into life-long friends.

His international reputation rests on his contributions to cancer epidemiology, which he took up at 42 years of age, when, in 1950, he became the first Professor of Public Health in Tohoku University, Sendai. Before then, however, he had already made two contributions which alone would have ensured a place for him in medical history.

One, which he made as a doctoral candidate in the Department of Anatomy in the Tokyo Imperial University Medical School, was the discovery of nests of granulated cells at the tips of the villi in the duodenum and jejunum of the 5 month old fetus. His beautiful figures illustrating these nests were subsequently overlooked until 1975, when they were rediscovered by Dr. Kobayashi and it gave Segi great pleasure that they were then very properly given the name of 'Segi's cap.'

The second was the introduction of "Pocket-books for the Health of Mother and Child" when he was administering maternal and child health in the Ministry of Health and Welfare. These books at first included only details of the mother's pregnancy and began to be issued to all pregnant women in 1942 with the aim of preventing toxaemia of pregnancy; but 5 years later they were extended to include details of the child's health, including records of medical examinations, preventive inoculations, and the child's physical mental development. These books now have more than 50 pages and include medical advice to mothers on the care of newborn children and I have often thought that they must have played a substantial part in bringing about the dramatic reduction in perinatal and infant mortality that has put Japan among the half dozen countries with the world's lowest rates.

Segi carried out a number of case-control studies seeking environmental causes for a variety of different cancers, both with other Japanese colleagues at home and with William Haenszel in Hawaii, at a time when these were less usual than they are today, but his major contributions were (i) the collection and presentation of international cancer mortality data in a form that was both convenient to use and allowed sensible comparisons to be made between mortality rates in different countries and (ii) the establishment of a model cancer registry in Japan. These contributions are discussed in detail by William Haenszel and John Higginson and I concur in everything they have said about the immense value that both have been to cancer research workers throughout the world. Few books can have been referred to more often that Segi and Kurihara's "Cancer

Mortality for Selected Sites in 24 Countries" (subsequently expanded to cover 43 countries) and there are certainly none that I have referred to more myself. All who are interested in seeking clues to aetiology from geographical differences in disease incidence owe a personal debt to Segi not only for the care with which he compiled his volumes, but also for benefactions which enabled the Segi Institute of Cancer Epidemiology in his home town of Nagoya to continue publishing further volumes after he retired from his University Chair. These volumes provided the stimulus and model for the publication of sister volumes on "Cancer Incidence in Five Continents" at first by the International Union against Cancer and subsequently by the International Agency for Research on Cancer and the International Association of Cancer Registries.

My last memory of Mitsuo Segi was a peculiarly happy one. It was through Segi's personal generosity that my wife was able to attend with me the first Conference on Cancer in Developing Countries that was held in Nagoya in the autumn of 1981 and we had the pleasure of being entertained by him and his wife in his own home. Segi had, by then, already suffered one myocardial infarction and was subject to frequent attacks of angina. He insisted, however, on showing us personally the sights of Nagoya and we remember with pleasure the quiet satisfaction he showed in the enormous improvement in the standard of living that had been made in Japan in his life-time, which was typified by the high standard and abundance of goods in so many large department stores.

Richard Doll
Oxford, United Kingdom

MITSUO SEGI, 1908–1982

I first met Professor Segi in 1954, when he presented a paper at the fifth conference of the International Society of Geographical Pathology in Washington, D.C.. During this visit he also gave a lecture at the National Institutes of Health, in which he reviewed the inter-country variation in site-specific cancer risks. His appraisal left little doubt about the important role of environmental factors in accounting for many of these differences. Dr. Segi spent several years in the Ministry of Health and Welfare as Head of the Maternal and Child Health Division and had a broad background of experience in vital statistics registration before he went to Tohoku University as Professor of Public Health in 1950. It was quite natural for him to tap his expertise in this area and to utilize cancer mortality data for descriptive epidemiology purposes. This led him to initiate the series of reports on cancer mortality first published under the title "Cancer Mortality for Selected Sites in 24 Countries" in the 1950 decade. To obtain comparable information on cancer death rates from many national vital statistics offices was a demanding chore and Dr. Segi rendered a useful service to the cancer research community by undertaking this assignment. Not only did he initiate the series, he also persevered in the collection and publication of the data in succeeding years. In this manner he assembled useful information on the time trends in site-specific mortality for these same countries. While cancer mortality data do not have the diagnostic accuracy and site specificity of reports collected by cancer registries, they do have the virtue of stability in methods of data collection and processing and thus are particularly valuable for describing time trends in cancer risks. Several papers reviewing the epidemiology of individual cancer sites have been published and many of the authors are indebted to Dr. Segi for his documentation of the mortality data which constitute a useful reference not readily available elsewhere.

After his arrival at Tohoku University Professor Segi soon realized the desirability of augmenting the mortality data for Miyagi prefecture with incidence data that could be collected by establishment of a prefectural population-based cancer registry. This was well before the concept of population-based registries came into vogue. At that time the best known registries were those in Denmark headed by Dr. Clemmesen and in the State of Connecticut by Dr. Griswold. At the inception of the Miyagi registry in 1952 there were no other registries in Asia. The Atomic Bomb Casualty Commission had attempted to establish registries in Hiroshima and Nagasaki, but it was not until 1958 that a registry in Nagasaki began operation. To initiate a registry in Miyagi prefecture in the face of very limited resources took courage and vision. Dr. Segi recognized very well the imperfections in the data produced in the initial years. However, he was a man to take the long view. He had faith that once established improvements in data quality would occur. What he might not have fully anticipated was that the existence of the Miyagi registry and the demonstration of its utility would provide a strong impetus to the creation of other population-based cancer registries in Japan. In the fourth edition of Cancer in Five Continents incidence data are published for Fukuoka, Nagasaki, and Osaka prefectures and several other prefectural registries have now been established in Japan. By virtue of his personal example in creating the Miyagi Registry and his counsel, encouragement and support to colleagues in other prefectures, Dr. Segi can be regarded as the father of cancer registration in Japan.

Professor Segi's influence on the development of cancer registration extended beyond Japan. He was active in promoting sessions on cancer registration and epidemiology at the quadrennial International Cancer Congresses. He recognized that this was not a popular topic with Congress organizing committees and he continued to promote the idea that cancer registries should take the initiative and sponsor their own sessions at a time immediately prior to the International Congresses. It is not known by many people that the original suggestion for the creation of an International Association of Cancer Registries (IACR) was made by Dr. Segi. At the 1966 Tokyo Congress he asked Dr. Cutler and me to propose the creation of an International Association at an informal gathering of cancer registry personnel. The proposal was not warmly received at the time and many reservations were expressed concerning the need for such an organization. At Dr. Segi's urging I consented to serve as Chairman of an Organizing Committee and with support from him and from members of the Organizing Committee the IACR came into being. This happy result owes much to the vision of Dr. Segi. Without his support it is doubtful that the IACR would exist today. With the pass age of time the need for the International Association has been demonstrated to everyone's satisfaction. It collaborates with the International Agency for Research on Cancer (IARC) in the production of revised editions of *Cancer in Five Continents*. The close working relationships between IACR and IARC are further enhanced by the designation of a staff member of IARC to serve as deputy secretary-general of IACR.

My second meeting with Professor Segi took place in Tokyo in 1960 at the inter-Congress planning session sponsored by the International Union against Cancer. By that time the cancer mortality experience of the Hawaiian Japanese was well documented and the changes in site-specific cancer risks of the migrant Japanese vis-a-vis those in Japan had become evident. Dr. Segi agreed that the time was ripe for case-control studies of Japanese in Hawaii and Japan to search for the underlying causes. We discussed plans and he consented to come to the National Cancer Institute as a Visiting Scientist in 1961 to participate in the development of case-control studies of stomach and large bowel cancer. During his stay in the United States he worked on the development of the questionnaires and contributed his expertise and knowledge of the situation in Japan that were critical in shaping the study design. He visited Hawaii with me and was influential in enlisting the support of local physicians. His major contribution was in the evaluation of possible study settings within Japan with attention to feasibility and indentification of the essential organizational and administrative components needed to ensure a successful outcome.

Professor Segi was a careful and conscientious collaborator. He always tried to brief me on the scientific and cultural context of his negotiations on behalf of the studies in Japan. In return, I tried to keep him appraised of the subtler aspects of research study gamesmanship within the United States. We both profited from this. To have had Dr. Segi as a collaborator I am sure kept me free from many mistakes that would have undermined work in Japan.

William HAENSZEL
Chicago, U.S.A.

APPRECIATION
Professor Mitsuo Segi

It is a great honor to be asked to write this appreciation in memory of the late Dr. Mitsuo Segi, Professor Emeritus of Tohoku University, who contributed so abundantly to the epidemiology and prevention of cancer. In 1954 Dr. Harold Stewart became chairman of the Committee of Geographical Pathology of the International Union Against Cancer. The program of this committee laid much of the foundation for what is now called environmental carcinogenesis and represented the first international approach to make a systematic multidisciplinary approach to the study of cancer causation in humans. The committee members came from many countries and included Dr. Hans Clemmesen of Copenhagen, Dr. Harold Dorn of the National Cancer Institute, and Professor Mitsuo Segi, all prestigious leaders in cancer epidemiology.

Today our recognition of the role of the environment and other factors responsible for cancer is largely based on the contributions of these earlier workers. It was they who emphasized that knowledge about the biology and distribution of human cancer was essential to the identification of cause(s).

I had the opportunity to meet Professor Segi for the first time at Washington in 1954 during the first post-war meeting of the International Society of Geographical Pathology. There he presented a careful analysis of the background and etiology of cancer of the breast. This presentation illustrated his workmanlike approach to all that he undertook. I learned at the same time of the important series of studies in descriptive epidemiology which was appearing from Sendai, at that time the hometown of Professor Segi.

That was a period when cancer statistics were widely dispersed and difficult to analyze; moreover comparisons between countries were often dependent on relative ratios. Although the World Health Organization was gradually collecting cancer mortality data, analysis lagged far behind. It was to overcome this lag that Professor Segi devoted his efforts. As a consequence he developed his famous monograph series on cancer mortality in 24 countries. These were first published from Tohoku University at Sendai and later were continued from the Segi Institute of Cancer Epidemiology at Nagoya.

Professor Segi's contribution made by descriptive epidemiology through his standardization of international data was a major accomplishment in that it facilitated comparisons between communities living under a wide range of environmental conditions. The use of a standard world population by Segi was a significant step in the presentation of comparable cancer data. Moreover, trends in cancer mortality in a number of countries over significant time periods were described for the first time. Soon, few publications on a specific cancer site and the causes of the cancers were considered to be complete without a Segi histogram. Such studies for the first time provided a clear picture of cancer as seen in industrial and industrializing countries and the monograph received world-wide recognition.

Professor Segi was fully aware of the limitations of mortality data and their biases. Accordingly, he proceeded at the same time to develop a cancer morbidity registry for the Miyagi province in Japan. The data in this registry provided background material to those interested in the impact of changing lifestyles and industrial conditions that were occurring in Japan in the post-war era and provided a useful comparison for the mortality data. Thus, to discuss epidemiology in the Asian region was to talk of Professor Segi in the same way as Professor Clemmesen was regarded as the doyen of descriptive epidemiology in Europe. Their studies of mortality and morbidity are still the recognized sources of material for any worker in this field. It was only natural at a later day that when, as chairman of the Committee of Geographical Pathology, I established a subcommittee under Sir Richard Doll to produce the first volume of "Cancer Incidence in Five Continents" under the auspices of the UICC, that Professor Segi was appointed a member.

During the UICC conference in 1960 at which the major contributions of Japanese workers to geographic pathology were presented, often for the first time, the work of Professor Segi dominated the epidemiological scene, as did the studies of Professor Yoshida in experimental carcinogenesis.

Professor Segi was a cultured and scholarly gentleman. He had many other interests which made him a pleasure to visit at Sendai. His erudition and kindnesses provided a unique insight for me, a young visiting scientist, into the world of Japanese accomplishments. My first opportunity to be a guest at a Japanese dinner was hosted by Professor Segi with extreme graciousness. I have many happy recollections of walking in the parks of his home town with the members of his staff and his colleagues. These remain for me experiences for which I shall always be grateful. I am sure the publication of this monograph will bring back similar memories to many others.

John HIGGINSON
Washington, D.C., U.S.A.

CONTENTS

INTERNATIONAL COMPARATIVE STUDY

CHANGING CANCER PATTERNS

CHANGING PATTERNS OF CANCER INCIDENCE IN FIVE CONTINENTS

C. S. MUIR and A. MALHOTRA

*International Agency for Research on Cancer**

The data published in successive volumes of "Cancer Incidence in Five Continents" are a relatively new resource for time trend analyses. They form the basis of this review of trends in the incidence of three cancers—stomach, breast, and prostate—in a fairly broad range of registration areas (27 in number). These trends are compared and contrasted with longer-term trends in mortality in 23 countries. For one of the cancers, stomach, incidence and mortality are close and substantial decreases are almost universal. For breast and prostate cancer, however, incidence and mortality are far apart and although both sites show generally increasing trends, there are large differences in the magnitude of the increases in some areas such that the impact of factors other than changing risks is an important consideration. Several of these are examined.

Some six million new cases of cancer occurred throughout the world in 1975 according to recent estimates (*44*) and in most parts of the world between one in four to one in five persons will develop cancer in their lifetime. International comparisons show that there are large variations in the risk of developing cancer and in the types of cancer that are common in different populations. Time trend studies, together with studies of migrants, have demonstrated that a population's cancer risk can undergo marked changes with the passage of time and after migration to a new environment, findings which strongly suggest that environmental rather than genetic factors cause most cancers and which provide the impetus to search for these environmental risk factors using epidemiological techniques of investigation.

Population-based cancer incidence and mortality data are central to the knowledge that has accumulated and to the continuing search for causes and the testing of hypotheses concerning causation, to monitoring changes and indicating if new cancer risks are occurring, and, increasingly, to predicting future trends so that rational planning of health services is possible (*45*). The data are invaluable but at the same time somewhat crude tools for the task at hand. They provide evidence of real differences in cancer risk but may, as will be illustrated later, also in part reflect differences and changes in factors which have nothing to do with risk of developing cancer and which can therefore make interpretation difficult.

Until comparatively recently the study of time trends relied entirely on mortality data. In some countries these data have been compiled for very long time periods, well over a century in England and Wales and since the beginning of this century for Japan

---

* 69372 Lyon Cedex 08, France.

and the U.S.A., for example, and data from many countries in the world have for several decades been made easily accessible to research workers through publications presenting them in a comparable form (54, 55). Mortality data are also, in spite of their well-recognized limitations (16), often considered to be more easily interpretable than incidence data. Nonetheless, it is generally acknowledged that incidence data provide, in principle, the most direct and complete information about cancer occurrence or cancer risk. They include all cancers, not only those that cause death; record the time of diagnosis, which may precede the time of death by many years for some cancers; and usually include detailed and reliable information about the diagnosis.

For some areas, incidence data have been available for quite a long time, over 50 years for Saskatchewan and Connecticut in North America, and for more than 20 years in the Nordic countries, and have been studied extensively. On a larger geographical scale, albeit one more limited in time, the cancer incidence data compiled for and published in successive volumes of "Cancer Incidence in Five Continents" (C15) (14, 15, 60, 61) are a resource that is growing in the number of time periods spanned and that has started to provide information about cancer incidence trends in many parts of the world. For three selected cancers, these recent trends, generally covering the period 1960–1962 to 1973–1977, will be reviewed here. Observations will be compared with those based on longer series of incidence data. Trends in cancer mortality, usually for the period 1955 to 1979, are also presented to permit a view of incidence trends within the broader and longer-term perspective they provide, and to compare the evidence of changing risks derived from the two sources of information.

Cancer Patterns and Time Trends in Selected Areas of the World

For the review of cancer incidence trends, 27 registration areas were selected, comprising 14 in Europe, 8 in America, 2 in Oceania, and 3 in Asia (Table IV). For some of the areas, New Zealand, California, and Hawaii, the selection included data for two ethnic groups. The continent of Africa as well as other parts of the less developed world are unfortunately not represented at all since comparable data for different time periods are not yet available. (Thus, despite the title this review covers but four continents). The few data that are available for these areas, usually based on special surveys or on relative frequency distributions rather than rates per population at risk, suggest that very different cancer patterns prevail (1, 18, 46).

Data for at least three time periods, 1963–1966, 1967–1972, and 1973–1977 are available from most of the selected areas as well as data for an earlier time span, 1960–1962, for about half of the registries. The years and range of years included in each time period do however vary between the registration areas. This irregularity of the data poses some difficulties in the comparisons of age-standardized rates and much greater problems when one wishes to examine the changes underlying the cross-sectional summary curves through birth cohort analysis. A procedure to estimate cohort rates from irregularly grouped cross-sectional data has recently been proposed (53) and was applied to the above data. Although observations for at most four time periods are as yet available, there are marked differences in incidence between different generations for some cancers and examples will be given. Study of these curves promises to reveal much valuable information as the data base grows and as techniques of analysis are refined to allow interpretation of the factors underlying the changes by separating the effects of age, period

TABLE I. Estimates of the Worldwide Frequency of Twelve Major Cancers in 1975: Incident Cases

Rank	Males		Females		Both sexes	
	Cancer site	Number of cases (in thousands)	Cancer site	Number of cases (in thousands)	Cancer site	Number of cases (in thousands)
1	Lung	464.3	Breast	541.2	Stomach	682.4
2	Stomach	421.7	Cervix	459.4	Lung	591.0
3	Colon/rectum	251.2	Stomach	260.6	Breast	541.2
4	Mouth/pharynx	232.9	Colon/rectum	255.6	Colon/rectum	506.9
5	Prostate	197.7	Lung	126.7	Cervix	459.4
6	Oesophagus	194.0	Mouth/pharynx	106.6	Mouth/pharynx	339.5
7	Liver	182.5	Oesophagus	102.3	Oesophagus	296.3
8	Bladder	130.7	Lymphatic	91.3	Liver	259.2
9	Lymphatic	129.5	Liver	76.7	Lymphatic	220.9
10	Leukaemia	100.3	Leukaemia	75.4	Prostate	197.7
11	—	—	Bladder	39.4	Bladder	170.1
12	—	—	—	—	Leukaemia	175.7
	All sites (excl. skin)	2,968.5	All sites (excl. skin)	2,901.8	All sites (excl. skin)	5,870.3

Source: Parkin *et al.* (1984).

of birth, and time of diagnosis (*10, 50*). Trends in mortality rates, usually for the period 1955 to 1979 are also presented. These rates are based on "Cancer Mortality Statistics in the World" (*31*) and on special tabulations from the WHO Data Bank (courtesy of Dr H. Hansluwka). Twenty-three countries, also representing all continents except Africa, were selected for this review (Table V). All age-standardized rates shown are based on the standard of the "world" population first constructed by Segi and Kurihara (*54*) and modified by Doll *et al.* (*14*). Comparisons between incidence and mortality trends will naturally be in very general terms only as the data are derived from different sources and there is direct correspondence neither of time periods reviewed nor of the geographic areas—the mortality data always cover an entire country whereas few of the incidence series do.

The cancers reviewed are those of the stomach, breast, and prostate. Their estimated worldwide frequency in 1975 is shown in Table I. Together these sites account for an estimated 21% and 28% of all cancers (excluding non-melanotic skin cancer) in males and females, respectively. The numerical importance and changing incidence of these cancers were the main considerations in their selection for review. Lung cancer was not included because it is reviewed elsewhere in this monograph. For stomach cancer incidence and mortality are close, unlike for breast and prostate so that the observed trends give rise to differing problems of interpretation. Also important in the choice of sites was the consistency of the evidence of changes in incidence that they provided; for the broad overview of time trends attempted here, the authors did not discuss unusual observations, perhaps arising from biases in the data, with the persons who know the data best, the registry staff.

Stomach Cancer

The estimates of worldwide incidence in 1975 indicate that cancer of the stomach is

TABLE II.   Stomach Cancer Incidence

Registration area	Males		Females	
	Rate[a] in 1973–1977	Average annual percentage change in rate[b]	Rate[a] in 1973–1977	Average annual percentage change in rate[b]
Japan, Miyagi	87.9	−0.52	43.0	−0.82
Colombia, Cali	44.6	0.05	26.9	3.26
Yugoslavia, Slovenia	42.0	−0.83	18.0	−1.99
New Zealand: Maori	41.7	−0.21	20.3	−5.15
Hungary, County Vas	37.4	−0.74	17.1	−1.03
U.S.A., Hawaii: Japanese	34.0	−2.55	15.1	−4.37
Poland, Warsaw City	31.4	−1.95	12.9	−3.42
Finland	29.3	−4.32	15.3	−4.75
Canada, Newfoundland	27.2	−2.69	11.1	−4.67
U.K., Mersey Region	23.4	−2.55	10.7	−2.91
U.S.A., Alameda: Black	18.5	−2.10	7.8	−0.42
Denmark	17.1	−3.13	8.9	−4.11
New Zealand: Non-Maori	16.3	−1.56	7.0	−2.95
Canada, Alberta	11.7	−2.48	5.1	−2.22
U.S.A., Alameda: White	10.5	−2.86	4.5	−3.79
U.S.A., Hawaii: Chinese	10.0	0.33	6.9	−5.37
India, Bombay	9.7	−0.37	5.9	−1.16

[a] Rates in selected registration areas in 1973-1977, age-standardized to the "world" population.

[b] Average annual percentage change in rates since 1960-1962 or 1962-1967, estimated from differences in log rates for the first and last time period divided by the number of years from the mid-year of the first to the mid-year of the last period. Time periods stated are approximations as they may vary slightly between registration areas.

TABLE III.   Stomach Cancer Mortality

Country	Males		Females	
	Rate[a] in 1978–1979	Average annual percentage change in rate[b]	Rate[a] in 1978–1979	Average annual percentage change in rate[b]
Japan	49.7	−1.53	25.2	−1.86
Chile	45.7	−2.15	20.4	−3.39
Portugal	30.8	0.41	15.3	−0.52
Uruguay	24.3[c]	−2.24	11.9[c]	−2.70
Finland	21.5	−4.21	11.2	−4.24
Spain	21.5	−1.17	10.8	−1.92
England and Wales	17.9	−1.96	8.1	−2.74
Norway	15.3	−3.51	7.6	−3.85
New Zealand	12.4	−2.16	5.4	−2.78
Canada	11.2	−3.20	4.8	−3.72
Australia	11.1	−2.65	5.2	−3.54
U.S.A.	6.3	−3.68	3.0	−4.07

Age-standardized rates in selected countries in 1978–1979, and average annual percentage change in rate since 1955.

[a] Rates age-standardized to the "world" population.

[b] Estimated as indicated in Table II. The period over which the change in rates is calculated may vary from that shown above for some countries.

[c] 1978 only.

globally still the most common cancer for both sexes combined although its continuing decline and the rapid rise in the incidence of lung cancer, which ranked second in 1975, may soon reverse the relative position of these two cancers (44).

Tables II and III show a selection of current patterns in stomach cancer incidence and mortality respectively as well as the changes in rates that have taken place.

Geographical variation in the incidence of stomach cancer is marked even within the limited range of registration areas reviewed. In the period 1973–1977, the highest age-standardized rates among the selected 27 cancer registration areas occurred in Miyagi Prefecture in Japan, for both males and females. These rates are nine times as high as in the areas of lowest incidence, Bombay in India for males, and the white population in Alameda County in California for females. The rates in Japan also far exceed those in other populations with a high incidence such as Cali in Colombia and Slovenia in Yugoslavia. Rates are generally low in North American registration areas and intermediate in most of Europe but higher in Eastern Europe than in the West or North. There are also large differences within countries and between different ethnic groups living in the same area. For example, rates in Newfoundland in Eastern Canada are more than twice as high as in Alberta in Western Canada; in California, rates for the black population in Alameda County are much higher than in the white population (1.8 and 1.7 times in males and females, respectively), and data for two of the ethnic groups in Hawaii show that incidence rates in the population of Japanese origin, while much lower than rates prevailing in Miyagi, exceed rates in those of Chinese origin by a factor of 3.4 in males and 2.2 in females. Similarly, in New Zealand, incidence of stomach cancer in Maoris is 2.5 to 3 times higher than in Non-Maoris.

Survival for cancer of the stomach is poor and mortality rates are generally not much lower than incidence rates. Data for the 1978–1979 period show a general pattern similar to the incidence data for comparable areas. Rates are highest in Japan and Chile and low in the U.S.A, Canada, Australia, and New Zealand.

The recent patterns in stomach cancer occurrence reflect the marked changes that have taken place in virtually all parts of the world for which data are available. Figure I and Tables II and III illustrate the decline in age-standardized stomach cancer incidence and mortality rates in several areas in the review period. Even within the relatively short time span of 1960–1962 to 1973–1977, that is some 15 years, stomach cancer incidence fell by about 25% in most areas. Comparatively small decreases, on average less than one percent annually, occurred in Miyagi Prefecture where indeed rates fell between 1962–1964 and 1968–1971 but then increased again. Japan has a relatively recent nationwide early detection programme for stomach cancer (28) which may explain the slow decline in incidence rates accompanied by larger decreases in mortality rates. The largest decrease in rates, more than 4% annually in both males and females, occurred in Finland. A review of longer-term trends in stomach cancer incidence in the Nordic countries shows that rates in these countries have been falling throughout the two or three decades for which incidence data are available (30).

Stomach cancer incidence rates in two populations stayed level (males in Cali, Colombia and Chinese males in Hawaii) or increased in one (females in Cali) and one might ask if this could be due to more complete registration. Although the last two volumes of CI5 included the ratio of mortality to new cases as an indicator of completeness of registration for most areas, this information was not available for the above registries. There is evidence that registration of cancer cases in the Hawaii registry

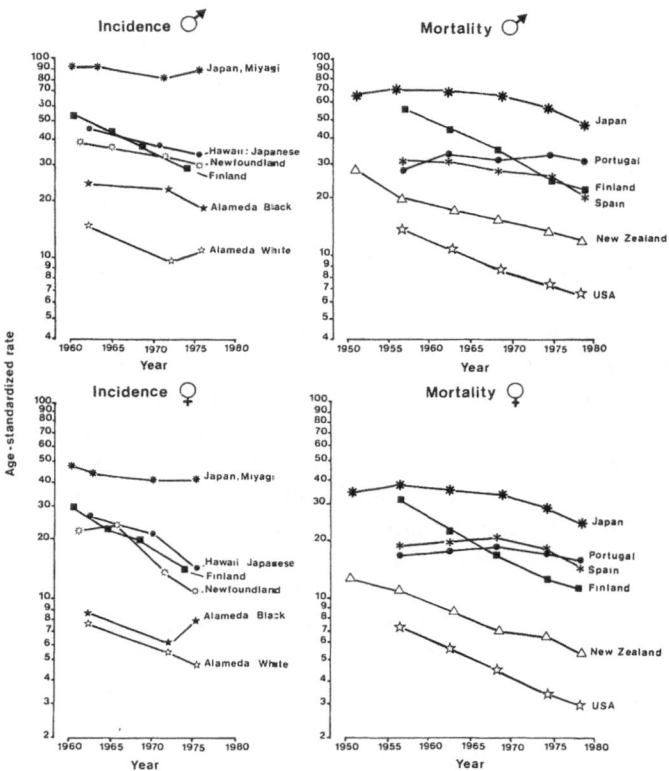

FIG. 1.   Trends in stomach cancer incidence and mortality in selected registration areas or countries

improved during the period (34). There is no evidence that this bias exists in Cali, but mortality data for other parts of South America (Chile, and Uruguay) show sizeable decreases for both males and females.

Mortality data have for some time demonstrated the decline in stomach cancer throughout the world and also reveal clearly that changes did not occur at the same time and at the same rate everywhere. Declines in rates were particulary rapid in Finland, as also shown by the incidence data, but started later and are occurring at a slower rate in Japan. Males in Portugal and Spain had very similar mortality rates in 1956–1957 and at that time age-standardized rates were still rising in both countries. The current pattern of higher rates in Portugal emerged because the eventual fall in rates took place later and at a slower pace there than in Spain. In females, on the other hand, rates rose in both countries until the late 1960's and then began to fall at a similar rate.

Stomach cancer rates in males are generally about twice as high as in females and both incidence and mortality data show that differences between the sexes have been widening in most areas as stomach cancer rates have fallen faster in females than males. The observed differences in stomach cancer incidence between the Maori and Non-Maori populations in New Zealand and between the black and white populations in Alameda County (where trends are somewhat irregular) also reflect widening differences since rates in Maoris as well as in Blacks have been decreasing more slowly. These differentials may be due to variation in socio-economic status and diet.

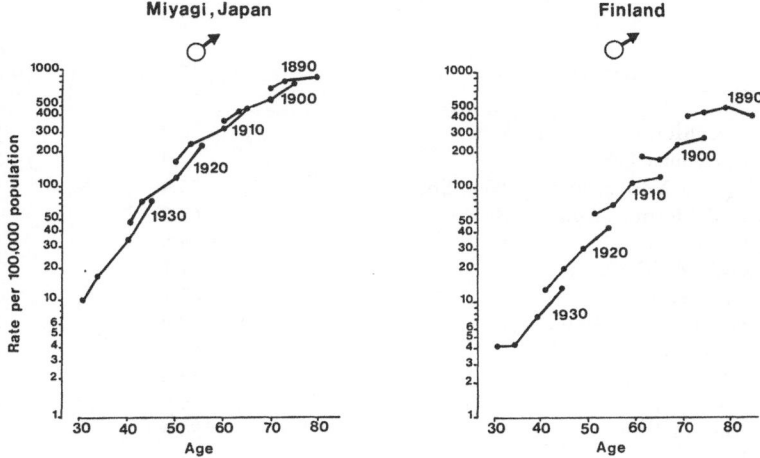

FIG. 2. Stomach cancer incidence for successive male birth cohorts in Miyagi, Japan and Finland in four time periods as published in CI5

It has been shown elsewhere that there are differences in the incidence patterns and trends for the two main histological types of stomach cancer: the intestinal type predominates in high-risk areas and the diffuse type in low-risk areas (40). It is largely the incidence of the intestinal type which is falling and this is therefore more likely to be related to environmental factors (21, 41).

Cohort curves of stomach cancer incidence show a clear pattern of declining rates for successively younger cohorts in some areas, as illustrated in Fig. 2 for Miyagi and Finland. The contrast between the rapid declines in Finland and the much slower changes in Miyagi is marked. A review of incidence trends in the last two or three decades in the five Nordic countries (30) demonstrates that in each of the countries and for both sexes, consecutive birth cohorts since the end of the 19th century experienced decreasing stomach cancer rates.

Although there have been suggestions that a major part of the decline in stomach cancer rates may be due to more precise diagnosis and that lack of accuracy previously resulted in other abdominal neoplasms being classified as stomach cancer, the observed falls in incidence and mortality have been so universal that the trend is generally accepted as real. A study of stomach cancer incidence trends in the Nordic countries (30) reviewed the available information about improvements in diagnostic practices and concluded that although these had indeed taken place, the evidence supported the view that there had been a true decline in the incidence of stomach cancer since the mid-1950s. In addition, data from the Danish cancer registry did not support the assumption that the decrease in stomach cancer incidence has been compensated by an increase in cancer of other digestive tract organs.

The large international differences and changes with time in the incidence of stomach cancer suggest environmental influences in the aetiology of this cancer. Studies of migrants from countries of high stomach cancer mortality in Europe to the U.S.A. have shown that rates tend to remain closer to those prevailing in the countries of origin (22, 56). This was also observed for Japanese migrants to the U.S.A. but rates in their offspring born in the U.S.A, while remaining above those in the native white population, were

TABLE IV. Breast Cancer Incidence

Registration area	Rate[a] in 1973–1977	Average annual percentage change in rate[b]
U.S.A., California, Alameda: White	78.2	1.76
U.S.A., Connecticut	77.9	2.01
U.S.A., New York State (less New York City)	75.4	2.90
U.S.A., California, Alameda: Black	67.2	4.36
Canada, Alberta	66.5	1.88
New Zealand: Maori	64.1	2.89
Canada, Quebec	63.1	2.51
New Zealand: Non-Maori	62.6	2.23
Israel: All Jews	59.4	2.58
U.K., Oxford Region	59.2	2.74
Denmark	58.8	1.53
U.K., Birmingham	56.4	1.40
F.R.G., Hamburg	55.7	2.80
U.S.A., Hawaii: Chinese	55.3	1.71
Sweden	55.2	1.55
U.K., Mersey Region	51.8	1.69
Norway	49.6	1.66
Canada, Newfoundland	49.6	2.15
U.S.A., Hawaii: Japanese	47.1	5.66
Finland	40.1	3.24
German Democratic Republic	37.4	2.72
Poland, Warsaw City	36.5	2.66
Yugoslavia, Slovenia	34.2	2.91
Colombia, Cali	32.6	2.34
Puerto Rico	29.5	4.95
Hungary, County Vas	29.2	2.88
Poland, Katowice District	23.8	4.31
India, Bombay	21.2	0.44
Hungary, County Szabolcs-Szatmar	20.6	1.61
Japan, Miyagi	17.4	1.82

[a] Rates in selected registration areas in 1973–1977, age-standardized to the "world" population.

[b] Average annual percentage change in rates since 1960–1962 or 1963–1967, estimated as indicated in Table II. Time periods stated are approximate and may vary slightly between registration areas.

lower than in the parents, suggesting that early exposures may be critical in the causation of stomach cancer (23). A number of dietary factors have been investigated and it has been shown that the consumption of dried / salted fish and pickled vegetables is associated with a high stomach cancer risk while the consumption of fresh fruits, vegetables and milk and milk products is associated with a reduced risk (24, 28). Differences in diet may also explain the inverse relationship between social class and stomach cancer which has been consistently observed in England and Wales since 1921 and which persists in spite of the general fall in mortality (32). Other causative factors, such as smoking, have been implicated as diet alone may not explain the generally higher incidence of stomach cancer in men (28).

Breast Cancer

Globally, breast cancer is estimated to be the leading cancer in females. Tables IV

TABLE V. Breast Cancer Mortality

Country	Rate[a] in 1978–1979	Average annual percentage change in rate[b]
England and Wales	27.7	0.61
Scotland	27.6	0.71
Netherlands	25.8	0.35
Israel	25.6	1.22
Belgium	25.5	0.74
Denmark	24.7	0.11
New Zealand	24.4	0.49
Switzerland	23.8	0.35
Uruguay	24.1[c]	0.53
Canada	22.8	0.04
U.S.A.	21.7	0.09
Federal Republic of Germany	20.5	1.11
Norway	19.1	−0.03
Australia	18.9	−0.08
Italy	18.8	1.23
France	18.1	1.08
Sweden	18.1	0.11
Finland	14.9	1.20
Portugal	14.5	1.37
Spain	13.3	2.60
Chile	11.4	1.25
Hong Kong	9.2	−0.20
Japan	5.2	1.16

Age-standardized rates in selected countries in 1978–1979, and average annual percentage change in rate since 1950.

[a] Rates age-standardized to the "world" population.

[b] Estimated as indicated in Table II. The period over which the change in rates is calculated may vary from that shown above for some countries.

[c] 1978 only.

and V show the current patterns in breast cancer incidence and mortality together with the average annual change in the rates during the review period. Incidence in the 1973–1977 period varies about 4.5-fold between high incidence areas in the U.S.A., Canada and New Zealand and low incidence areas in Asia and Eastern Europe. In other parts of Europe rates are intermediate. Rates in Japanese and Chinese women in Hawaii are more than twice as high as in women in Miyagi and Chinese woman in Singapore.

The relationship between incidence and mortality is not straightforward and mortality rates do not reflect occurrence of this cancer well. Reported incidence data, on the other hand, are not easy to interpret as they are suspected of being more sensitive to international differences in diagnostic practices and access to medical care and changes with time in these factors. In contrast to the pattern of the incidence data, breast cancer mortality rates in 1978–1979 are highest in some European countries while rates in the U.S.A. and Canada, although still high, rank lower. There is concordance between incidence and mortality data for the low rates in Asia.

In all of the registration areas reviewed breast cancer incidence rates are increasing. Annual rates of increase range from a high of 5.7% in Japanese in Hawaii to a low of 0.4% in Bombay. Rates in Miyagi Prefecture increased by 1.8%. In Alameda County

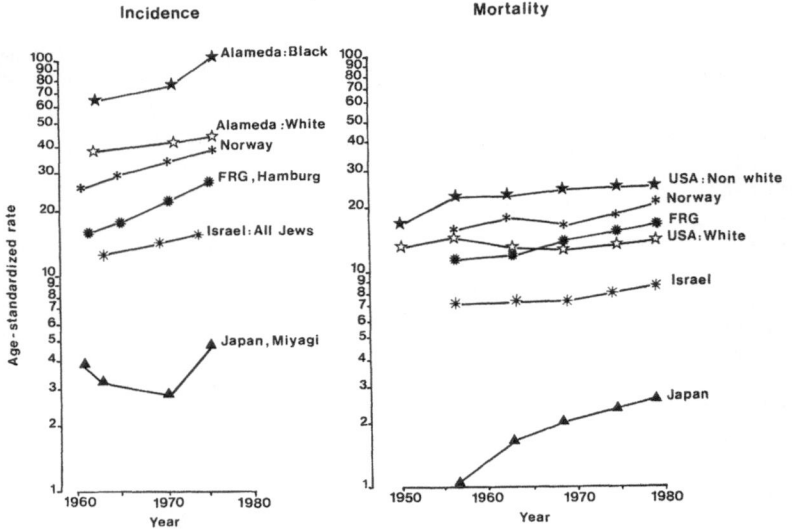

FIG. 3. Trends in breast cancer incidence and mortality in selected registration areas or countries

the increase of 4.4% annually in black women was more than twice as high as in white women.

A study of trends in breast cancer incidence (34) included a review of CI5 data for the four major ethnic groups in Hawaii and the investigator suggested that too much should not be read into the recent trends in Hawaii. The reasons included, first, evidence that completeness of registration in the Hawaii Cancer Registry improved between 1960–1964 and 1968–1972 and, second, that from 1968–1972 to 1973–1977 breast cancer rates increased as much among the Caucasians as among the Orientals, so that although Oriental women in Hawaii have in the past acquired a higher breast cancer incidence than prevailing in their country of origin, it would, in the author's opinion, be difficult to attribute the most recent increase to further westernization.

Breast cancer mortality rates in the 23 countries, seen over a longer time span, 1950 to 1982 for most countries, also generally increased but at a much lower rate. Small decreases occurred in Australia, Norway, and Hong Kong. The only country in which the annual increase exceeded 2% was Spain. Virtually no rise in mortality rates occurred in the U.S.A. and Canada, although incidence rates in north american registration areas have risen, by an average of 2% annually. Figure 3 illustrates the trends in incidence and mortality in some of these areas.

Greater efficiency of diagnosis and perhaps the tendency to label more conditions as cancer have been suggested as possible explanations for the pattern of rising incidence rates but stable mortality rates, which have been observed in North America as well as in other parts of the world (36). A study of the interrelationship of incidence, survival and mortality and their effects on time trends, based on data from Connecticut (42) found that breast cancer incidence increased by 1% per year in the period 1949 to 1973 while mortality rates hardly changed. This pattern was judged to be consistent with an observed increase in survival. Major improvements in breast cancer treatment have, however, not been demonstrated and it has been proposed that incidence is rising because

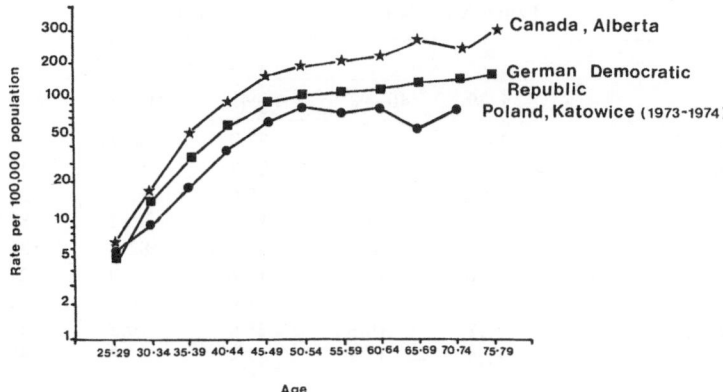

FIG. 4. Age-specific breast cancer incidence rates in three registration areas in 1973–1977.

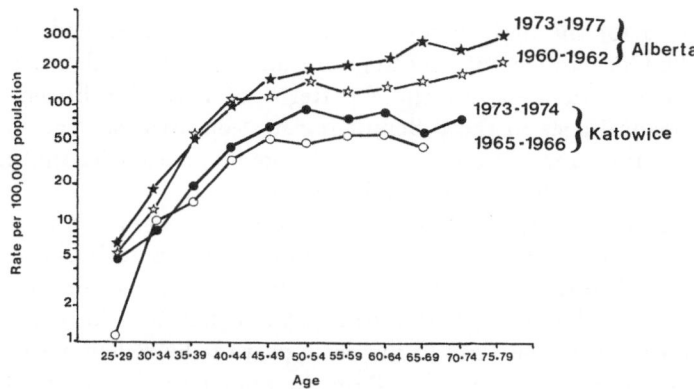

FIG. 5. Age-specific breast cancer incidence rates in Alberta, Canada and Katowice District, Poland in two time periods.

changes in diagnostic practices have led to the inclusion of more borderline cancers that do not cause death. This would lead to an increase in survival rates even in the absence of improvements in the methods of treatment (8, 16, 52). Screening for breast cancer may have a similar effect by detecting potentially fatal cancers at an early, more curable stage.

The shape of the age-specific incidence curve for breast cancer has unusual features and has generated hypotheses concerning hormonal influences, nutrition and obesity (12, 33, 57). It generally rises sharply with age up to the years of menopause, levels off and then rises again more slowly. Comparisons of age-specific incidence curves from areas of high, medium, and low incidence of breast cancer have shown that the pattern of rapidly increasing rates up to about the age of menopause is very similar. The age-specific rates then diverge in post-menopausal years: rates in low incidence areas decline and, in areas of medium and high rates, stay level or increase slowly respectively, resulting in greater variation in incidence rates in post- than pre-menopausal women. Moreover, it has been observed that rises in incidence over time in Iceland followed a similar pattern of increases affecting primarily postmenopausal women (4, 37).

TABLE VI.   Breast Cancer Incidence

Registry	Age group					
	35–39	40–44	45–49	50–54	55–59	60–64
USA, New York State	52.7	46.6	52.9	62.9	63.1	57.5
Canada, Alberta	−1.4	−12.0	24.7	15.0	44.3	54.1
U.K., Oxford Region	20.6	6.6	55.6	37.3	25.2	44.9
FRG, Hamburg	65.1	27.1	33.7	85.2	85.9	49.4
Hawaii: Japanese[a]	36.9	14.2	101.0	182.4	181.4	158.0
German Democratic Republic	32.0	18.7	15.6	37.9	27.3	40.3
Colombia, Cali	7.6	1.9	2.6	6.8	9.3	47.6
Poland, Katowice	27.2	10.5	25.9	70.3	31.3	47.7
Japan, Miyagi	−11.3	13.4	12.4	44.7	49.8	64.0

Percentage change in age-specific rates in selected registration areas between the first (1960–62 or 1963–67) and last (1973–77) of period of data, as published in CI5.

[a] Registration may have been incomplete in first time period.

Data from CI5 for the high incidence area of Alberta in Canada, the medium incidence area of the German Democratic Republic and the low incidence area of Katowice District in Poland also demonstrate these patterns of diverging breast cancer rates at older, post-menopausal ages in the different registration areas seen at the same point in time (Fig. 4). The larger increases in rates at post-menopausal ages that may occur over time are shown for two of these registries in Fig. 5.

Changes observed at younger ages may be an early signal of changing risks and there has been some discussion about the direction of trends in breast cancer incidence in younger women. A review of longer-term trends in breast cancer incidence in Saskatchewan for the period 1951 to 1975 (36) indicated that rates for pre- and peri-menopausal women did increase but only in the early part of the review period and rates appeared to be falling in more recent years. Rates in women in their post-menopausal years were increasing throughout the period. Data for other Canadian registries for a shorter period, 1971 to 1976 or 1966 to 1971, indicated that rates were only increasing in post-menopausal women. Similarly, a study of Connecticut data for the period 1935 to 1978 (34), although showing a different pattern than observed in Saskatchewan for the first half of the period, indicated that, in the second half of the period, rates were rising in the older age groups while rates in the younger age groups (under 45) appeared to have levelled off or decreased in the latest years. A study of incidence data for Scotland over the period 1960 to 1979 (5) found a decreasing breast cancer incidence in younger cohorts, indicating that overall incidence rates might fall in two or three decades. Table VI is based on CI5 data and shows how rates at ages 35–39, 40–44, 45–49, 50–54, 55–59, and 60–64 changed in selected registries between the first and last period of publication. In contrast to the above observations of falling or stable breast cancer rates in younger women, rates at premenopausal ages (35–44) increased in 8 of the 9 registries shown, although increases at older ages were always larger.

Migrant studies have shown that breast cancer rates of migrants and their descendents move, although slowly, towards those prevailing in the new environment (7, 19, 33) suggesting environmental causation. The two groups of factors considered most likely to explain the large differences in breast cancer risk in different populations and the changes that are occurring over time are related to diet and reproduction. Many investi-

TABLE VII. Prostate Cancer Incidence

Registration area	Rate[a] in 1973–1977	Average annual percentage change in rate[b]
U.S.A., Alameda: Black	100.2	3.35
U.S.A., Alameda: White	44.5	1.21
Sweden	44.4	4.04
U.S.A., Connecticut	42.7	1.67
New Zealand: Maori	39.8	−0.11
Norway	38.9	2.98
U.S.A., Hawaii: Japanese	36.0	7.51
Canada, Quebec	31.9	4.04
New Zealand: Non-Maori	30.7	−2.61
U.S.A., Hawaii: Chinese	25.8	7.68
Puerto Rico	25.0	3.35
U.K., Oxford Region	20.8	0.69
German Democratic Republic	18.1	3.66
Israel: All Jews	15.1	1.73
Hungary, Szabolcs-Szatmar	10.1	6.49
India, Bombay	6.7	0.52
Japan, Miyagi	4.9	1.58

[a] Rates in selected registration areas in 1973–1977, age-standardized to the "world" population.

[b] Average annual percentage change in rates since 1960–1962 or 1963–1967, estimated as indicated in Table II. Time periods stated are approximate and may vary slightly between registration areas.

gators have concluded that the principal reproductive risk factors, early menarche, late menopause and late first full-term pregnancy, cannot explain the major international differences in breast cancer patterns (12, 33) or the observed increases in incidence (2, 59) and that other aetiologic factors such as dietary differences are likely to play a role. A model based on the concept of "breast tissue age" is able to provide an explanation of much of the international variation in the age-incidence pattern of breast cancer in terms of these known risk factors (49).

Prostate Cancer

Worldwide cancer incidence estimates in males show prostate cancer ranking fifth. Table VII shows that geographical differences in incidence are very large for this cancer: rates vary about 20-fold for the registration areas shown, Incidence is highest in North America and low in East Asia and Eastern Europe, a distribution which at the extremes of the range strongly resembles that for breast cancer. The similarity is not observed for areas of intermediate incidence, however. For example, prostate cancer incidence rates in Israel and the U.K. are relatively low whereas breast cancer rates are not. Rates in men of Japanese and Chinese origin in Hawaii are at least five times higher than in Miyagi and in Chinese in Singapore (not shown). In Alameda County, rates in black men, which are by far the highest of all, are also more than twice as high as those in white men in the same County.

Mortality rates shown in Table VIII confirm the very low rates in Asia. As was also observed for breast cancer, however, in contrast to the pattern shown by incidence rates, mortality rates in many European countries, particularly those in the North, are higher than rates in Canada and the U.S.A.

TABLE VIII. Prostate Cancer Mortality

Country	Rate in[a] 1978–1979	Average annual percentage change in rate[b]
Sweden	20.7	1.07
Norway	20.3	1.37
Switzerland	18.2	1.19
Netherlands	15.8	0.92
New Zealand	15.1	0.59
U.S.A.	14.8	0.18
Canada	14.7	0.47
France	14.6	0.62
England and Wales	12.3	0.29
Italy	10.7[c]	1.70
Israel	8.7	0.01
Hong Kong	2.7	0.90
Japan	2.6	3.56

Age-standardized rates in selected countries in 1978–1979, and average annual percentage change in rate since 1955.

[a] Rates age-standardized to the "world" population.

[b] Estimated as indicated in Table II. The period over which the change in rates is calculated may vary from that shown above for some countries.

[c] 1978 only.

Tables VII and VIII also indicate the changes in incidence and mortality that have occurred. Incidence rates have increased in all but four of the registration areas reviewed. The only sizeable decreases occurred in New Zealand and in County Vas in Hungary (not shown). The reasons for these exceptions to the trend are unknown. Very large increases in rates, over 7% annually, were reported for Japanese and Chinese populations in Hawaii. As noted before, there is evidence that completeness of registration at the Hawaii cancer registry improved between 1960–1972 and, indeed, in this period the average annual change in the rate was slightly larger than from 1968–1972 to 1973–1977. Changes in the second period were, however, also large so that most of the reported increase may be real. Rates in Blacks in Alameda County increased by 3.4% annually, a rate of increase that is close to three times higher than in Whites in that area. It has been observed elsewhere (9) that an epidemic of prostate cancer may also be taking place in some Caribbean Islands and, perhaps, among African Blacks. Higher than average annual increases in incidence rates, over 3%, generally occurred in North America, Northern Europe, Germany, and Puerto Rico. A study of prostate cancer incidence in the Nordic countries from 1953–1977 (26) found clear increases in all countries.

Mortality rates rose in all but one of the countries reviewed but the rate of increase, less than 1% in eight countries and less than 2% in all but one country, was generally much lower than that observed for incidence in the same parts of the world. Japan is an exception, however. Compared with other countries, prostate cancer mortality rates remain very low but steep increases in rates, 3.6% annually, occurred which were furthermore much higher than the uneven increases in incidence reported for Miyagi.

Marked differences in prostate cancer mortality trends between the White and Nonwhite population of the U.S.A. occurred in the early part of the period 1950–1951 to

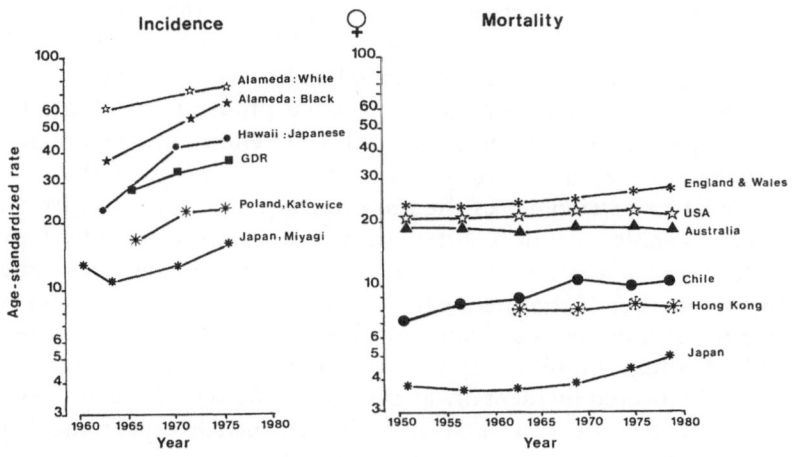

FIG. 6. Trends in prostate cancer incidence and mortality in selected registration areas or countries.

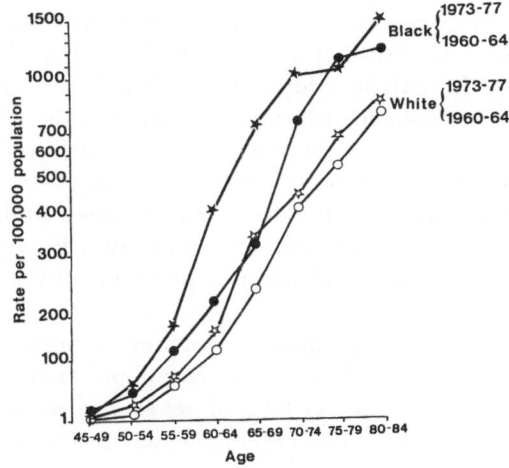

FIG. 7. Age-specific prostate cancer incidence rates in two time periods in Blacks and Whites in Alameda County, California, U.S.A.

1978. Between 1950–1951 and 1962–1963, mortality rates in Whites decreased slightly while rates in Nonwhites increased by 30%. In the latter part of the period, up to 1978, rates increased in both racial groups and although the increases were larger among Nonwhites, the differences were slight compared with the earlier years. Figure 6 illustrates some of the above changes. An examination of cohort-specific prostate cancer mortality rates in U.S. Nonwhites in the period 1930 to 1970 (20) found that rates reached a peak at every age in the cohort of 1896–1900 and declined thereafter, suggesting that age-adjusted rates among Nonwhites might decline in future years.

An examination of trends in age-specific incidence rates in Whites and Blacks in Alameda County (Fig. 7) shows the steeply rising incidence with age that is typical for this cancer as well as the higher rates in Blacks than in Whites at all ages. With the exception of a small decrease in Blacks aged 75–79 years, rates increased at all ages between 50 and 84 years and in both racial groups between 1960–1964 and 1973–1977. Increases in black men were particularly large between 60 and 69 years of age.

Prostate cancer incidence data present particular problems of interpretation. Latent carcinomas of the prostate are estimated to be three to eight times commoner than clinically apparent cancers (17) and a study based on autopsies (6) has shown that the frequency of larger latent carcinomas of the prostate varies with age and from area to area in a pattern that resembles that of reported incidence and mortality rates for clinical cancers. The discovery of latent cancers and, *pari passu*, reported incidence rates is greatly influenced by the number of routine medical checkups, prostatectomies for prostatic hypertropy and autopsies performed. Donn and Muir (17) have described the effect of an exceptionally high autopsy rate on reported incidence: in 1981, the proportion of prostate cancer cases discovered incidentally at autopsy in Malmö, Sweden, was 34.5% compared with 7.6% nationally and age-standardized prostate cancer incidence rates in Malmö were some 50% higher than in other areas of Sweden.

As for breast cancer, the observed relatively large increases in incidence compared with small increases in mortality have been attributed to the inclusion of nonfatal "cancers" in the incidence data since clinical trials have failed to demonstrate any major advances in the treatment of cancer of the prostate in recent years (8). A number of investigators, however, feel that real increases in prostate cancer incidence may also have taken place. For example, in both an examination of incidence data from CI5 (62) as well as one of the trends in the incidence of prostatic cancer in the Nordic countries (26), at least part of the observed increases were attributed to better diagnosis—the "Nordic study" included evidence of a shift to a higher percentage of localized cases—but it was also conceded that a real increase in incidence was a strong probability. Improvements in diagnostic practices are also an insufficient explanation for the very different trends in incidence and mortality in black and white populations in the U.S.A. (11, 17, 20, 27, 35).

The reasons for the marked geographical variation of prostate cancer, its increasing incidence and mortality and the "epidemic" in black populations are not clear but hormonal and genetic factors as well as dietary fat and venereal diseases have been implicated, while consumption of green and yellow vegetables may reduce the risk (29).

CONCLUSION

In view of the relatively short period in time spanned by the incidence data from CI5 and the fact that they are frequently based on small populations, the clarity with which they nonetheless show the general direction of the trends is noteworthy and can be interpreted as providing further evidence of the standards of quality applied by the editors in their selection of the data.

Not so clear are some aspects of the trends such as the magnitude of the increases in the incidence of breast and prostate cancer. It appears that the recording of cancers with good survival, for which incidence data, in principle, reflect occurrence so much better than mortality data, may be subject to the largest distortions and the question of which of the data sources provides more accurate estimates of changes in risk can be raised. For breast and prostate cancer, the generally much smaller increases in mortality rates may provide a more reliable indication of the real trends, at least in some areas.

This may be so notwithstanding the inaccuracies of death certification, the significant, and often ignored, international differences in death certificate coding (47) and the possibility that large artefactual changes in mortality could occur due to physicians changing their method of recording diagnoses when they fill out death certificates (48). Although not considered in this broad review, indicators of reliability of registration published in CI5, as well as several of the studies on trends in cancer incidence in the Nordic countries, show that cancer registries can provide much information, including that on changes in methods of diagnosis, autopsy rates and stage of the tumour at time of diagnosis, which permit some assessment of the effects of better diagnosis, changes in the definition of a cancer and improvements in completeness of registration of cancer cases on reported incidence.

The contributions that cancer incidence and mortality data can make to the knowledge of cancer have been described (13, 39) and trend analyses of the CI5 data are likely to play an increasingly important role in three main areas. First, observations of the time trends, not only for longer periods but also for a broader range of geographical areas and cancer sites than considered in the past, can be expected to be increasingly applied in the search for risk factors. Particularly fruitful may be a greater emphasis on the study of trends by histological types of cancer. Berg (3) wrote in 1970 that "the time is ripe for introducing histology systematically into the study of cancer epidemiology". Volumes II and IV of CI5 (15, 61) presented information on histological type for several cancer sites and many cancer registries have now collected histological information long enough to allow time trend analyses of these data. There appears to be an increase in such studies in recent years which may signal a growing exploitation of this information. Second, time trends in incidence play a major part in validating aetiological hypotheses as well as showing that measures of intervention are working: to demonstrate a causal relationship, the time trend in incidence of the cancer, taking induction period into account, has to correlate with changes in the prevalence of the suspected causes. The third area in which information on time trends in incidence can make a growing contribution is in the planning of health services. Investigators working with incidence data of the Nordic countries have shown what can be done in the way of forecasting future incidence based on observed trends (25, 58) and how the accuracy of these forecasts can be improved by taking knowledge of risk factors (e.g., smoking and lung cancer) or of the natural history of the cancer (e.g., cervix) or of intervention (e.g., fewer starting to smoke, lower tar content of cigarettes, screening for precancerous lesions of the cervix) into consideration. Requirements for different diagnostic and therapeutic services and for medical and surgical specialists of differing training are clearly indicated by the decreasing incidence of some cancers, such as stomach, and the increasing incidence of others, such as lung, breast, and prostate.

In all of the above endeavours, the contribution of incidence as well as mortality data can be enhanced by the systematic use of cohort analyses. Although the separation and interpretation of cohort, calendar year and age effects is difficult, it has been demonstrated that these analyses can shed much light on the nature of the factors underlying the observed trends and may thus suggest or confirm possible risk factors (37, 38) as well as possible biases of the data (10, 43) and that they are the preferred tool in predictions of the future burden of cancer (25, 51, 58).

Time trends are but one avenue of cancer research, but to quote Seneca "*Veritatem dies aperit*" (Time discovers the truth).

Acknowledgment

It is a pleasure to acknowledge the help of Mme A. Romanoff and Mlle O. Bouvy in the preparation of the manuscript.

REFERENCES

1. Aoki, K., Tominaga, S., Hirayama, T., and Hirota, Y. (eds.) "Cancer Prevention in Developing Countries," (1982). The University of Nagoya Press, Nagoya.
2. Armstrong, B. Recent trends in breast cancer incidence and mortality in relation to changes in possible risk factors. *Int. J. Cancer*, **17**, 204–211 (1976).
3. Berg, J. Some intercountry and intergroup differences in histological types of cancer. *J. Chron. Dis.*, **23**, 325–334 (1970).
4. Bjarnason, O., Day, N., Snaedal, G., and Tulinius, H. The effect of year of birth on the breast cancer age incidence curve in Iceland. *Int. J. Cancer*, **13**, 689–696 (1974).
5. Boyle, P. and Robertson, C., Age-time-cohort models of breast cancer and colon cancer in females in Scotland, 1960–1979. *J. Natl. Cancer Inst.* (in press).
6. Breslow, N., Chan, C. W., Dhom, G., Drury, R.A.B., Franks, L. M., Gellei, B., Lee, Y. S., Lundberg, S., Sparke, B., Sternby, N. H., and Tulinius, H. Latent carcinoma of prostate at autopsy in seven areas. *Int. J. Cancer*, **20**, 680–688 (1977).
7. Buell, P. Changing incidence of breast cancer in Japanese-American women. *J. Natl. Cancer Inst.*, **51**, 1479–1483 (1973).
8. Cairns, J. The treatment of diseases and the war against cancer. *Sci. Am.* **253**, 31–39 (1985).
9. Correa, P. and Londoño, J. Time trends in the Americas. *In* "Trends in Cancer Incidence: Causes and Practical Implications," ed. K. Magnus, pp. 335–344 (1982). Hemisphere Publishing Corporation, Washington, New York, and London.
10. Day, N. E. and Charnay, B., Time trends, cohort effects, and aging as influence on cancer incidence. *In* "Trends in Cancer Incidence: Causes and Practical Implications," ed. K. Magnus, pp. 263–270 (1982). Hemisphere Publishing Corporation, Washington, New York, and London.
11. Devesa, S. S. and Silverman, D. T. Cancer incidence and mortality trends in the United States: 1935–74. *J. Natl. Cancer Inst.*, **60**, 545–571 (1978).
12. DeWaard, F. Breast cancer trends in Europe and Israel: Implications for the nutritional etiology of breast cancer. *In* "Trends in Cancer Incidence: Causes and Practical Implications," ed. K. Magnus, pp. 263–270 (1982). Hemisphere Publishing Corporation, Washington, New York, and London.
13. Doll, R. The epidemiology of cancer. *Cancer*, **45**, 2475–2485 (1980).
14. Doll, R., Payne, P., and Waterhouse, J. (eds.) "Cancer Incidence in Five Continents," Vol. I (1966). Springer-Verlag, Berlin.
15. Doll, R., Muir, C., and Waterhouse, J. (eds.) "Cancer Incidence in Five Continents," Vol. II (1970). Springer-Verlag, Berlin.
16. Doll, R. and Peto, R. The Causes of Cancer, (1981). Oxford University Press, Oxford.
17. Donn, A. S. and Muir, C. S. Prostatic cancer: Some epidemiological features. *Bull. Cancer* **72**, 381–390 (1985).
18. Dunham, L. J. and Bailar, J. C., III. World maps of cancer mortality rates and frequency ratios. *J. Natl. Cancer Inst.*, **41**, 155–203 (1968).
19. Dunn, J. Breast cancer among American Japanese in the San Francisco Bay area. *Natl. Cancer Inst. Monogr.*, **47**, 157–160 (1977).
20. Ernster, V., Selvin, S., and Winkelstein, W. Cohort mortality for prostatic cancer among United States nonwhites. *Science*, **200**, 1165–1166 (1978).

21. Fujimoto, I. and Hanai, A. Trends of cancer incidence by site and histological type in Osaka, Japan, 1963–1982. This volume, pp. 25–31.

22. Haenszel, W. Cancer mortality among the foreign-born in the United States. *J. Natl. Cancer Inst.*, **26**, 37–132 (1961).

23. Haenszel, W. and Kurihara, M. Studies of Japanese migrants. I. Mortality from cancer and other diseases among Japanese in the United States. *J. Natl. Cancer Inst.*, **40**, 43–68 (1968).

24. Haenszel, W., Kurihara, M., Segi, M., and Lee, R. Stomach cancer among Japanese in Hawaii. *J. Natl. Cancer Inst.*, **49**, 969–988 (1972).

25. Hakulinen, T. and Pukkala, E. Prediction of cancer incidence by utilization of risk factors and the effect of intervention. *In* "Trends in Cancer Incidence: Causes and Practical Implications," ed. K. Magnus, pp. 111–123 (1982). Hemisphere Publishing Corporation, Washington, New York, and London.

26. Harvei, S. and Johansen, A. Incidence trends in the Nordic countries. *In* "Trends in Cancer Incidence: Causes and Practical Implications," ed. K. Magnus, pp. 325–334 (1982). Hemisphere Publishing Corporation, Washington, New York, and London.

27. Henschke, U., Leffall, L., Mason, C., Rheinhold, A., Schneider, R., and White, J. Alarming increase of the cancer mortality in the U.S. Black population (1950–1967). *Cancer*, **31**, 763–768 (1973).

28. Hirayama, T. Changing patterns of cancer in Japan with special reference to the decrease in stomach cancer mortality. *In* "Origins of Human Cancer," Book A., eds. H. H. Hiatt, J. P. Watson, and J. A. Winston, pp. 55–75 (1977). Cold Spring Harbor Laboratory, New York.

29. Hirayama, T. Epidemiology of prostate cancer with special reference to the role of diet. *Natl. Cancer Inst. Monogr.*, **53**, 149–155 (1979).

30. Jensen, O. M. Trends in the incidence of stomach cancer in the five Nordic countries. *In* "Trends in Cancer Incidence: Causes and Practical Implications," ed. K. Magnus, pp. 127–142 (1982). Hemisphere Publishing Corporation, Washington, New York, and London.

31. Kurihara, M., Aoki, K., and Tominaga, S. (eds). "Cancer Mortality Statistics in the World," (1984). The University of Nagoya Press, Nagoya.

32. Logan, W.P.D. Cancer mortality by occupation and social class 1851–1971. IARC Scientific Publications No. 36. Studies on medical and population subjects No. 44 (1982). Her Majesty's Stationery Office, London, and IARC, Lyon.

33. MacMahon, B., Cole, P., and Brown, J. Etiology of human breast cancer: A review. *J. Natl. Cancer Inst.*, **50**, 21–42 (1973).

34. MacMahon, B. Incidence trends in North America, Japan and Hawaii. *In* "Trends in Cancer Incidence: Causes and Practical Implications," ed. K. Magnus, pp. 249–261 (1982). Hemisphere Publishing Corporation, Washington, New York, and London.

35. Mandel, J. and Schuman, L. Epidemiology of cancer of the prostate. *In* "Reviews in Cancer Epidemiology," ed. A. M. Lilienfeld, Vol. 1, pp. 2–83 (1980). Elsevier / North-Holland, New York.

36. Miller, A. B. Cancer of the breast. *In* "Trends in Cancer Incidence: Causes and Practical Implications," ed. K. Magnus, pp. 231–234 (1982). Hemisphere Publishing Corporation, Washington, New York, and London.

37. Muir, C. S., Choi, N. W., and Schifflers, E. Time trends in cancer mortality in some countries: Their possible causes and significance. *In* "Medical Aspects of Mortality Statistics," eds. H. Bostrom and N. Ljungstedt, pp. 269–309 (1981). Skandia International Symposia. Almquist & Wiksell International, Stockholm.

38. Muir, C. S. Time trends as indicators of etiology. *In* "Trends in Cancer Incidence: Causes and Practical Implications," ed. K. Magnus, pp. 89–102 (1982). Hemisphere Publishing Corporation, Washington, New York, and London.

39. Muir, C. S., Démaret, E., and Boyle, P. The cancer registry in cancer control: An overview. *In*: "The Role of the Registry in Cancer Control," eds. D. M. Parkin, G. Wagner, and C. S. Muir. IARC Scientific Publications No. 66, pp. 13–26 (1985).

40. Muñoz, N., Correa, P., Cuello, C., and Duque, E. Histologic types of gastric carcinoma in high- and low-risk areas. *Int. J. Cancer*, **3**, 809–818 (1968).

41. Muñoz, N. and Asvall, J. Time trends of intestinal and diffuse types of gastric cancer in Norway. *Int. J. Cancer*, **8**, 144–157 (1971).

42. Myers, M., Hankey, B., Steinhorn, S., and Flannery, J. Interrelationship of incidence, survival and mortality and their effects on time trends. *In* "Trends in Cancer Incidence: Causes and Practical Implications," ed. K. Magnus, pp. 79–87 (1982). Hemisphere Publishing Corporation, Washington, New York, and London.

43. Osmond, C., Gardner, M. J., Acheson, E. D., and Adelstein, A. M. Trends in cancer mortality 1951–1980: analyses by period of birth and death. Series DHI No. 11 (1983). Her Majesty's Stationery Office, London.

44. Parkin, D. M., Stjernswärd, J., and Muir, C. S. Estimates of the worldwide frequency of twelve major cancers. *Bull. WHO*, **62**, 163–182 (1984).

45. Parkin, D. M., Wagner, G., and Muir, C. S. (eds.). "The Role of the Registry in Cancer Control," IARC Scientific Publications, No. 66 (1985). IARC, Lyon.

46. Parkin, D. M. (ed.). "Cancer Occurrence in Developing Countries," IARC Scientific Publications, No. 75. IARC, Lyon (in press).

47. Percy, C. and Dolman, A. Comparison of the coding of death certificates related to cancer in seven countries. *Public Health Reports*, **93**, 335–350 (1978).

48. Percy, C., Stanek, E., and Gloeckler, L. Accuracy of cancer death certificates and its effect on cancer mortality statistics. *AJPH*, **71**, 242–250 (1981).

49. Pike, M. C., Krailo, M. D., Henderson, B. E., Casagrande, J. T., and Hoel, D. G. 'Hormonal' risk factors, 'breast tissue age' and the age-incidence of breast cancer. *Nature*, **303**, 767–770 (1983).

50. Roush, G., Schymura, M., Holford, J., White, C., and Flannery, J. Time period compared to birth cohort in Connecticut incidence rates for twenty-five malignant neoplasms. *J. Natl. Cancer Inst.*, **74**. 779–788 (1985).

51. Sandstad, B. Prediction of cancer incidence based on cohort analysis. *In* "Trends in Cancer Incidence: Causes and Practical Implications," ed. K. Magnus, pp. 103–110 (1982). Hemisphere Publishing Corporation, Washington, New York, and London.

52. Saxén, E. Trends: Facts or fallacy. *In* "Trends in Cancer Incidence: Causes and Practical Implications," ed. K. Magnus, pp. 5–16 (1982). Hemisphere Publishing Corporation, Washington, New York, and London.

53. Schifflers, E., Smans, M., and Muir, C. Birth cohort analysis using irregular cross-sectional data: A technical note. *Stat. Med.*, **4**, 63–75 (1985).

54. Segi, M. and Kurihara, M. "Cancer Mortality for Selected Sites in 24 Countries," Nos. 1–5 (1960, 1962, 1964, 1966, 1969). Tohoku University School of Medicine, Sendai.

55. Segi M. and Kurihara, M. "Cancer Mortality for Selected Sites in 24 Countries," No. 6 (1972). Japan Cancer Society, Tokyo.

56. Staszewski, J. and Haenszel, W. Cancer mortality among the Polish-born in the United States. *J. Natl. Cancer Inst.*, **35**, 291–297 (1965).

57. Thomas, D. Epidemiologic and related studies of breast cancer etiology. *In* "Reviews in Cancer Epidemiology," ed. A. M. Lilienfeld, Vol. 1, pp. 153–217 (1980). Elsevier / North-Holland, New York.

58. Teppo, L., Hakama, M., Hakulinen, T., Pukkala, E., and Saxén, E. Planning and evaluating preventive measures. *In* "The Role of the Registry in Cancer Control," eds. D. M. Parkin, G. Wagner, and C. Muir, IARC Scientific Publications, No. 66, pp. 27–44 (1985). IARC, Lyon.

59. Tulinius, H. and Sigvaldason, H. Trends in incidence of female breast cancer in the Nordic countries. *In* "Trends in Cancer Incidence: Causes and Practical Implications," ed. K. Magnus, pp. 235–247 (1982). Hemisphere Publishing Corporation, Washington, New York, and London.

60. Waterhouse, J., Muir, C., Correa, P., and Powell, J. (eds.) "Cancer Incidence in Five Continents," Vol. III, IARC Scientific Publications, No. 15 (1976). IARC, Lyon.

61. Waterhouse, J., Muir, C., Shanmugaratnam, K., and Powell, J. (eds.) "Cancer Incidence in Five Continents," Vol. IV, IARC Scientific Publications, No. 42 (1982). IARC, Lyon.

62. Waterhouse, J. Cancer of the prostate. *In* "Trends in Cancer Incidence: Causes and Practical Implications," ed. K. Magnus, pp. 321–324 (1982). Hemisphere Publishing Corporation, Washington, New York, and London.

TRENDS OF CANCER INCIDENCE BY SITE AND HISTOLOGICAL TYPE IN OSAKA, JAPAN, 1963–1982

Isaburo Fujimoto and Aya Hanai

*Department of Field Research, Center for Adult Diseases**

The cancer incidence of many sites changed in Osaka during the period from 1963 to 1982. A decrease was observed in cancers of the esophagus, stomach, larynx, and uterus. An increase in both sexes was noticed in cancers of the colon, rectum, pancreas, liver (male), gallbladder, lung, breast (female), and in leukemia. Distribution of histological type has also changed in cancers of the stomach and lung.

Age-adjusted incidence rates were calculated for three histological types of stomach cancer, so-called intestinal, diffuse, and other types, according to Lauren's criteria, for the periods of 1966–1971 and 1972–1977. Estimated incidence rates of the intestinal type decreased markedly in both sexes in the latter period. The rate of the diffuse type decreased slightly among males and remained fairly constant among females.

Relative frequencies of major histological types of lung cancer in the 1971–1975 period were compared to those in the 1976–1980 period. The proportion of adenocarcinoma and undifferentiated carcinoma increased in the latter period, while the proportion of squamous cell carcinoma decreased.

Further studies are necessary to observe the sequence of these phenomena and to clarify factors associated with these changes.

The first population-based cancer registry in Japan, the Miyagi Tumor Registry, was established in 1951 and was operated for 3 years by the late Mitsuo Segi, Honorary Professor of Tohoku University. After an interval it was started again in 1959 under his hand and has continued as one of the most reliable cancer registries in Japan. Professor Segi was a pioneer in cancer epidemiology, especially in the field of descriptive epidemiology and had published a series of "Cancer mortality for selected sites in 24 countries," commonly known throughout the world as Segi's book. He pointed out that cancer mortality was markedly different by country.

The population-based Osaka Cancer Registry (OCR) began in 1962 and has reported remarkable changes in the incidence rates of many cancer sites in these 20 years. These changes have encouraged us to develop analytical studies as well as descriptive epidemiological studies. The registry data has also been utilized for planning and evaluating cancer control programs and for information services to the participating hospitals and physicians in Osaka.

In this report, results of descriptive studies in the OCR are introduced.

---

* Nakamichi 1-chome, Higashinari-ku, Osaka 537, Japan (藤本伊三郎, 花井 彩).

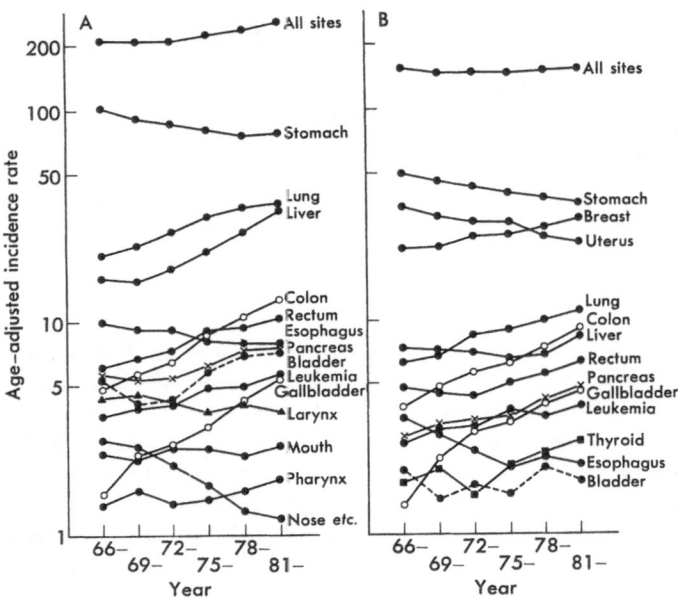

FIG. 1.   Trends of age-adjusted incidence rates
A: male. B: female, Osaka.

Time Trends of Cancer Incidence of Major Sites in Osaka

The OCR now has incidence data of more than 20 years. Details of the background of the registration areas and activities of the OCR are described elsewhere (3, 4).

The observation time of 1966–1982 was divided into six periods; five 3-year periods between 1963 and 1980 and a 2-year period, 1981–1982. Figure 1 shows the age-adjusted incidence rates in each period by sex and site. The world population presented by Doll et al. (1) was used as a standard population.

A decrease of incidence rates was observed in cancers of the stomach and esophagus for both sexes, of the larynx in males and of the uterus in females. An increase was noticed in cancers of the lung, colon, pancreas, gallbladder and biliary passage, leukemia for both sexes, liver cancer for males, and breast cancer for females.

Similar changes were observed in other cancer registries in Japan (7), suggesting that these changes would be seen in all areas of the country and were caused by changes of living conditions, life styles such as dietary, and smoking habits, etc. in Japan after the Second World War.

Stomach Cancer

The age-adjusted incidence rate of stomach cancer in 1972–1977 decreased by 15% from the 1966–1971 period in both sexes. The data were examined to determine whether or not the histological distribution of stomach cancer had also changed during the observation periods.

The histological diagnoses described in cancer reports which were sent by the participating medical doctors in Osaka were analysed. Cancer cases with histological diagnoses were classified into three types, so-called intestinal, diffuse, and others, according

TABLE I. Time Trend of the Estimated Age-adjusted Incidence Rates of Each Histological Type of Stomach Cancer in Osaka

Period	Male			Female		
	Actual	Estimated		Actual	Estimated	
	All stomach	Intestinal	Diffuse	All stomach	Intestinal	Diffuse
(I) 1966–1971	93.7	58.5	35.0	46.5	23.8	22.6
(II) 1972–1977	79.4	47.3	32.4	39.7	17.8	21.9
Ratio II/I	0.85	0.81	0.93	0.85	0.75	0.97

Standard population for age-adjusting is the world population.

to Lauren's criteria (5). Age-adjusted incidence rates of these types were calculated based on the age-specific rates. The latter were estimated by multiplying the total stomach cancer age-specific incidence rates with relative frequencies (%) of each histological type in each age-group (Table I). The rates for "other types" were very small, so these are not given in Table I.

Estimated incidence rates of the intestinal type decreased markedly in both sexes during the period 1966–1977. The rate for the diffuse type decreased slightly among males and females (Table I). Although the data are not shown in this paper, the incidence rate of the intestinal type decreased more in the younger age-groups than in the older ones (5).

It was reported that the frequency of the intestinal type was higher in high-incidence areas (9), and decreased when the incidence decreased (10). The findings in Osaka were in agreement with these results.

It is commonly known that the diffuse type of carcinoma of the stomach is more difficult to diagnose in the earlier stages than the other type and shows less favourable survival. Therefore, it is urgent to develop methods to diagnose diffuse type of carcinoma in the earlier stages.

Lung Cancer

Analysing hospital-based materials, an increase in the relative frequency of adenocarcinoma was observed among lung cancer cases in U.S.A. (14) and in Tokyo, Japan (13). The population-based materials in the OCR were examined to see whether or not similar changes could be observed (6).

Table II shows the relative frequencies of the major histological types of lung cancer, according to the description of histological diagnosis in cancer reports. Among males, proportions of adenocarcinoma and undifferentiated carcinoma (small cell carcinoma and large cell carcinoma) increased in the period 1976–1980 as compared with the period 1971–1975. The proportion of squamous cell carcinomas decreased between these periods. These changes were observed more markedly in the younger age group (under 59 years old) than in the older age group (over 60 years old). Although the data for females are not shown in this paper, similar trends were observed.

It has been reported that the increase in the lung cancer incidence rate is associated with the increase of squamous cell carcinoma or Kreyberg I type of carcinoma due to the increasing risks of environmental factors such as smoking, air pollution, etc. (8). However, in Osaka and also in Tokyo, a marked increase of lung cancer incidence was

TABLE II.   Time Trend of the Distribution of Each Histological Type
of Lung Cancer among Males in Osaka

Age group	All ages		Age less than 59		Age more than 60	
Observing period	1971–75	76–80	71–75	76–80	71–75	76–80
No. observed	1,185	2,852	443	808	742	2,044
Adenocarcinoma	33.0%	26.6%	34.3%	43.4%	32.2%	33.9%
Squamous cell ca.	49.6	41.7	47.2	32.9	51.1	45.2
Undifferentiated ca.	16.5	20.7	17.6	22.4	15.9	20.0
Small cell ca.	8.8	13.6	8.8	14.2	8.8	13.3
Large cell ca.	3.6	4.9	4.5	5.7	3.1	4.5
Unclassified	4.1	2.2	4.3	2.5	4.0	2.1

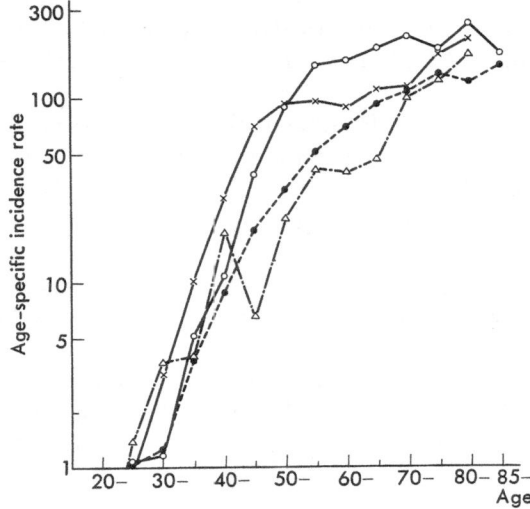

FIG. 2.   Trends of age-specific incidence rates for liver cancer and death rates for
liver cirrhosis among males in Osaka, Japan
● liver cancer, 1966–1969 (155 and 197.8 ICD-8); ○ liver cancer, 1981–1982 (155
in ICD-9); △ liver cirrhosis, 1965; × liver cirrhosis, 1980.

observed with the increase of the relative frequency of adenocarcinoma. Detailed studies
are now necessary for clarifying the effects of active as well as passive smoking, air pollution, dietary habits, life style, *etc.*, on each histological type of lung cancer.

Liver Cancer

Figure 2 shows age-specific incidence rates for male liver cancer in 1966–1969
and in 1981–1982 in Osaka. A noticeable increase was observed in age-groups 35–74.
Figure 2 also shows age-specific mortality for male liver cirrhosis in 1965 and 1980 in
Osaka. A marked increase was observed in age groups 35–69. Both risks for live cancer
and for liver cirrhosis seemed to increase in recent years.

Reasons for the increase of male liver cancer and male liver cirrhosis are not completely clear at present. The hepatitis B antigen positive carrier rate was assumed to be

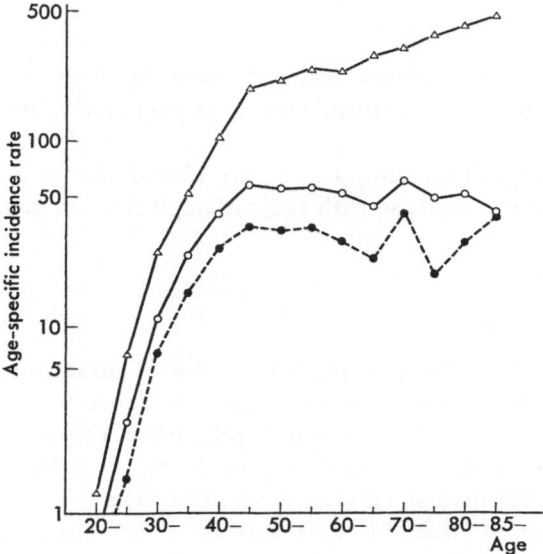

FIG. 3.   Age-specific incidence rates for female breast cancer in Osaka and in Connecticut
● Osaka, 1966–1968; ○ Osaka, 1981–1982; △ Connecticut, 1973–1977.

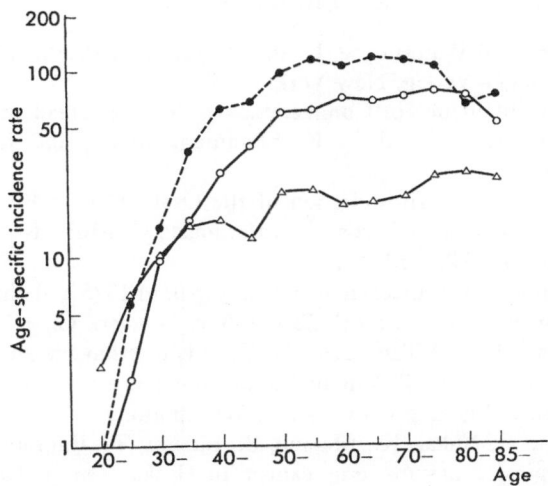

FIG. 4.   Age-specific incidence rates for uterine cancer in Osaka and for cervical cancer in Connecticut
● Osaka, 1966–1968; ○ Osaka, 1981–1982; △ Connecticut, 1973–1977.

constant (around 2%) in the observation period (11, 12). Epidemiological studies are urgently needed to clarify the factors associated with the increase of these two related diseases.

Breast Cancer

Figure 3 shows the age-specific incidence rates of breast cancer from 1966–1968 and 1981–1982 in Osaka. The increase was more remarkable in age-groups above 45 years of age.

Incidence rates for Connecticut, U.S.A. are also shown in the figure (*2*). This incidence curve continued to increase with age, although such an increase has not yet been observed in Osaka.

Uterine Cancer

Figure 4 shows the age-specific incidence rates of invasive uterine cancer (ICD-9 code, 179–182). In 1982, invasive uterine cancer incidence was 933, consisting of 692 cervical cancer (ICD-9 code, 180), 2 chorioepithelioma (code 181), 99 corpus cancer (code 182), and 140 unspecified uterine cancer (code 179). Most uterine cancer cases (85% or more) were classified as cervical cancer in Osaka.

The incidence rate in Osaka has decreased in all age groups except for age groups 80–89 (Fig. 4). Compared with the incidence rates of cervical cancer (ICD-9 code 179) in Connecticut, U.S.A., (*2*), Osaka in 1981–1982 had lower incidence rates in age-groups 20–29, and higher rates in age-groups 40–89.

REFERENCES

1. Doll, R., Payne, P., and Waterhouse, J. eds. Cancer Incidence in Five Continents, p. 236 (1966). UICC, Springer-Verlag, New York.
2. Flannery, J. Cancer incidence in Connecticut. *In* "Cancer Incidence in Five Continents, IV," eds. J. Waterhouse, C. Muir, K. Shanmugaratnam, and J. Powell, pp. 320–323 (1982). IARC, Lyon.
3. Fujimoto, I. and Hanai, A. Introduction of the Osaka Cancer Registry. *In* "Cancer Incidence in Five Continents, IV," eds. J. Waterhouse, C. Muir, K. Shanmugaratnam, and J. Powell, pp. 430–431 (1982). IARC, Lyon.
4. Hanai, A. and Fujimoto, I. Cancer incidence in Japan in 1975 and changes of epidemiological features for cancer in Osaka. *Natl. Cancer Inst. Monogr.*, **62**, 3–7 (1982).
5. Hanai, A., Fujimoto, I., and Taniguchi, H. Trends of stomach cancer incidence and histological types in Osaka. *In* "Trends in Cancer Incidence," ed. K. Magnus, pp. 143–154 (1982). Hemisphere Publishing Corporation, Washington.
6. Hanai, A., Hiyama, Y., Nakai, K., Matsuo, S., Suzuki, T., Fujimoto, I., and Tateishi, R. Trends of histological types of lung cancer in Osaka. *Jpn. J. Cancer Clin.*, **28**, 1589–1596 (1982) (in Japanese).
7. Hanai, A., Kitamura, H., Fukuma, S., and Fujimoto, I. Cancer incidence in Japan 1975–1979, pp. xii and 8–17 (1984). The Research Group for Population-based Cancer Registration in Japan, Chiba and Osaka.
8. Higginson, J. and Jensen, O. M. Epidemiological review of lung cancer in man. *In* "Air Pollution and Cancer in Man," eds. U. Mohr, D. Schmahl, and L. Tomatis, pp. 169–189 (1977). IARC, Lyon.
9. Munoz, N., Correa, P., Cuello, C., and Duque, E. Histologic types of gastric carcinoma in high- and low- risk areas. *Int. J. Cancer*, **3**, 809–818 (1968).
10. Munoz, N. and Asvall, J. Time trends of intestinal and diffuse types of gastric cancer in Norway. *Int. J. Cancer*, **8**, 144–157 (1971).

11. Oshima, A., Hiyama, T., Fujimoto, I., Song, K., Yamano, H., and Tanaka, M. Epidemiology of liver cancer in Japan. *Jpn. J. Cancer Clin.*, **28**, 962–971 (1982) (in Japanese).
12. Oshima, A., Tsukuma, H., Hiyama, T., Fujimoto, I. Yamano, H., and Tanaka, M. Follow-up study of HBs Ag-positive blood donors with special reference to effect of drinking and smoking on development of liver cancer. *Int. J. Cancer*, **34**, 775–779 (1984).
13. Tsuchiya, E., Concetti, H. F., Wakimoto, J., Kitagawa, T., Nakagawa, K., Kinoshita, I., and Sugano, H. Time trend data of histological subtypes of lung cancer cases operated and non-operated at the Cancer Institute Hospital from 1961 to 1978. *Jpn. J. Cancer Clin.*, **28**, 196–203 (1982) (in Japanese).
14. Vincent, R. G., Pickren, J. W., Lane, W. W., Bross, I., Takita, H., Houten, L., Gutierrez, A. C., and Rzepka, T. The changing histology of lung cancer. *Cancer*, **39**, 1647–1655 (1977).

CHANGES IN MORTALITY OF ALL FORMS OF MALIGNANT NEOPLASMS AMONG JAPANESE FOR THE LAST DECADES

Kunio Aoki, Ryuichiro Sasaki,
and Shoichi Mizuno

*Department of Preventive Medicine,
Nagoya University School of Medicine**

The changing pattern of malignant neoplasms, all forms, among Japanese was examined using vital statistics for the period 1950 to 1983. Number of deaths from this cause has increased annually but the trends in age-adjusted death rates for the last two decades are stable in males and show a slight decline in females. Age-specific death rates indicate a stable trend in the middle-aged and an increasing trend in the elderly aged. Little geographical difference in mortality was observed between prefectures.

Although remarkable changes in mortality were seen in some types of malignant neoplasms, overall changes were small. There was little difference in overall cancer mortality between Japanese in Hawaii and in Japan, despite the quite different environments.

Cumulative death rates of all forms of malignant neoplasms up to the age of 84 in several populations were similar which may suggest some threshold of cancer mortality in these populations. Interaction of host-agent-environment in carcinogenesis should therefore be more carefully studied to clarify this epidemiological description.

All things are in flux and nothing is permanent. The epidemiology of cancer is no exception. Japanese have experienced extraordinary changes in the component of causes of death in quantity and quality during the four decades after World War II (*4*). This paper is to examine changing patterns of all forms of malignant neoplasms, in relation to time-space-person, and discusses key factors affecting the incidence of disease.

Deaths from All Causes and All Forms of Malignant Neoplasms (ICD 140-209)

Figure 1 shows the proportion of deaths from malignant neoplasms to those from all causes, and the age-adjusted death rates of all forms of malignant neoplasms and of all causes in 1935, 1950, 1965, 1975, and 1980. The percentage of malignant neoplasms in all causes of death was only 4.2% in 1935, but began to increase rapidly around 1950 and in 1980 reached 22.3%, three times higher than that in 1950 (*4, 7, 13*).

Age-adjusted death rate from all forms of malignant neoplasms (using the Japanese population in 1935 as a standard) was 72 per 100,000 in 1935, 76 in 1950, after which it gradually increased to 98 in 1980. Meanwhile, the death rate for all causes has continu-

---

* Tsurumai-cho 65, Schowa-ku, Nagoya 466, Japan (青木國雄, 佐々木隆一郎, 水野正一).

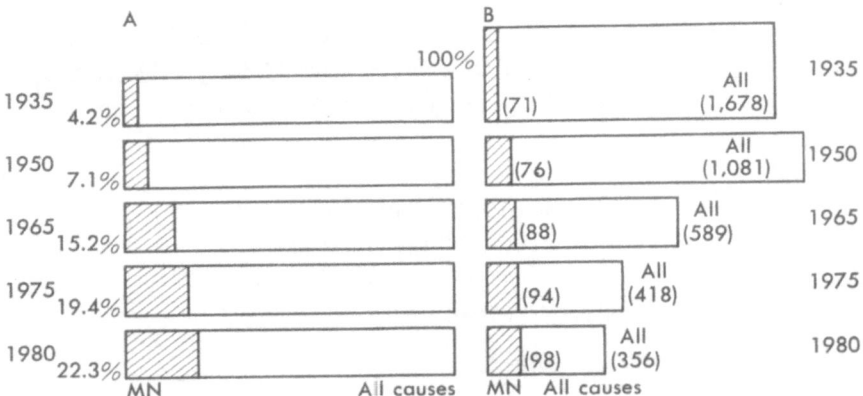

FIG. 1. Deaths from malignant neoplasms (MN) of all forms and all causes in
Japan, 1935–1980
A: proportion of deaths from MN to deaths from all causes. B: age-adjusted death
rates of MN and all causes per 100,000.

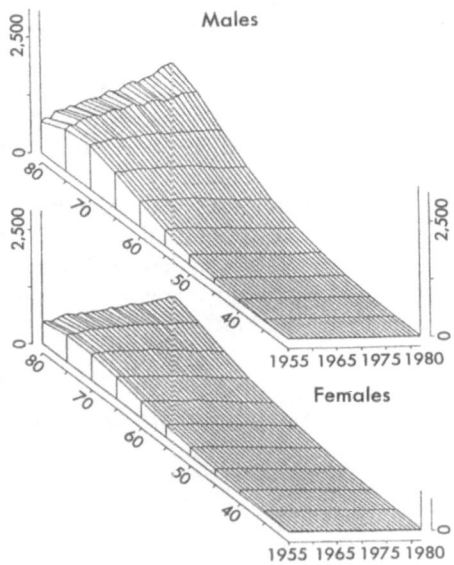

FIG. 2. Trends in age-specific death rates of malignant neoplasms of all forms in
Japan, 1955–1983

ously decreased from 1,081 in 1950 to 356 per 100,000 in 1980 (4, 13). Therefore, the
relative frequency of malignant neoplasms to all causes rose about 3-fold during the last
three decades, although the increase in the age-adjusted rate for this disease was about
15%.

Figure 2 shows a bird's eye view of trends in age-specific death rates of malignant
neoplasms at 30 years and over between 1955 and 1983 (10). Very stationary trends in
age-specific death rates were observed in groups of under 70 years in both sexes, although
the frequency differed between the sexes. However, the rates in the age groups over 70

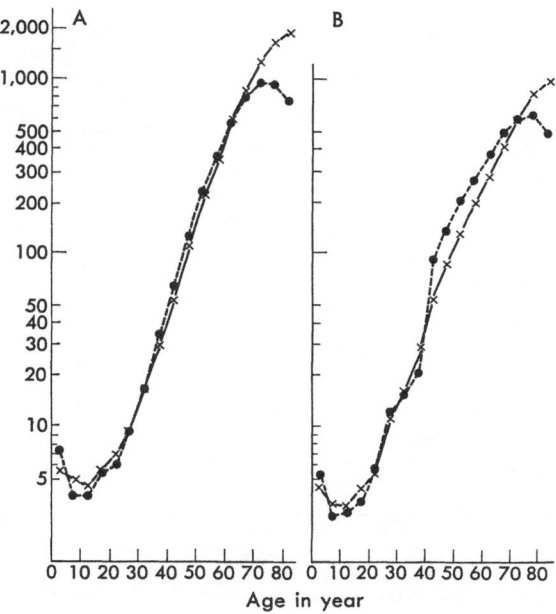

FIG. 3.   Changes in age-specific death rates of cancer of all sites in Japan, 1950–
1951 (●) and 1981–1982 (×)
A: male, B: female.

show a slow and smooth increase. The same stable trends in age-specific death rates
from all causes were observed in the middle and younger age groups, but uneven and
fluctuating trend curves were observed in the aged groups, which suggest very mild
changes in cancer mortality compared with those for all causes of death.

Trends in Age-specific Death Rates (4)

The changes in age-specific death rates of all forms of malignant neoplasms between
1950–1951 and 1981–1982 are shown in Fig. 3. The curves for age-specific death rates
were superimposed on male age groups of 30 to 60 years; a marked increased in the
rates was observed in the more elderly groups for both sexes. In females, a reduction in
rates was observed in the 40 to 64 year age-groups. At younger than 20 years, a slight
increase in the rates was observed except for the 0–4 year group. However, the overall
death rates for malignant neoplasms at ages less than 20 have been quite stable for the
last four decades (7).

Trends in age-specific death rates of all forms of malignant neoplasms by birth cohort
are shown in Figs. 4 and 5. In males, the birth cohort curves of ages 30 to 64 for those
born from 1900–1904 to 1935–1939 overlapped; that is, there was little difference in
rate among birth cohorts. In older ages, a gradual increasing rate trend by birth cohort
between 1875 and 1900 was observed but levelled off in those born after 1900. The curves
reflecting the rates in younger ages are trough-shaped, and variations among birth cohorts
did not show regular changes, although the rates were low. In females, marked changes
in age-specific death rates were seen among birth cohorts. In more recent cohorts the

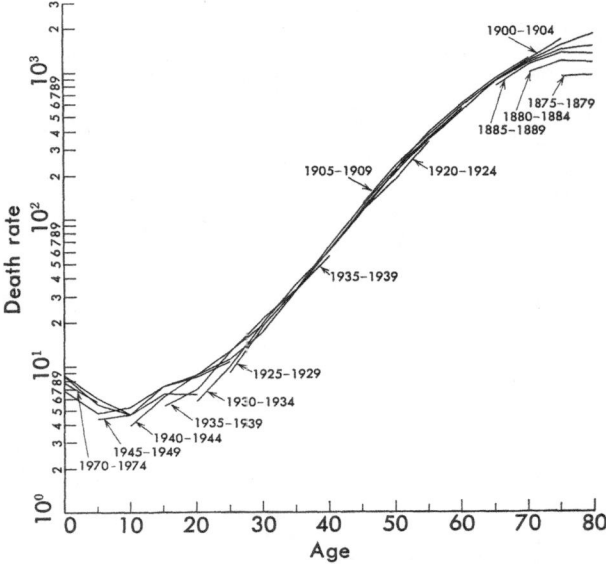

FIG. 4. Age-specific death rates of malignant neoplasms of all forms by birth co-hort born 1875 to 1974 in Japan (males)

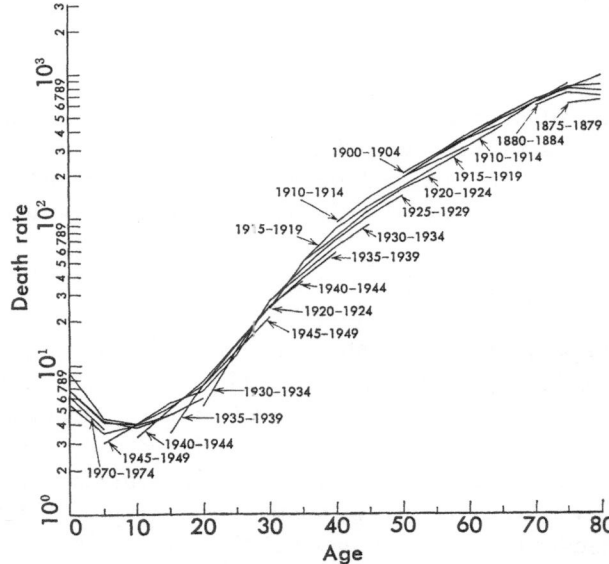

FIG. 5. Age-specific death rates of malignant neoplasms of all forms by birth co-hort born 1875 to 1974 in Japan (females)

rates decreased between the ages of 35 to 64. The changes in old and young ages were not so remarkable in females as in males, although the patterns were similar.

Geographical Distribution

Figure 6 shows the geographical distribution of the standardized mortality ratio

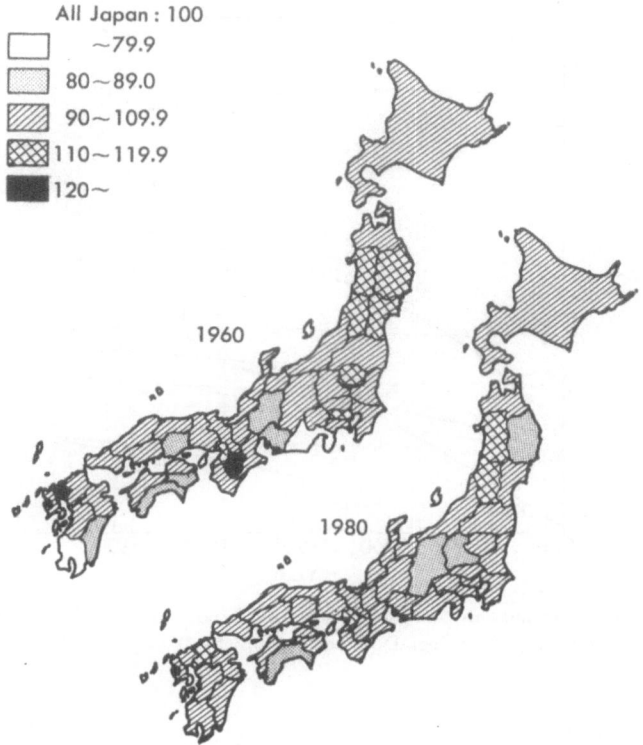

All Japan : 100

☐   ~79.9
▨   80~89.0
▨   90~109.9
▨ 110~119.9
■ 120~

FIG. 6.   Standardized mortality rates of malignant neoplasms by prefecture in Japan, 1960 and 1980 (males)

(SMR) for all forms of malignant neoplasms by prefecture. In 1960, there were two prefectures with SMRs of more than 120, three with SMRs of less than 80 and the remaining 42 prefectures had moderate SMRs for males. In 1980, the difference in mortality among prefectures became smaller, and very high- or very low-rate areas disappeared in this period. The difference in female rates by prefecture was smaller than that of males. The geographical difference in mortality from malignant neoplasms seems to be decreasing, despite considerable environmental differences among prefectures, such as climatic, geological, industrial, economical, and other conditions.

Changes in Death Rates of Malignant Neoplasms by Site (4)

The age-adjusted death rates for all forms of malignant neoplasms show a stationary trend with a slight recent increase in males (3.0%, 1960–1980) and a decreasing trend in females (13.4%, 1960–1980), as depicted in Figs. 7 and 8.

The most remarkable changes in rate by site were observed in cancers of the stomach, lung, and uterus (all forms); of these, uterus cancer showed the most striking reduction. The reduction of esophageal cancer in females is also remarkable. Stomach cancer has been gradually decreasing since around 1965 while lung cancer has shown a steep and continuous increase since 1947 in both sexes. The trend curves for stomach and lung cancers are expected to cross between 1995 and 2000. Cancers of the intestine, rectum,

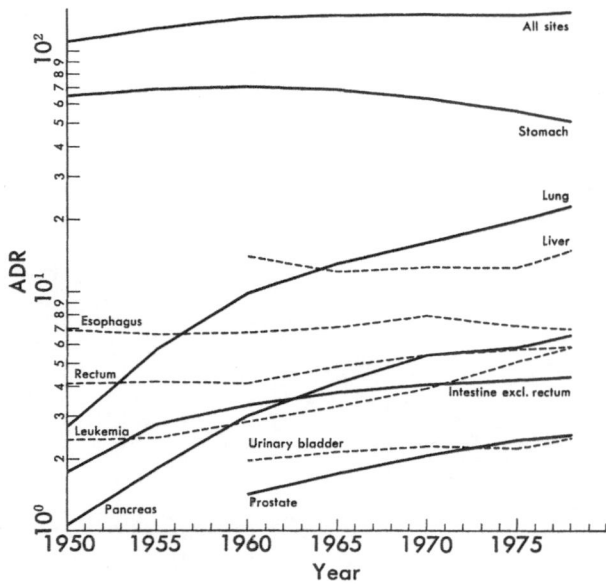

FIG. 7. Trends in age-adjusted death rate from cancer for selected sites in Japan, 1950–1978 (male) (based on Segi-Doll world population)

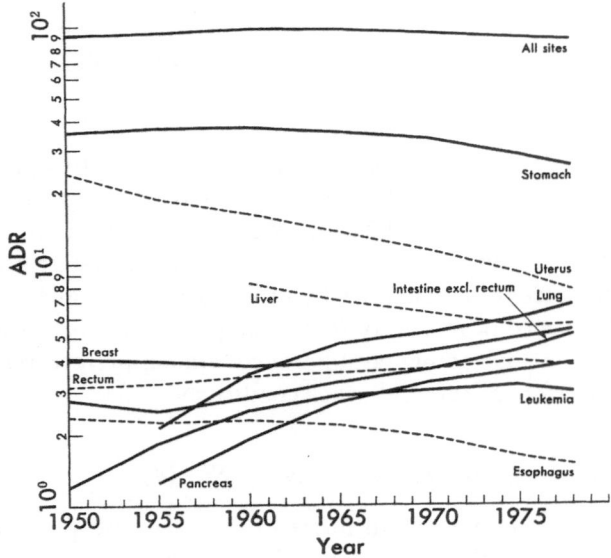

FIG. 8. Trends in age-adjusted death rate from cancer for selected sites in Japan, 1950–1978 (female) (based on Segi-Doll world population) (6)

pancrease, and sexual organs show an increasing tendency for both sexes. The rate of leukemia has increased in males but is levelling off in females.

Table I shows the rates of change (percent per year) in age-adjusted death rates for malignant neoplasms of selected sites between 1954–1955 and 1976–1977 (7). Marked

TABLE I. Rate of Change in Age-Adjusted Death Rates for Cancer of Selected Sites between 1954-1955 and 1976-1977 in Japan (percent per year)

	Males	Females
All sites	0.5	−0.4
Gallbladder and bile ducts	5.6	6.1
Lung	5.3	4.0
Pancreas	5.3	4.4
Intestine	4.0	3.0
Prostate	3.7	—
Ovary	—	3.4
Thyroid gland	3.4	2.5
Leukemia	2.0	1.9
Breast	—	1.4
Rectum	1.7	0.9
Bladder	1.3	−0.1
Esophagus	0.4	−1.6
Liver	−0.4	−2.6
Larynx	−0.7	−4.5
Stomach	−1.2	−1.4
Uterus (all)	—	−3.7

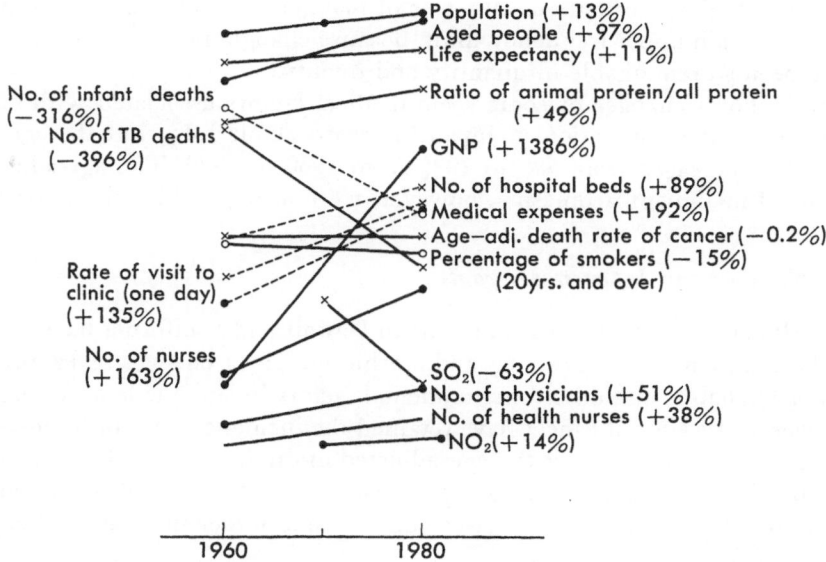

FIG. 9. Changes of social-medical factors between 1960 and 1980 in Japan.

changes of more than 4% per year were observed in mortality from cancers of the gallbladder, lung, and pancreas in both sexes, followed by cancers of the intestine, prostate, ovary, and thyroid gland. Leukemia showed about 2% increase per year, but the trend in mortality rate is regarded as stable in the last decade. A relatively marked reduction was recorded in mortality from cancer of the stomach for both sexes, and the larynx, liver, and esophagus for females. However, it is interesting that overall changes in the death rate of malignant neoplasms were very small, being 0.5% for males and −0.4% for females. Rate of change per year in age adjusted death rates of all forms of malignant

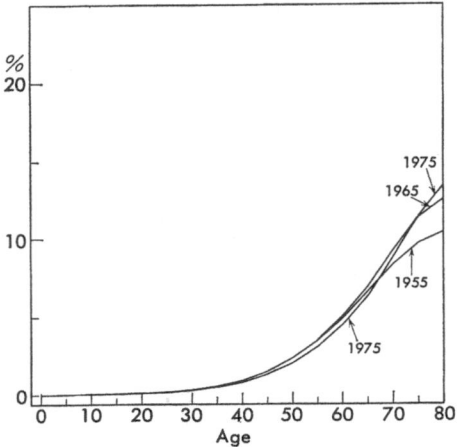

FIG. 10. Cumulative death rates of malignant neoplasms of all forms from birth to
84 years in Japan, 1955, 1965, and 1975 (females)

neoplasms in 15 developed countries of the world ranged −0.2∼1.0 for males and −0.9 ∼0.0 for females.

This suggests that mortality of all forms of malignant neoplasms in large population might have a certain upper frequency limit, because changes in environmental factors in Japan have been so remarkable in quantity and quality.

Figure 9 shows changes of some socio-medical factors associated with cancer frequency (6). The total population in Japan increased about 13%, but the aged population (above 65) increased from 5% to 10% from 1960 to 1980. The age-adjusted rates for all forms of malignant neoplasms, however, were nearly stable for the period.

Malignant Neoplasms in Japanese Migrants

It is well known that Japanese migrants in Hawaii and California have experienced substantial changes in cancer mortality and morbidity. These changes reveal the potential effect of lifestlye habits and other environmental factors in site incidence of various cancers. However, some sites of cancer have retained the incidence rates of indigenous Japanese. Another interesting figure is the age-adjusted mortality from all forms of malignant neoplasms in Hawaii Japanese during the last decades. The rates were similar to those of Japanese in Japan, and the trends were quite stable under markedly different living conditions (5, 12).

This suggests that cancer mortality by site might be determined by environmental background, but that ethnic characteristics remain even after different external exposure for several decades.

Lifelong Cumulative Mortality of Malignant Neoplasms

Cumulative mortality of all forms of malignant neoplasm up to the age of 84 for Japanese was estimated in 1955, 1965, and 1975 using age-specific population figures and death rates in a respective year. The calculation was carried out by a modified life table method (3) assuming that birth cohorts born in 1960 died from malignant neoplasms

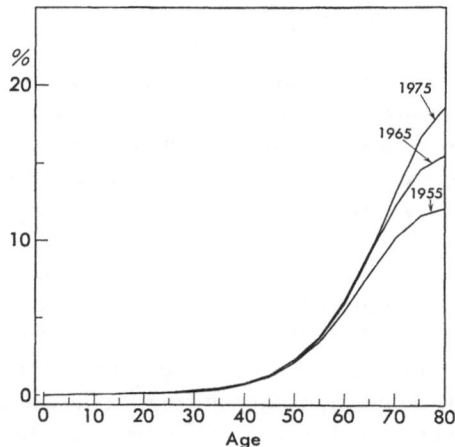

FIG. 11. Cumulative death rates of malignant neoplasms of all forms from birth to 84 years in Japan, 1955, 1965, and 1975 (males)

from birth to 84 years at the same cancer age-specific death rates prevailing in 1960. The same estimation was dose for 1965 and 1975, making general comparison possible.

In females, the cumulative death rates of all forms of malignant neoplasms increased from 1955 to 1975, approaching 15% of the total population (Fig. 10), although the age-adjusted death rates for all forms of malignant neoplasms decreased (Fig. 8). Thus, lifelong mortality in birth cohorts has tended to rise with increasing age, and the age-adjusted death rate based on a standard population with fixed age construction in a certain year has not always indicated a figure applicable throughout life, where the age construction of a population and the causes of death do change considerably over a short period of time as they do in Japan.

In males, the cumulative death rates of all forms of malignant neoplasms has gradually increased from 16.9% in 1955 to 21.3% in 1975 (Fig. 11), while the age-adjusted rates have shown a relatively stable trend (Fig. 7). The cumulative rates of recent birth cohorts are lower in the middle-ages and higher in the older ages; this is more prominent in females since 1965.

Cumulative death rates of all forms of malignant neoplasms plus tuberculosis up to 85 years were calculated in England and Wales, Scotland, New Jersey (9), and Japan (2). The rates ranged between 16% and 21% with no remarkable differences in the trend. The death rate from tuberculosis has steadily decreased in the last few decades and became very low in 1975; the rate of increase in cumulative cancer mortality has recently levelled off. In England-Wales, it is estimated that this threshold is about 18–20% for both sexes (2, 9).

DISCUSSION

Mortality statistics are very useful for epidemiological study because of the homogeneous data in the large population. Examination of the increase in cancer deaths showed it was largely due to the increasing age of the population, that is, the annual age-adjusted incidence rate of this disease has not markedly increased.

The increase trend in mortality from malignant neoplasms with age between 30 and 64 years is quite stable, and in males over 70 the rate of incerase is remarkable. But, in older females, the increase has gradually been levelling off. There has been little geographical difference in mortality of all forms of malignant neoplasms for the decades, and even this difference, if any, has decreased in recent years.

Remarkable changes in cancer mortality by site have been observed, but the increase trend has levelled off in many sites during the last decade, especially in females.

Japanese migrants to Hawaii showed considerable changes in cancer mortality by site, but the patterns are still similar to those of indigenous Japanese and overall death rates of cancer are not greatly different between Japanese in the two countries. Cumulative death rates from cancer up to 84 years in many areas were similar (2, 9) and appear to have an upper threshold, such as 20% of the birth cohort population. Considering the substantial changes in environmental factors observed in each country, one may say that the changes in overall cancer mortality during the last decades have been small.

As the etiology of cancer is believed to differ from site to site and cancer mortality has been changing in time and space, it may be fruitless to discuss overall cancer incidence. However, each animal species has its own specific sensitivity to this disease, and genetic traits with high susceptibility to cancer are well-known. Familial aggregation of cancer and ethnic susceptibility are also acknowledged. Strong correlations between cancer frequencies of various sites in many areas might be considered from this aspect (8). Further analysis and more detailed discussion of overall cancer mortality, as proposed earlier (11, 14), therefore seems appropriate. If the cumulative death rates from all forms of malignant neoplasmas are similar in many populations, further consideration should be given to the interaction of environmental factors and other carcinogenetic factors.

Each cause of death is more or less related to other diseases, and the array of causes of death also depends on the life expectancy in each population. Careful and continuous observation of the frequency and distribution of malignant neoplasmas may give us more information with which to explain changes in the variety of mortality in human populations.

REFERENCES

1. Aoki, K. Mortality of childhood cancer, unpublished data.
2. Aoki, K., Kuroishi, T., and Ohno, Y. An epidemiologic approach to host factors in the etiology of cancer. Second Symposium on Epidemiology, and Cancer Registries in the Pacific Basin. *Natl. Cancer Inst. Monogr.*, **53**, 17–23 (1979).
3. Day, N. E. A new measure of age standardized incidence, the cumulative rate, Cancer Incidence in Five Continents, eds., J. Waterhouse, C. Muir, P. Correa, and J. Powell, Vol. III, pp. 443–445 (1976). IARC, Lyon.
4. Health and Welfare Statistics and Information Department, Ministry's Secretariat, Ministry of Health and Welfare. Vital Statistics, Japan, 1947–1983, Kosei-Tokei Kyokai, Tokyo, 1949–1984 (in Japanese).
5. Hirohata, T. Mortality experience of various ethnic groups in Hawaii—with particular reference to the comparison with their mother populations. *Jpn. J. Public Health*, **21**, 17–26 (1974).
6. Kokumin-Eisei No Doko (Trends in Hygiene among Japanese), 1965, 1975, 1985, Kosei-No-Shihyo, Vols. 12, 22, 32, Suppl. (1965, 1975, 1985). Kosei-Tokei Kyokai, Tokyo (in Japanese)

7. Kurihara, M., Aoki, K., and Tominaga, S. (eds.) Cancer Mortality Statistics in the World (1984). Univ. Nagoya Press, Nagoya.

8. Kurihara, M. Geographic pathology of cancer. *Igaku No Ayumi*, **96**, 330–346, 1977 (in Japanese).

9. Mercer, A. J. Risk of dying from tuberculosis or cancer: Further aspects of a possible association. *Int. J. Epidemiol.*, **10**, 371–380 (1981).

10. Mizuno, S. and Aoki, K. Unpublished data.

11. Oeser, H., Laeppe, P., and Rach, K. Die Konstang der Krebsgetahrdung des Menschen. These und Folgerungen. *Dtsch. Med. Wochenschr.*, **99**, 273–277 (1974).

12. Rellahan, W., Reshad, M. N., Burch, T. A., and Okinaga, N.S.G., eds. Cancer Patterns in Hawaii 1960–1964 and 1968–1972, The Cancer Center of Hawaii, Hawaii State Department of Health.

13. Segi, M., Tominaga, S., Aoki, K., and Fujimoto, I. (eds.) Cancer Mortality and Morbidity Statistics. Japan and the World (1981). Japan Sci. Soc. Press, Tokyo.

14. Zdeb, M. S. The probability of developing cancer. *Am. J. Epidemiol.*, **106**, 6–16 (1979).

TRENDS IN LUNG CANCER MORTALITY IN 24 COUNTRIES

Minoru KURIHARA

*Department of Epidemiology and Social Medicine, Research
Institute for Nuclear Medicine and Biology,
Hiroshima University**

Observation of the yearly trends in lung cancer death rates in 24 countries has shown that a decrease has begun to appear in young adults in many countries and it is expected that this decrease will extend gradually into the upper ages. Such a decrease is also observed in lung cancer incidence rates in some regions, suggesting that the causative factors of this cancer are decreasing. A review of reports on descriptive epidemiology of this decrease in lung cancer has shown an almost consistent view that reduced cigarette consumption and improvement of tobacco quality have contributed to this decrease. Views are divided as to the magnitude of the contribution being made by other factors such as air pollution.

It is well known that the incidence of lung cancer has increased in many countries since the Second World War, but in recent years a decrease in lung cancer mortality among young males has been pointed out in the U.K., U.S.A., Netherlands, and others. Based on "Cancer Mortality in 24 Countries" by Segi and Kurihara (*18*) for the period from 1950 to 1967 and on the mortality statistics compiled by Kurihara *et al.* (*12*) for the period from 1968 to 1979, the international trend in lung cancer mortality was comparatively observed together with a review on the association of lung cancer mortality and incidence to cigarette smoking from the standpoint of descriptive epidemiology.

Trends in Age-adjusted Death Rates

Trends in age-adjusted death rates for lung cancer from 1950 to 1979 in 24 countries examined on a 2-year basis are shown in Fig. 1. Among males, the rates showed a consistent elevation until about 1970, but, after peaking in 1970–1971 in Finland and in 1974–1975 in England and Wales, Australia, and Austria, they began to decline and even in Ireland, Northern Ireland, Norway, *etc.* began to show signs of decreasing in 1978–1979. Among females, the rates in many countries showed a yearly variation due generally to the low rates, but an increasing trend has continued. In recent years in particular, there are some countries such as England and Wales, Scotland, U.S. whites, Canada, *etc.* in which the rates among females have demonstrated a more rapid increase than those among males.

To observe the slope of the increasing trend in death rates in a more simplified form, the increase rate per year was computed. On the assumption that the logarithm of age-adjusted death rates would change linearly with time—that is, the rate at which the

---

* Kasumi 1-2-3, Minami-ku, Hiroshima 734, Japan (栗原　登).

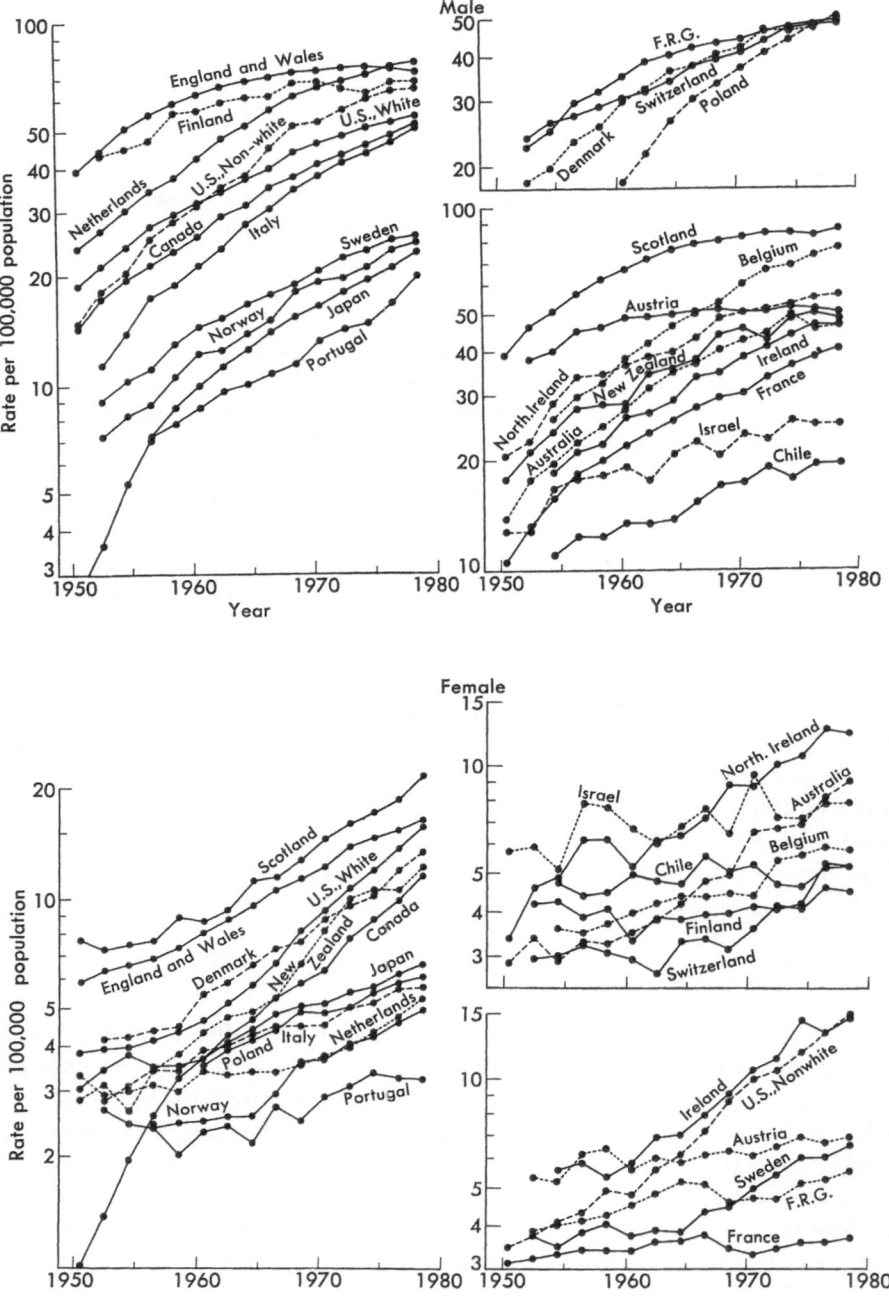

FIG. 1.   Trends in age-adjusted death rates for lung cancer from 1950–1951 to
1978–1979 in 24 countries
Standard population is Segi's World Population.

TABLE I. Annual Percentages of Increase in Age-adjusted Death Rates for Lung Cancer from 1954–1955 to 1978–1979 in 24 Countries

	Male			Female		
	From 1954–1955 to 1978–1979	From 1954–1955 to 1968–1969	From 1970–1971 to 1978–1979	From 1954–1955 to 1978–1979	From 1954–1955 to 1968–1969	From 1970–1971 to 1978–1979
Australia	3.5	5.3	1.1	5.2	4.0	3.9
Austria	0.7	1.5	0.1	0.9	0.6	1.4
Belgium	4.4	5.3	2.9	2.3	2.0	2.9
Canada	4.0	4.8	2.8	6.0	4.2	7.6
Chile	2.2	2.5	1.3	0.4	1.0	0.4
Denmark	3.6	5.0	2.3	5.2	4.8	5.6
Finland	1.3	2.5	−0.1	1.2	−0.3	3.7
France	3.7	4.3	3.5	0.2	0.6	1.2
F.R.G.	2.3	3.7	1.2	1.0	1.4	2.0
Ireland	3.9	4.8	2.4	5.0	3.8	4.1
Israel	1.8	2.0	0.9	0.9	0.3	−1.2
Italy	5.1	6.4	3.6	2.4	2.8	2.8
Japan	5.1	6.9	4.5	3.9	6.0	3.2
Netherlands	3.7	5.1	2.0	2.4	1.2	4.7
New Zealand	3.0	4.2	1.3	6.5	5.7	4.3
Norway	4.5	5.4	3.5	1.6	2.6	3.8
Poland	5.3[a]	7.8[c]	4.0	2.9[a]	4.2[c]	3.1
Portugal	4.4[b]	3.9[d]	7.0	2.0[b]	2.6[d]	1.2
Sweden	3.7	4.2	2.7	2.8	1.4	3.3
Switzerland	2.8	3.0	2.1	2.1	0.3	2.8
United Kingdom						
England and Wales	1.3	2.4	−0.2	4.1	4.4	3.2
Northern Ireland	2.7	3.3	1.5	4.2	3.4	4.5
Scotland	1.9	3.3	0.3	4.7	4.1	5.2
United States, white	3.2	4.1	1.9	6.6	5.5	6.5
United States, nonwhite	4.5	6.2	2.7	6.0	5.7	5.3

Estimated by maximum likelihood method on the assumption of log-linear function.
[a] From 1960–1961 to 1978–1979.
[b] From 1956–1957 to 1978–1979.
[c] From 1960–1961 to 1968–1969.
[d] From 1956–1957 to 1968–1969.

adjusted death rates would change would be constant—the slope of the straight line was obtained by maximum likelihood method and this slope was converted into annual rates of increase. The results thus obtained are shown in Table I.

The annual rate of increase from 1954–1955 to 1978–1979 among males was the highest in Poland, being 5.3%, and the rate in Japan and Italy was also more than 5%. Austria showed the lowest rate of 0.7%, and it was low in Finland, England and Wales, Israel, and Scotland, being less than 2%. Among females, the annual rate of increase was more than 6% in U.S. whites and New Zealand and about 6% in U.S. nonwhites and Canada, but it was the lowest in France, being 0.2% and was less than 1% in Chile, Israel, Austria, and the F.R.G. In comparing the sexes, there were many countries in which the rate of increase was higher among males than females particularly in Chile, France, the F.R.G., and Israel this was remarkably true. However, there were 10 countries in which the rate of increase was higher among females: it was 2-fold that of males in England and Wales, Scotland, New Zealand, and U.S. whites.

As shown in Fig. 1, there were many countries in which the increase in age-adjusted death rates for lung cancer among males after 1970 was small and in some countries these rates have levelled off. On the contrary, there were many countries in which the rate rapidly increased among females. Therefore, the annual rate of increase was computed for two periods, the former period (16 years from 1954–1955 to 1968–1969) and the latter period (10 years from 1970–1971 to 1978–1979), and these results are also presented in Table I.

Among males, only in Portugal among the 24 countries was the annual rate of increase higher in the latter period than in the former; in all other countries, the annual rate of increase was lower in the latter period. In particular, England and Wales and Frence showed a slight decreasing trend in the latter period, it being −0.2% and −0.1%, respectively. In Austria, Scotland, and Israel the annual rate of increase in the latter period was less than 1%. In examining the annual rate of increase in the latter period, an excess of 3% was observed only in Portugal, Japan, Poland, Italy, France, and Norway. In all of these countries, the death rates were relatively low.

Among females, the annual rate of increase in the latter period was smaller than the former period in eight countries including Japan, Portugal, and England and Wales and in U.S. nonwhites as in was true males. Particularly in Israel, the rate of increase showed a decrease to −1.2%, but in the other 15 countries and U.S. whites the annual rate of increase was higher in the latter period. In Finland, the rate in the former period was −0.3%, but in the latter period the rate of increase showed a value of 4.8%. In examining the latter period, the increase rate was large in Canada, U.S. whites, Denmark, U.S. nonwhites, and Scotland.

In examining the annual rate of increase in the latter period by sex, the increase was greater among males in Chile, France, Israel, Italy, Japan, Poland, and Portugal, but in the other countries the rate was higher among females. In many of these advanced countries, lung cancer among males rapidly increased until about 1970, but in recent years this increase has levelled off and in some of the countries, the rate has decreased. On the contrary, among females it is noteworthy that there is a greater increase than among males.

Doll and Peto (7) have pointed out that lung cancer death rates in England and Wales can be utilized from 1941 but the data prior to 1950 are weak in reliability, and that the same can be said for the U.S.A.. Kobayashi et al. (10) reported that the accurate diagnosis rate of lung cancer in Japan was 51.3% in 1948–1951, which rose 1.4-fold in about 10 years to 70.7% in 1958–1963. During this period, the adjusted death rate for lung cancer increased about 3.6-fold. They pointed out that this increase includes an apparent increase due to elevation of accurate diagnosis rate. As shown in Table I, the rate of increase in the foimer period in Japan is larger than that in the latter period and, furthermore, the level of changes is almost the same for both sexes. These suggest that the increased rate in the former period is affected by the elevation in the rate for accurate diagnosis.

Trends in Mortality by Age Group

It has recently been reported in many countries that the lung cancer death rates in

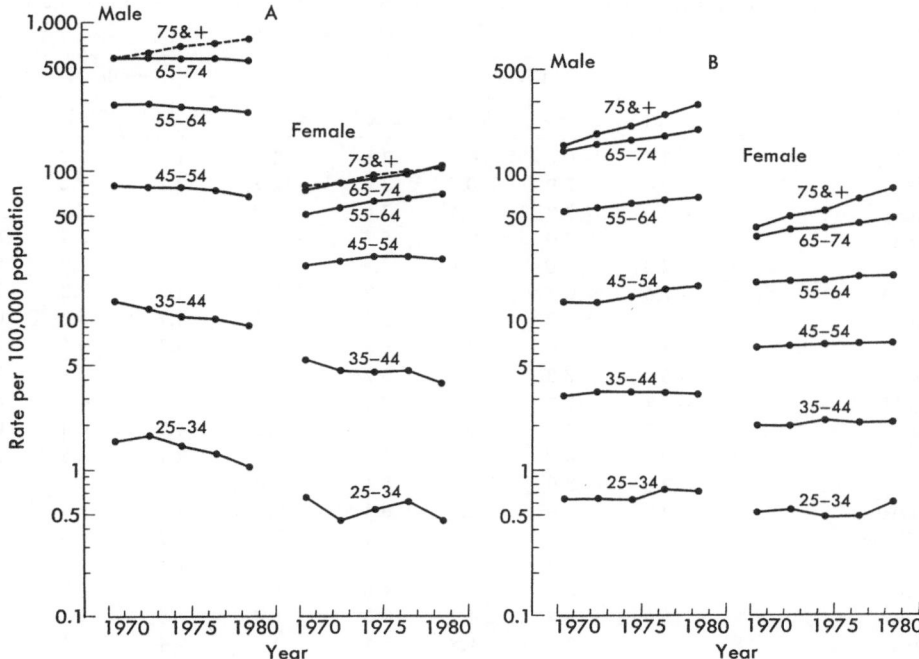

FIG. 2. Trends in age-specific death rates for lung cancer from 1950–1951 to 1978–1979 in England and Wales (A), and Japan (B)

younger males have begun to decline. Shown in Fig. 2 are the trends in death rates by 10-year age-groups for lung cancer during a 10-year period from 1970–1971 to 1978–1979 in England and Wales and Japan. In Japan, except for the almost horizontal curves for both males and females in the 35–44-year old group, a rising trend is observed with the rising slope becoming more steep with age. In England and Wales the rates among males have decreased in all age-groups under 75 and this decline is steeper, the younger the age. Among females, a declining trend is observed in the 25–34-year old group and in the 35–44-year old group and even in the 45–54-year old group a declining trend has recently been observed, but in the groups over 55 an apparent increase can be seen.

In order to examine the trends in age-specific death rates in countries other than the foregoing two, the annual percentages of increase in death rates in 24 countries for a 10-year period from 1970–1971 to 1978–1979 by four age-groups (25–34, 35–54, 55–74, and 75 and over) were computed by the same method as described earlier and the results are shown in Table II.

In the 25–34-year old group, only the males of England and Wales and U.S. whites showed a statistically significant decrease in rate, the number of deaths in this age-group being small. However, it can be assumed that there is a decreasing trend in many of the countries. A decrease can be observed in both sexes in Australia, Austria, Chile, New Zealand, Sweden, England and Wales, and U.S. whites, and an increase was seen among both sexes in only Finland, Japan, and Switzerland.

In the 35–54-year old group, a decrease is seen among males in six countries and among females in two. In not only the U.K. but also Australia, Finland, and Ireland an increase is seen among females and a decrease among males. In many of the countries,

M. KURIHARA

TABLE II. Annual Percentages of Increase in Age-specific Death Rates for Lung Cancer from 1970–1971 to 1978–1979 in 24 Countries

	Male				Female			
	25–34	35–54	55–74	75 &+	25–34	35–54	55–74	75 &+
Australia	−3.5	−0.6	0.6	3.8	−2.6	1.9	5.7	4.8
Austria	−2.4	2.9	−0.8	3.6	−12.7	−1.1	1.8	4.1
Belgium	−4.0	3.7	2.1	7.6	3.0	3.9	3.7	1.3
Canada	2.3	2.0	2.6	5.3	−2.3	6.6	8.7	6.4
Chile	−2.3	1.0	0.9	3.9	−7.4	0.1	1.0	0.2
Denmark	−7.6	0.3	2.2	5.2	1.3	4.2	7.2	2.1
Finland	16.3	−1.2	0.0	3.1	6.2	4.7	5.2	0.0
France	3.7	6.6	2.7	6.1	−9.5	5.3	0.6	1.1
F.R.G.	−0.0	3.3	0.6	5.2	5.3	1.5	2.1	3.3
Ireland	−6.1	−2.1	2.1	9.2	0.5	1.8	4.2	6.5
Israel	3.7	5.7	0.4	1.7	−12.0	−4.7	0.4	0.1
Italy	−0.8	4.7	3.5	8.0	0.5	2.1	3.5	3.9
Japan	2.0	3.9	3.9	8.1	1.0	1.4	2.6	7.4
Netherlands	−2.1	0.9	1.5	6.4	8.5	4.8	5.4	3.1
New Zealand	−8.2	0.2	1.0	4.4	−7.8	3.2	4.9	4.5
Norway	−16.7	1.7	3.1	7.3	...	2.4	4.9	1.7
Poland	0.3	8.5	3.6	4.6	−1.1	4.0	3.7	3.2
Portugal	11.6	5.8	4.1	8.0	−1.8	1.8	1.4	2.3
Sweden	−1.4	2.5	1.8	5.6	−4.5	2.4	4.1	2.0
Switzerland	20.8	2.2	2.0	3.6	2.0	5.3	2.1	2.7
United Kingdom								
England and Wales	−5.0	−2.2	−0.5	3.7	−2.3	0.4	4.7	4.0
Northern Ireland	4.3	−0.2	0.5	7.1	−11.5	1.3	6.7	6.4
Scotland	−3.3	−1.9	0.3	3.9	4.0	2.4	6.9	4.0
United States, white	−3.7	0.3	1.7	4.5	−0.9	3.8	8.1	6.0
United States, nonwhite	−3.7	0.6	3.3	5.3	4.8	3.3	6.4	7.1

Estimated by same method as Table I.
... not available by reason of few deaths.

an increase is observed among both sexes. In Belgium, Canada, and Denmark the increase among females was remarkably higher than that among males.

In the 55–74-year old group, only the males in England and Wales, and in Austria showed a decrease. In this age-group, it was characteristic that the increase among males was remarkably larger than that among females in many countries such as Canada, the U.S.A., Scotland, and Denmark.

In the age-group 75 years or over, an increasing trend was observed among both sexes in all countries. In many countries the increase among males markedly exceeded that among females, but in the U.S.A., England and Wales, Canada, and Australia the increase observed in females of this age-group was larger than that of males.

During this 10-year period, an increase in all four age-groups among both sexes was observed only in Japan and Switzerland. It may be concluded that a decrease in lung cancer death rates has begun in the younger age-groups in many countries. The phenomenon observed in England and Wales that the decrease in lung cancer begins in young males and later extends to females and gradually to the higher age-groups is considered to have commenced in many countries.

TABLE III. Age-adjusted Incidence Rates for Lung Cancer of Two Age-classes
(25–49 and 50 &+ Years of Age) in Some Registries in the World
for Previous and Recent Periods

Registry	Year	Male		Female	
		25–49	50 &+	25–49	50 &+
Canada, Alberta	1960–1962	4.6	102.0	2.5	19.3
	1973–1977	9.4	162.0	5.0	37.3
Newfoundland	1960–1962	18.3	80.6	1.8	15.9
	1973–1977	16.6	185.6	3.1	19.7
Colombia, Cali	1962–1966	4.8	77.3	2.0	15.6
	1972–1976	4.3	89.0	2.2	23.2
Denmark	1953–1957	8.7	108.1	1.9	19.1
	1973–1976	10.4	242.1	6.3	50.2
Finland	1959–1961	17.8	294.5	1.8	17.0
	1971–1976	14.4	349.0	2.5	24.7
Germany, Hamburg	1960–1962	12.3	273.1	3.9	31.7
	1973–1977	13.9	299.5	3.6	44.0
Japan, Miyagi	1959–1960	4.2	63.0	2.1	23.1
	1973–1977	4.3	120.6	2.4	33.5
New Zealand: Non-Maori	1962–1966	12.0	206.2	3.1	25.6
	1972–1976	9.5	250.4	5.2	48.6
Norway	1959–1961	4.5	60.1	0.9	12.5
	1973–1977	6.9	115.9	2.9	22.0
Sweden	1959–1961	4.6	72.7	1.8	16.5
	1971–1975	5.4	110.4	2.4	24.6
England, Birmingham Region	1960–1962	21.7	322.4	4.9	29.3
	1973–1976	17.8	371.0	5.6	59.6
Liverpool Region	1959–1963	24.2	348.7	5.8	38.5
	1975–1977	17.9	411.9	7.1	85.2
U.S., Connecticut	1960–1962	13.1	191.5	4.8	25.8
	1973–1977	18.6	274.8	10.1	74.0
New York State	1959–1961	10.6	169.9	3.3	18.9
	1973–1977	17.8	296.2	10.7	78.5
Yugoslavia, Slovenia	1956–1960	7.7	135.2	1.8	18.0
	1973–1976	18.8	247.8	2.7	26.5

Trends in Incidence Rates

As the foregoing mortality statistics are influenced also by advances made in medical care, it is necessary to observe the trends in morbidity rates in order to examine the trends in incidence. Fortunately, it is possible to use the morbidity rates in many regions of the world published in "Cancer Incidence in Five Continents," (6, 20) to compute the age-adjusted incidence rates for lung cancer of the two age-classes of 25–49 and 50+ in a number of major registries in the world for the earliest and latest periods. The results are presented in Table III. The interval between the earliest period and the latest period varies by country from 10 to 20 years.

The morbidity rate among males belonging to the 25–49 age class has decreased in six registries of Newfoundland in Canada, Cali in Colombia, Finland, New Zealand, and the Birmingham and Liverpool regions in England, and that among females only in Hamburg, Germany. The morbidity rates in the age class of 50+ have increased among both sexes in all the registries.

Due to the paucity of cases in the younger age-groups, computation was made on the broad age-group of 25–49. Thus, the trends in the younger age-groups cannot necessarily be well observed, but there are regions in the world in which the incidence of new cases among young males has declined. This suggests that the decrease in lung cancer mortality among the younger groups is attributable not only to the elevation in cure rate but also to the decrease in the incidence of new patients and that internationally the causes of lung cancer development are already decreasing.

Relationship to Changing Patterns of Smoking

Smoking is regarded to be the most important risk factor of lung cancer. In examining the yearly trend of the smoking amount per adult in the U.K. (14), a decline has been observed among males from the 1960s, but among females an increase has continued up to the present. The decrease in lung cancer among young males in England and Wales may well be explained by the decrease in the amount of smoking.

There are many reports which explain the recent decrease in lung cancer incidence among young males and the increase among females as being associated with the change in smoking habits. The coincidence of the rapid elevation in death rates among females to the increase in the amount of smoking among females has been pointed out in the U.S.A. by Burbank (3) and in Denmark by Jensen. (9) Higginson and Jensen (8), in pointing out the rapid increase in lung cancer mortality among females in many countries, reported that the carcinogenic stimulus affecting males is now beginning to act on females, that this finding is consistent with available information on cigarette smoking habits among females, and that the presence of a non-specific carcinogenic factor which would affect both males and females equally, such as air pollution, is not suggested.

Doll and Peto (7) have stressed that in carcinogenesis there is a long delay between the cause and its full effect and that cancers which develop in advanced age are strongly influenced by exposure to causative factor(s) during younger age. They have called this a "successive generation effect." Using as a measure of the causative agent of smoking the tar intake per adult which takes into account presence or absence of filter, tar yields and method of smoking, the trend in age-specific death rates for lung cancer in the U.S.A. and England could be well explained by the trends in smoking. Though cigarette consumption in the U.S.A. has not decreased, lung cancer has begun to decrease in the younger population. Though the mean sales of cigarettes per adult between 1925 and 1940 were similar in the U.S.A. and England, the death rate of U.S. males born in about 1910 was only about one-half that of England. Though both the sales of cigarettes and tar intake in the U.S.A. since 1945 have been remarkably larger than those in England, the age-adjusted death rates for the same period have been markedly higher in England. These findings could be well explained by a successive generation effect and tar intake per adult. They have concluded that the most important parts of the pattern of trends in lung cancer death rates can be explained by plausible assumptions about the effects of smoking.

According to Devesa et al. (5), the changing pattern in lung cancer incidence rates seems consistent with what we know about smoking patterns, how they differ between males and females, and how they have changed over time.

Also in Italy, Mastrandrea et al. (15) have reported that the signs of leveling off of death rates among males born after 1925 are attributable to the increase of low-tar and filter-tipped cigarettes from 1950.

On the other hand, there are reports published in the literature that the yearly trends in lung cancer death rates cannot be explained only by smoking. Beamis *et al.* (1) pointed out that though lung cancer among females has suddenly increased in the U.S.A., there has been no change in the proportion by cell type and that the low incidence of lung cancer among females is not attributable only to smoking but is also related to the low air contamination in homes. Based on mortality statistics in Italy, Saracci (17) has reported that the findings among males can be readily explained by smoking but not those among females and that the trend in lung cancer mortality among females may indicate the operation of some general environmental agents. According to Blot and Fraumeni (2), smoking has played an important role in shifting the patterns of lung cancer in the U.S.A., but the difference in lung cancer incidence between the white and nonwhite populations and the geographical distribution of the disease cannot be explained only by smoking. They consider that such factors as industrial exposures and nutritional deficiencies are also involved in the development of lung cancer.

Cuello *et al.* (4) have assumed that the adoption of the smoking habit among young females in Cali, Colombia is associated with elevation of lung cancer morbidity, but histologically the absence of a decrease in the proportion of adenocarcinoma which is only weakly associated with smoking history suggests the involvement of factors other than smoking.

The lung cancer death rate in Hong Kong (12) was the highest among 39 countries in 1978–1979 and was characterized by a low male:female ratio of 2.3:1. According to Kung and his colleagues (11), though the death rate in Hong Kong has suddenly risen among both sexes, in view of the increase in the proportion of adenocarcinoma and the relatively high incidence among females, lung cancer in Hong Kong Chinese can be explained by factors other than smoking.

Also, in Japan Mori and Sakai (16) in their observation of autopsy cases have pointed out an increase in lung cancer incidence in both smokers and non-smokers with the increase being larger in the latter and have emphasized that the relative importance of smoking as a cause of this cancer has decreased and that factors other than smoking have assumed greater importance.

Waterhouse (19) reported that cigarette smoking constitutes the highest single factor of lung cancer and has a synergistic effect with other factors such as air pollution, but the effect of smoking cannot be evaluated separately from other factors except by means of *ad hoc* surveys which are expensive and seldom comprehensive. Also, in the report of Lawther and Waller (13), smoke concentration has been remarkably reduced in the atmosphere in England during the last 20 years, but it would be difficult to disentangle any effects from those of changing smoking habits.

It is the consistent view of many reporters that the decrease in cigarette consumption and improvement of tobacco quality have contributed to the decrease in lung cancer and will continue to so contribute in the near future, but views are divided on the magnitude of involvement of other factors such as air pollution. As it is relatively simple to quantitate the national cigarette consumption and the improvement in cigarette quality, a number of studies from the standpoint of descriptive epidemiology have been made on the relationship to lung cancer incidence. In view of the difficulty involved in quantitating national exposure to environmental factors such as air pollution, only a few discussions based on concrete data have been offered on the association of these factors to lung cancer incidence.

Regardless of the reasons involved, lung cancer incidence has begun to decline in early adult life and it is expected that decrease will extend into the upper ages. This presents an optimistic prospect to the control of lung cancer.

REFERENCES

1. Beamis, J. F., Jr., Stein, A., and Andrews, J. L., Jr. Changing epidemiology of lung cancer, increasing incidence in women. *Med. Clin. N. Am.*, **59**, 315–325 (1975).
2. Blot, W. J. and Fraumeni, J. F., Jr. Changing patterns of lung cancer in the United States. *Am. J. Epidemiol.*, **115**, 664–673 (1982).
3. Burbank, F. U.S. lung cancer death rates begin to rise proportionately more rapidly for females than males: A dose response effect? *J. Chron. Dis.*, **25**, 473–479 (1972).
4. Cuello, C., Correa, P., and Haenszel, W. Trends in cancer incidence in Cali, Colombia. *J. Natl. Cancer Inst.*, **70**, 635–641 (1983).
5. Devesa, S. S., Pollack, E. S., and Young, J. L., Jr. Assessing the validity of observed cancer incidence trends. *Am. J. Epidemiol.*, **119**, 274–291 (1984).
6. Doll, R., Payne, P., and Waterhouse, J. (eds.) Cancer Incidence in Five Continents (1966). Springer-Verlag, Berlin.
7. Doll, R. and Peto, R. The causes of cancer. *J. Natl. Cancer Inst.*, **66**, 1191–1308 (1981).
8. Higginson, J. and Jensen, O. M. Epidemiological review of lung cancer in man. *In* "Air Pollution and Cancer in Man," ed. U. Mohr, D. Schmähl, and L. Tomatis, pp. 169–189 (1977). IARC, Lyon.
9. Jensen, O. M. Lung cancer and smoking in Danish women. *Int. J. Cancer*, **15**, 954–961 (1975).
10. Kobayashi, H., Miyashita, T., and Takeda, K. Present state of deaths by lung cancer in Japan. *Gann*, **58**, 101–104 (1967).
11. Kung, I.T.M., So, K. F., and Lam, T. H. Lung cancer in Hong Kong Chinese: Mortality and histological types, 1973–1982. *Br. J. Cancer*, **50**, 381–388 (1984).
12. Kurihara, M., Aoki, K., and Tominaga, S. (eds.) "Cancer Mortality Statistics in the World" (1984). The University of Nagoya Press, Nagoya.
13. Lawther, P. J. and Waller, R. E. Trends in urban air pollution in the United Kingdom in relation to lung cancer mortality. *Environ. Health Perspect.*, **22**, 71–73 (1978).
14. Lee, P. N. (ed.) "Statistics of Smoking in the United Kingdom," Tobacco Research Council Research Paper I, 7th edition, pp. 16–20 (1976). Tobacco Research Council, London.
15. Mastrandrea, V., La Rosa, F., and Cresci, A. Trends of lung cancer mortality in Italy in relation to consumption of tobacco products. *Am. J. Epidemiol.*, **120**, 257–264 (1984).
16. Mori, W. and Sakai, R. A study on chronologic change of the relationship between cigarette smoking and lung cancer based on autopsy diagnosis. *Cancer*, **54**, 1038–1042 (1984).
17. Saracci, R. Epidemiology of lung cancer in Italy. *In* "Air Pollution and Cancer in Man," ed., U. Mohr, D. Schmähl, and L. Tomatis, pp. 205–215 (1977). IARC, Lyon.
18. Segi, M. and Kurihara, M. "Cancer Mortality for Selected Sites in 24 Countries," No. 6 (1966–1967) (1972). Japan Cancer Society, Tokyo.
19. Waterhouse, J.A.H. Epidemiology of lung cancer in England and Wales. *In* "Air Pollution and Cancer in Man," ed. U. Mohr, D. Schmähl, and L. Tomatis, pp. 229–240 (1977). IARC, Lyon.
20. Waterhouse, J., Muir, C., Shanmugaratnam, K., and Powell, J. (eds.) "Cancer Incidence in Five Continents," Vol. IV. IARC Scientific Publications, No. 42 (1982). UICC, Lyon.

CANCER REGISTRATION

CANCER REGISTRATION IN THE NEAR FUTURE

John A. H. Waterhouse

*Department of Social Medicine, Queen Elizabeth Medical Centre, University of Birmingham**

From the series of publications by Professor Mitsuo Segi which compared world cancer mortality rates, and from the successive volumes of "Cancer Incidence in Five Continents" which used cancer registry data to compare morbidity rates, a composite picture has been built up of the geographical distribution of cancer by site throughout the world, and of changes in this pattern over time. The quality and reliability of cancer registration data depend very much on the use that is made of them: the more they are used, the more readily errors and omissions are discovered and corrected. It is urged herein that, to survive as useful entities, cancer registries should extend both the range of their clinical data set and their action participation in related fields, such as clinical trials, screening, environmental and industrial hazard investigations, teaching, and research. Each additional activity interacts with others and with the basic function of data collection to improve the efficiency and accuracy of the data base, and thus the value of the enterprise as a whole.

The ways in which Cancer Registries have originated in various parts of the world have been many. Those that are territorially-based—the so-called population-based registries which endeavour to include every cancer diagnosed within their boundaries—have been made increasingly aware of their importance in descriptive epidemiology. For example, at approximately quinquennial intervals the successive volumes (*1, 2, 8, 9, 10*) of "Cancer Incidence in Five Continents" have gathered together the records of many of those registries attaining to reasonable degrees of quality and completeness of data. It has always been the first intention of those volumes to bring together in compact form basic descriptive epidemiological data on the incidence of cancer, from as wide a field as possible, suitable for subsequent analysis and presentation in any manner considered appropriate. It was in fact Professor Segi (*6*) who presented analyses of this material, following similar patterns to his pioneering series (*5*) of volumes on cancer mortality data from various countries. He it was also who developed the notion of a "world standard population," as a construct intermediate in its age structure between the developing countries with their preponderance at the younger ages and the developed countries which contain rather more in the middle and older age-groups. This world population, with only very slight modification, has now been very widely adopted as a basis for directly-standardised mortality or morbidity rates.

Whatever their original *raison d'être* therefore, the theme of descriptive epidemiology now is the most significant link between cancer registries on a world scale. There are already available several variations on that basic theme, provided for instance by tabula-

---

* Birmingham B15 2TH, U.K.

tions of standardised rates by site and sex, such as are given in the "Cancer Incidence in Five Continents" series, and also in more directly visual form as maps, coloured to indicate high and low risk areas. Most of the published atlases of cancer refer to mortality, but recently one based on morbidity rates has been published, for Scotland (4). It is likely to be followed by others mapping cancer morbidity, though there are few countries where cancer registration is as widespread or as consistently efficient as is death certification. Such maps are more informative, however, than the division of incidence rates into urban and rural, when the bases of that division are as various in definition as they are in different countries, thus largely invalidating any possible aetiological inferences that might be drawn from them. But we have now got the basis for a general, if approximate, world picture of the distribution of cancer.

In that picture we see the variations by site of tumour: breast rates increasing when going from the Far East to the West; stomach the reverse; oesophagus showing high rates in South African blacks, in the Caspian littoral, and in certain adjacent provinces of China. The very high incidence of stomach cancer in Japan (the world's highest), with the high surgical survival rates have led to question whether it is the same disease as that seen in the West, though few would now seriously maintain it. Knowledge of major differences in incidence has, however, facilitated clinical exchanges, both of personnel and of techniques, and sometimes has demonstrated marked alterations in response—to chemotherapeutic agents, for instance, in terms of the haemolytic-uraemic syndrome following the use of mitomycin-C. Useful as this knowledge is, and will continue to be, the general outline of the world distribution of cancer is now reasonably well established. This is so, despite the fact that there are many parts of the world where it would be very desirable to obtain knowledge of cancer morbidity but no cancer registries exist. In the course of time perhaps some of these gaps may be filled, to give a fuller illustration than before and one that may include some unexpected features.

However complete the picture may become, it does not remain static, but exhibits time trends, some of them widespread, like the falling incidence of stomach cancer, the rising rates of lung cancer, especially among women, and the increase of skin cancers in whites; others are of more limited or localised distribution. Trends based on morbidity rates, taken together with population age projections, are of course more useful in predicting health service requirements than those based on mortality rates. They can also be used to indicate areas for investigation or preventive action, and to assess their results. But the trends themselves require careful statistical assessment to prevent the adoption of misleading inferences: if in fact they are to be used as monitors of changes in rates, there are more appropriate and sensitive tests to be applied to data from successive years, especially where the magnitude of the change is small.

Progression

The uses described above of the descriptive epidemiological data derived from cancer registries have depended only upon records of the site, sex and age of each cancer case occurring in the registry's territory, combined with the year of occurrence and set against the population at risk to yield an incidence rate. In what directions are developments likely to come about?

The establishment of new cancer registries in some parts of the world is an ongoing process. But in those parts of the world where the information they can supply would be of especial value, such as in parts of Africa, Southeast Asia, India, South America, *etc.*, the setting-up of new registries is slow or non-existent. It is difficult to predict whether they would in fact lead to any major advances, other than of geographical distribution, in the knowledge of cancer. But they do constitute an unknown and therefore "grey area" where knowledge, even from mortality data, is very deficient.

Existing registries, however, may well be asked to supply a wider range of data in future than the basic site, sex and age grouping, for publications such as the Cancer Incidence in Five Continents series. An obvious extension is to histology, especially of certain sites where there are several common types of different behaviour. There are known grographical differences in the pattern of histology which could be much more firmly quantified by the publication of such data. It generates simultaneously, however, a number of additional problems. First is the consistency, between different registries, of the histological diagnosis and of the descriptive terminology; these aspects are currently of particular importance in the classification of the leukaemias and lymphomas. To extend the tabulations of rates to include histological breakdowns of each site would greatly increase the size of compendium publications such as "Cancer Incidence in Five Continents," necessitating its issue in separate volumes, perhaps by site groupings or by geographical areas.

To reduce the bulk, implied by publication in the form of large volumes, it would be perfectly feasible to provide the tabulations as microfiches. Many books that regularly include extensive tables have now shrunk in overall size because the tables are on microfiches, but they are not completely satisfying to all users. A much more versatile form would be on magnetic tape, as a cassette or a reel, or a flexible disc. Given the wide dispersal of computers, including micros, there should be no major difficulty in reading from any of those forms.

Computerisation

Given, in fact, the very rapid developments in the computer field, of the micro and the mini as dedicated machines, many cancer registries now possess them, and record all their data on them. This situation has been reflected, for instance, in the numbers of registries despatching their entries for "Cancer Incidence in Five Continents" on magnetic tape. The tabulations have been generated from the data in the registry's computer, processed to provide the required rates and layout, and the results transmitted in the standard format. But the system has been extended further by the acceptance of tapes of the registry's data bank, unsorted and untabulated, but stripped only of identifying items. Not only is it a saving of time and effort at the contributing registry for the processing to be done centrally, it forms part of a plan to store "raw" registry data at Lyon, to set up there a data bank—with the agreement of each participating registry, of course. Such a data bank would have many advantages in making available at one centre a potentially very large quantity of material for analysis. Moreover, depending on the extent of selection when transcribing such tapes from the registry's master files— and, of course, on the range of data normally recorded by the registry—other items than the basic site, sex, age, and date could well be made available. In particular, they could include detailed histology, and might extend to fuller descriptions of the tumour, its size and more precise location, involvement of local or regional nodes, sites of metastases, results of investigations made, details of treatment given, follow up information, date and causes of death.

Many registries would not normally collect all the items listed above, and of those that did so, many again would not readily agree to deposit what would amount to a replica of their entire data-base, to be available for general use, even if subject to regulation and requiring specific permission. There could be facets of interpretation of the data which were peculiar to one registry and different from others, while there are always the problems which local knowledge can solve—indeed, does not recognise as problems because of their familiarity—but which can confuse the uninitiated. Of this species was the apparent excess—statistically significant—of cancer cases born in July, which resulted from the practice of placing the birthdate of all those where only a birth year was known, at the centre of the year. Furthermore, the registry's own data base will diverge from that held at the centre because of the addition of new cases (referring to those same calendar years for which the original list was prepared, *i.e.*, late registrations), because of amendments or correction of individual data-items, and because of the addition of follow up information, including death. Updating tapes, sent at regular intervals, could of course remedy the divergence, if it were considered to be appropriate.

Clinical Data

It is, however, unlikely that central accumulation of data on such an extensive scale would be feasible, especially for a wide and representative spread of registries. A good deal of clinical data about individual cases has been collected for some years on an international scale by the UICC's CICA programme from comprehensive cancer treatment centres in Europe and in America. It has been limited to certain selected sites of the disease, and also has no territorially-defined catchment area from which epidemiological rates could be derived. Nonetheless it is an important data source for detailed clinical information from a number of different countries. But centralised publication of epidemiological data, territorially based, seems unlikely in the near future to go beyond the inclusion of histological information.

Future Developments

What future developments are there for the population-based cancer registry? For those that are limited to a minimal data set of site, sex, age, date, but including also perhaps histology, there may be little or none without extending the data set. Population-based registries obtain their data primarily from hospitals; as more hospitals computerise their patient records, the same data will be available directly, together with further items in addition, probably. Some circumspection is required to avoid duplicate registrations for patients admitted more than once for the same condition, or to different hospitals in the area, and to ensure that out-patients, as well as in-patients, are included. Other sources may exist, such as private clinics, or patients not referred to hospital, where copies of histology reports and death certificates mentioning cancer can contribute towards completeness.

If the registry records more clinical details, or extends its previous data set to include them, then it becomes a much more valuable resource to clinicians. The longer the period for which such data have been collected the more valuable they become. They can serve as sources for retrospective analysis as a preliminary to forward planning of clinical programmes; they can provide a base line for clinical trial design, and they can also summarise contemporaneously the behaviour of those patients not included in the trial, neither in the experimental nor in the control groups, to contrast with both those groups; they can aid in the design and evaluation of screening programmes. An exhaustive study (3) of 13,000 cases of stomach cancer in the Midlands of England, for instance, showed that for the small proportion (less than 1%) of very early cases the age-adjusted survival rate was good (70%) at 5 years, approaching some of those from Japan. This result has led to setting up a screening clinic for high risk groups (age over 40, in areas of known raised risk, presenting with persistent dyspepsia) which has already yielded an encouraging number of early cases.

Research Interests

Whether a registry normally collects a large or a small range of data, to publish in an annual report the returns by site, sex, and age serves only to emphasise the extent of numerical variation, and thence its misinterpretation as trends. More useful is a compendium of the registrations of a number of adjacent years. The Cancer Handbook of Epidemiology and Prognosis (7), based on the data of the Birmingham and West Midlands Cancer Registry, exemplifies the stability of a longer period, in both incidence and survival figures, as well as in detailed subsite distributions. The same Registry has embarked on a series of Clinical Cancer Monographs, the first of which is soon to be published. Their aim is to present, for a single site or group of sites, the extensive clinical data normally collected by the Registry, analysed both by a clinician specialising in that group of sites and by an epidemiologist from the Registry. Frequently the data have been augmented by reference back to the original charts or case notes, or have been carefully re-examined and reassessed for the purposes of the monograph. Not only do they cover a significant period of time (a quarter century) but they cover the whole of a large and representative region, not being confined only to a hospital series. As a result, they represent an unbiased picture of the pattern of a cancer, in terms of both incidence and survival, free from the distortion of the usual journal presentations referring to a single hospital. Because also of the long and stable period of data collection, even rare cancers may accumulate in number to admit further analysis, and may thereby reveal previously unsuspected relationships.

Follow Up

Incidence data from a registry can well illustrate the onset of cancer in a community, and if, as is the common practice, the registry records tumours rather than patients, it will show also the incidence of multiple primaries. But the subsequent fate of each case, from the time of diagnosis forward, represents also an important characteristic of the disease. Follow up of patients can exhibit wide differences between registries, from those that do not undertake it in any form, through those that record death only, either passively or actively, to those that attempt a full and complete record of all subsequent events, such as the development of recurrences or metastases, or of subsequent primaries, and of treatments given, to the ultimate cause of death, together with autopsy findings when applicable. For a registry that has been in existence for a long period, even the simplest follow up will provide examples of long term survival for some cancers. Not enough use has been made in terms of publicity of the fact that a diagnosis of cancer is not the death sentence it is so often imagined to be, but that there are many who survive for a great many years afterwards.

Other Activities

The activities of a cancer registry may extend further, either directly or in association with other bodies, into the field of publicity and public relations. The data from the registry can supply the backing for campaigns of prevention and of screening, by utilising local statistics which are always more persuasive than national or international. Even if not closely involved with putting over such campaigns as anti-smoking and dietary propaganda, cervical smears or mammography, its epidemiological expertise can be of value in designing suitable methods of evaluation and assessment of the efficacy of the schemes. Participation in as wide a range of activities as possible is always advantageous to the registry, by getting itself better known and thus improving its rate of data capture, and by the resulting cross-fertilisation of interests between different bodies with a common general interest.

Future Trends

The provision of incidence rates has for long been regarded as one of the chief activities of a population-based cancer registry, and indeed it has been of inestimable importance to the epidemiology of cancer, based on morbidity rather than mortality. Although there are many parts of the world where registries do not exist and their data would be valuable, much of the general worldwide pattern of cancer is known. While it is still of importance that registries should continue to collect and process their data since it can serve a valuable monitoring function, there are many further activities, such as some that have been outlined above, in which they should engage, in order to avoid stagnation and degeneration. The "minimalist" registry, collecting only the basic requirements for incidence, is frequently left on the periphery of all other activities in the field of cancer, and thus neglected, its quality and efficiency tend quickly to diminish. It is active participation and involvement in related fields which maintains an alert and progressive attitude, leading to continual improvement of function. The more data normally collected, the wider the range of contributions a registry can make: they can include investigations of industrial hazards, or of differences attributable to environmental features; or they can take the form of studies within the field of medicine itself, such as of multiple primaries or of the enhanced cancer risk in certain chronic diseases.

The cancer registries most likely to survive and flourish will be those that advance with clinical advances, that regularly analyse and monitor their own data, and that extend their involvement in the wider field of cancer studies.

REFERENCES

1. Doll, R., Payne, P., and Waterhouse, J. (eds.) "Cancer Incidence in Five Continents" (1966). Springer-Verlag, Berlin.

2. Doll, R., Muir, C., and Waterhouse, J. (eds.) "Cancer Incidence in Five Continents," Vol. II (1970). Springer-Verlag, Berlin.
3. Fielding, J.W.L., Ellis, D. J., Jones, B. G., Paterson, J., Powell, D. J., Waterhouse, J.A.H., and Brookes, V. S. Natural history of "early" gastric cancer: Results of a 10-year regional survey. *Br. Med. J.*, **281**, 965–968 (1980).
4. Kemp, I., Boyle, P., Smans, M., and Muir, C. "Atlas of Cancer in Scotland 1975–1980: Incidence and Epidemiological Perspective" (1985). IARC, Lyon.
5. Segi, M. and Kurihara, M. "Cancer Mortality for Selected Sites in 24 Countries," No. 6 (1966–1967) (1972). Japan Cancer Society, Tokyo.
6. Segi, M. "Graphic Presentation of Cancer Incidence by Site and by Area and Population" (1977). Segi Institute of Cancer Epidemiology, Nagoya.
7. Waterhouse, J. "Cancer Handbook of Epidemiology and Prognosis" (1974). Churchill Livingstone, Edinburgh and London.
8. Waterhouse, J., Muir, C., Correa, P., and Powell, J. (eds.) "Cancer Incidence in Five Continents," Vol. III (1976). IARC, Lyon.
9. Waterhouse, J., Shanmugaratnam, K., Muir, C., and Powell, J. (eds.) "Cancer Incidence in Five Continents," Vol. IV (1983). IARC, Lyon.
10. Waterhouse, J., Muir, C., Powell, J., and Mack, T. (eds.) "Cancer Incidence in Five Continents," Vol. V. IARC, Lyon (in preparation).

THE CANCER REGISTRY AND THE STUDY OF OCCUPATIONAL CANCER IN DENMARK

Ole Møller JENSEN, J. H. OLSEN, and E. LYNGE

*Danish Cancer Registry, Institute of Cancer Epidemiology, Danish Cancer Society**

The Danish Cancer Registry records information on occupation. All cancer cases reported between 1970 and 1980 have been linked with occupational information from the national census in 1970, and with the occupational information available from a national pension fund. Examples are provided of the use of these three sources for the routine description of occupational cancer risks in Denmark. Such routine information systems may provide a first attempt to identify high-risk groups. The comparison of risks emerging from different health information systems may be helpful in setting priorities for *ad hoc* investigations of the case-control or cohort type. Due to the limitations of the routine information systems, which are normally based on broad occupational groups and contain no information on potential confounding factors, such information systems cannot be used to demonstrate absence of risk.

The study of occupational cancer has attracted substantial interest during the past decade for several reasons. First, there is a widespread demand that occupational activities should not involve hazards to human health, and it is realized that the prevention of occupational cancer may to a large extent be accomplished by way of legislation. Secondly, the interest in occupational cancer is related to the recognition of chemicals as human carcinogens. This naturally focuses attention on the workplace, where people are likely to be exposed first and most heavily. Thirdly, it is the privilege of epidemiology studies to evaluate public health aspects of occupational risks.

Cancer registry and death certificate data are useful for the calculation of incidence and mortality rates for occupational groups. The study of occupational cancer for England and Wales is the classic example in which the number of deaths is related to the number of persons at risk known from the census (*12*). There are, however, difficulties with such risk estimates, for example, those related to the possible lack of comparability between the numerator and the denominator.

Some of these problems have been solved in Scandinavia, where information from population censuses in Denmark, Finland, Norway, and Sweden has been linked both with cancer registry material and with mortality data. In Denmark, it has also been possible to link cancer registry data with occupational records of individual members of a national pension fund. This paper gives examples of the use of occupational information recorded by the Danish Cancer Registry, and the Registry's use of linked studies of occupational risk.

---

* DK-2100, Copenhagen Ø, Denmark.

Recording of Occupation by the Cancer Registry

Since the start of the Danish Cancer Registry in 1942, information on the occupation of cancer patients has been transmitted from the reporting hospital departments. In a registration system based on reports from hospital departments (8) it is difficult to maintain consistency and the high quality of information which is generally not of major interest to the diagnosing and reporting physicians, *e.g.*, occupation. Nevertheless, the Danish Cancer Registry records "main occupation," though little use has been made of this information which, by its nature, is most likely to reflect the "occupational history" only of skilled persons who spend a major part or all of their working life in a given trade.

In spite of these limitations, and as no denominator information is available to match the numerator information on occupation derived from the Registry, we have previously shown that a proportional or case-control analysis may provide useful information (6). We used information from the Danish Cancer Registry, as routinely reported to us by the clinical departments, to evaluate the risk of nasal cancer for the 3-year period, 1978–1980, in relation to occupations involving possible exposure to wood-dust. A total of 7, *e.i.*, 7.9%, of 89 men with a specific occupation and a malignant tumor of the nasal cavities were woodworkers. This contrasts with 3.7% woodworkers among 3,662 colorectal cancer patients selected as controls, which means that the relative risk after age adjustment is 2.2 for the development of nasal cancers among woodworkers compared with other occupations, There were 14 adenocarcinomas, with a relative risk of 7.1 for nasal cancer development among woodworkers. Two men were furniture makers, representing 14.3% of the nasal adenocarcinomas.

Although numbers are small, and the study was done after the demonstration of the association between wood-dust exposure and nasal cavity cancer, 3 years of data were sufficient to indicate an unusual situation. In addition, the population-based Cancer Registry addresses an aspect which is of importance in public health: nasal adenocarcinomas are rare, and the increased risk in woodworkers makes little difference to the approximately 23,000 new cancer cases in Denmark each year. For the furniture makers, however, nasal adenocarcinomas represent a sizeable problem, accounting for approximately 10% of all their malignant neoplasms during the 3-year period examined.

Linkage of Occupational Records and Cancer Registry

In Denmark the universal personal identification number has been used to link individual records from census returns and pension funds with death certificates and registered cancer cases. The resulting information systems on occupational mortality and cancer morbidity provide the potential for identifying moderately elevated risks for more common types of tumours among occupational groups spread throughout the country. Generation of clues from such information systems have been called "automatized case reports" (4), which supplement clues that emerge from observations by alert physicians.

1. Census—Danish Cancer Registry Linkage Study

The first census after the introduction of the personal identification number in Denmark was held in 1970. Occupation on the census date was recorded and then classified. Persons aged 20–46 years have been followed up for death through record-linkage with all death certifications in the country, and census records have then been linked with the records of cancer cases of which the Cancer Registry has been notified between 1970 and 1980.

From this linked file, relative risk of cancer in various occupational groups may be calculated using all economically active perons as a reference category. Such risks form the basis for the description of cancer occurrence by occupation. Clues concerning cancer aetiology must be followed up by *ad hoc* cohort studies of groups with defined exposures, or by case-control studies examining risk in relation to the exposure under suspicion. A close collaboration between the epidemiologist and the industrial hygienist is necessary for the creation of such hypothesis, which may be supported by a laboratory research working with animals, who should be encouraged to examine the carcinogenic effect of suspect chemicals or exposures in *in vivo* or *in vitro* systems.

The selection of associations for further investigation may be facilitated by comparing the results from various information systems (7). To exploit the full potential of the existing systems for the identification of occupational groups at high risk of cancer and for hypothesis generation, it would be advantageous for each system to undertake tabulations for detailed occupational and diagnostic groups, as has been suggested previously and is now being attempted on a limited scale in North America (1). The detection of an increased risk of lung cancer among butchers may serve as an example of such an approach. All else being equal, it strengthens the validity of the association that it was observed in parallel in Denmark, Sweden, and England and Wales (3). Excess tobacco smoking among butchers does not seem to explain the risk in Denmark (9) and further studies are now being undertaken to identify the possible risk factors.

The existence of such information systems also provides the basis for the testing of hypotheses which have been generated outside the data set. Several studies have raised suspicion that exposure to silica dust increases the risk of lung cancer, although some of the dust-exposed groups have also been exposed to identified carcinogens. In spite of the fact that the information on occupation in the census refers to one point in time only, and the classification used is often broad, it is interesting that the results of the linkage between census records and cancer incidence data in the Nordic countries with regard to lung cancer are in line with previous results for occupational groups where in-depth epidemiology studies are available (10). An increased risk of lung cancer is thus found among foundry workers and Swedish miners. Such consistencies strengthen the results emerging for occupations in which an excess risk of lung cancer has not previously been noticed. With regard to the possible carcinogenic effect of silica dust, it is of interest that the risk of lung cancer is increased among stone cutters in both Denmark and Finland but not in Norway and Sweden (Table I), since this group is probably not exposed to known lung carcinogens at the workplace. A more detailed study of the lung cancer risk in this group seems needed.

TABLE I. Relative Risk of Lung Cancer among Stone Cutters in the Nordic Countries[a]

Country	Number of persons exposed	Obs	RR	95% CI
Denmark	532	13	1.98	1.06–3.39
Finland	820	15	1.75	0.98–2.89
Norway	781	3	0.83	0.17–2.44
Sweden	3,275	37	0.98	0.83–1.16

[a] After Lynge et al. (10).

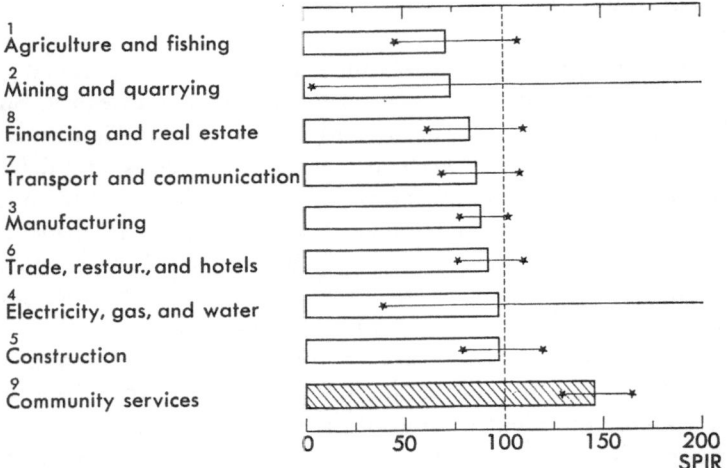

FIG. 1.   Risk of malignant melanoma among male employees
★—★ 95% confidence interval (Figs. 1–4).

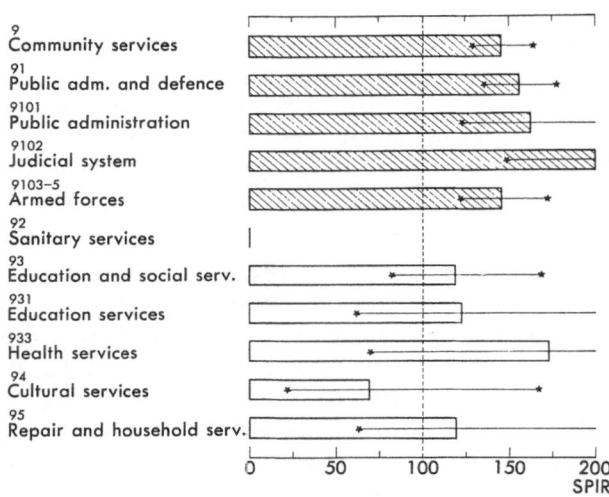

FIG. 2.   Risk of malignant melanoma among males employed in community services

2.   The Supplementary Pension Fund—Danish Cancer Registry Linkage

The Danish Supplementary Pension Fund was established on 1st April 1964 for all wage earners aged 16–66 years. Contributions are paid by the employers to a national fund which retains all information on contributors, pensioners, and on deceased persons. The occupational history of each employee can thus be reconstructed from 1st April 1964, coded as it is by means of five-digit numbers (2) that closely correspond to the International Standard Industrial Classification of all Economic Activities.

The Danish Central Population Registry comprises information on all persons who have resided in Denmark since 1st April 1968. It retains the most recent job title, which indicates whether an employee is likely to be among the persons exposed in the process of production (blue collar worker) or not (white collar worker.)

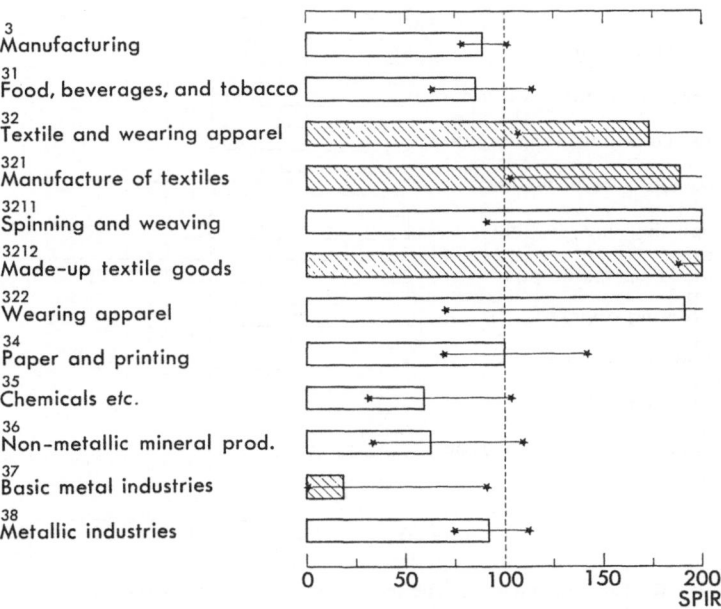

FIG. 3. Risk of malignant melanoma among males employed in manufacturing

Altogether 153,427 cases of cancer recorded by the Cancer Registry in the decade 1970–1979 were linked with these two data sources (*14*). For these patients more than 2.8 million items of information on employment were recorded in the Supplementary Pension Fund varying from no employment at all (*e.g.*, self-employed, housewives, students, unemployed) to 152 different types of employment dating back to 1964.

1) *Screening for occupational risks*

In the absence of population denominators a proportional incidence analysis has been carried out to estimate Standardized Proportional Incidence Ratios (SPIR), which are similar to the standardized incidence or mortality ratios (SIR; SMR), when the cancer under investigation constitutes a minor part of all the malignancies included in the study, and when exposure has no effect on cancer risk in general (*11*, *14*).

Risk estimates have till now been calculated for some 130 industries, specifying 31 defined categories for males and females separately.

As an example, malignant melanoma accounts for 2.1% of all incident cancers in Denmark and a dramatic rise in incidence has been observed over the last 40 years (*16*). A total of 2,296 persons with melanoma (1,076 males and 1,220 females) had membership in the Supplementary Pension Fund. Figure 1 shows the risk of melanomas among men in the nine main branches of industry. In the branch of Community, Social & Personal Services there were 276 cases observed compared to 190.0 expected (SPIR=145; 95% confidence interval (CI)=129–164) and a slight excess of melanomas was also seen among females (SPIR 113; 95 CI=104–124) with 513 observed cases *versus* 452.3 expected.

The increased risk of melanoma among employees in the Community, Social & Personal Services, who are mostly indoor workers, is mainly due to significant excesses in Public Administration & Defence with SPIR=156 among males and SPIR=119 among females (Fig. 2). The most pronounced excesses are seen among male employees

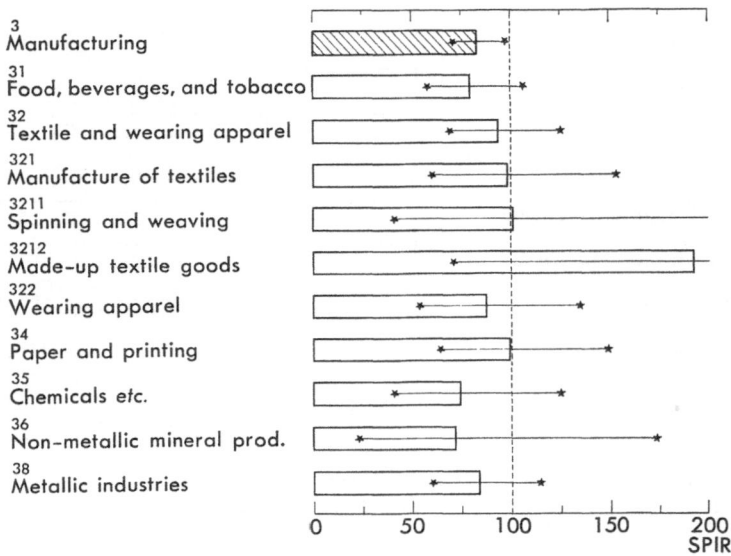

FIG. 4.   Risk of malignant melanoma among females employed in manufacturing

in the public administration associated with government (SPIR=163; 95% CI=125–211), in the judicial system, including the police (SPIR=223; 95% CI=152–327), and in the armed forces (SPIR=146; 95% CI=123–172). Outside Public Administration & Defence the excesses observed are more questionable; however, the cases are fewer. This finding is in line with the increased risk of melanoma seen in middle and high social classes with indoor occupations (*12*), and is possibly related to peak exposure to sunshine in leisure time (*5*). Figure 3 gives the relative risk estimates for skin melanoma among males in selected industries of manufacturing. The risk is 11% below the national average in manufacturing, but an excess of malignant melanoma is seen in the textile industry (SPIR=173; 95% CI=110–172) (Fig. 3), including the manufacture of made-up textile goods (SPIR=590; 95% CI=221–1572). Among females, only those with employment in made-up textile goods show an increased risk (SPIR=192) (Fig. 4). Such findings may warrant further study in order to evaluate whether the risk is related to the working or social environments prevailing in these industries.

2)   *Hypothesis testing*

The approach described above may provide clues concerning aetiology, but to evaluate cancer risk in relation to a defined chemical exposure additional information is necessary. Suspect exposures often fall into different occupational groups and risk may best be evaluated by means of a case-control approach, where cases and controls are selected from the linked data set and where the job information on relevant exposures is obtained from complementary sources, such as measurements in the working environments, questionnaires to the workplaces involved, or exposure evaluation made by industrial hygienists.

The latter method was used in the assessment of sino-nasal cancer after occupational exposure to formaldehyde, wood-dust, and other specified compounds or working processes. The occupational histories from the linked file were used to confirm the role of wood-dust in nasal cavity cancer in Denmark—in particular, adenocarcinomas—and to indicate an aetiological role of formaldehyde in human cancer (*13, 15*). It is important to note that for such investigations carried out within the framework of the linkage study, ascertainment of employment is uninfluenced by memories of cases and controls, and exposures are assessed without disclosing case-control status.

CONCLUSION

In conclusion then, the Cancer Registry serves an important purpose in identifying occupational groups at increased risk of cancer. There are limitations due to the quality of information of reports to the Cancer Registry, but nevertheless such information may serve as a point of departure for a first look into high-risk groups, in particular for persons in long-term jobs. In the absence of corresponding numerator information, alternative methods of analysis should be considered such as proportional analysis or case-control studies within the Cancer Registry material.

The Nordic experience shows that the Cancer Registry material may be enhanced considerably for the study of occupational risks of cancer by record-linkage between external data sources, such as census returns or pension funds, and cancer registry data. In this way information systems may be created which are easily available for the routine description of occupational risks, and for rapid checks when suspicion of such risk arises.

A number of potential limitations must be kept in mind when interpreting the results of such studies. For the census-Cancer Registry linkage the results refer to the industry and job title at a given time, whereas the pension fund—Cancer Registry linkage has limited information on the type of job held within the industry. Common to all such linked information systems is the possible attenuation of risk due to heterogeneous job categories. Such systems are thus likely to reflect the individual's exact type of work compared with the information which may be obtained in *ad hoc* epidemiologic studies. Confounding may be a further problem in such linked materials where information on other risk factors is rarely if ever available. However, there is reason to believe that confounding is unlikely to explain major deviations in risk, and any relative risk above 1.5 which seems biologically possible should be explored by additional investigations.

An insoluble problem for individual studies is the phenomenon of mass significance resulting from the large number of comparisons normally undertaken. It is a strength of the Danish situation that two independent data sources provide information on cancer risks. The plausibility of an occupational cancer risk is thus strengthened if it emerges from both information systems. Furthermore, it is of value to be able to compare risks across national boundaries. Such comparisons of results between information systems are particularly important for setting priorities concerning associations to be more closely studied by *ad hoc* studies, be they of the case-control type taking individual occupational exposure histories, or of the cohort type in which industrial groups are identified on the basis of their occupational exposures, and follow-up for cancer risk is performed. The Cancer Registry in such follow-up studies may prove of particular value due to the specific information available on tumour type. Such follow-up studies still provide the strongest evidence that can be obtained on cancer risk in humans. It is important to stress that the limitations mentioned above make the routine information systems of little value in providing evidence of the absence of occupational risks.

Acknowledgments

The authors wish to thank Ms. Marianne Harnek for help with the preparation of the manuscript. This work has been performed with support from the Danish Cancer Society (Grant No. M 1/81).

REFERENCES

1. Dubbrow, R. and Wegman, D. H. Setting priorities for occupational cancer research and control: Synthesis of the results of occupational disease surveillance studies. *J. Natl. Cancer Inst.*, **71**, 1123–1142 (1983).
2. Erhvervsgrupperingskode af 1. april 1977. Danmarks statistik.
3. Fox, A. J., Lynge, E., and Malker, H., Lung cancer in butchers. *Lancet*, **ii**, 399 (1982).
4. Hogstedt, C. Paper presented at IARC meeting on the use of available statistical sources for the detection of occupational cancer. The City University, London (1982).
5. Holman, C.D.J., Armstrong, B. K., and Heenan, P.J. A theory of etiology and pathogenesis of human cutaneous malignant melanoma. *J. Natl. Cancer Inst.* **71**, 651–656 (1983).
6. Jensen, O. M. The Cancer Registry as a tool to detect industrial risks. *Bull. Cancer*, **70**, 423–428 (1983).
7. Jensen, O. M. and Lynge, E. The contribution of epidemiology to the study of occupational cancer. *J. Cancer Res. Clin. Oncol.*, **108**, 257–263 (1984).
8. Jensen, O. M., Storm, H. H., and Jensen, H. S. Cancer registration in Denmark and the study of multiple primary cancers, 1943–80. *Natl. Cancer Inst. Monogr.*, **67**, 245–251 (1985).
9. Lynge, E. and Andersen, O. Lung cancer in Danish butchers. *Lancet*, **i**, 527–528 (1983).
10. Lynge, E., Kurppa, K., Kristofersen, L., Malker, H., and Sauli, H. Silica dust and lung cancer. Results from the Nordic occupational mortality and cancer incidence registers. *J. Natl. Cancer Inst.*, **77**, 883–889 (1986).
11. Monson, R. R. Analysis of relative survival and proportional mortality. *Comp. Biomed. Res.*, **7**, 325–332 (1974).
12. Office of population censuses and surveys. Occupational mortality. The Registrar General's decennial supplement for England and Wales, 1970–72. A publication of the Government Statistical Service (1978).
13. Olsen, J. H. and Asnæs, S. Formaldehyde and squamous cell carcinoma of the sinonasal cavities in humans. *Br. J. Industr. Med.*, **43**, 769–774 (1986).
14. Olsen, J. H. and Jensen, O. M. Occupation and risk of cancer in Denmark: An analysis of 98,810 cancer cases, 1970–1979. *Scand. J. Work Environ. Health*, Suppl. (1987) (in press).
15. Olsen, J. H., Jensen, S. P., Hink, M., Faurbo, K., Breum, N. O., and Jensen, O. M. Occupational formaldehyde exposure and increased nasal cancer risk in man. *Int. J. Cancer*, **34**, 639–644 (1984).
16. Østerlind, A. and Jensen, O. M. Trends in incidence of malignant melanoma of the skin in Denmark, 1943–1982. *In* "Recent Results in Cancer Research, Vol. 102. Epidemiology of Malignant Melanoma," ed. R. P. Gallagher, pp. 8–17 (1985). Springer-Verlag, Berlin.

CHANGES IN FREQUENCY OF LESS COMMON CANCERS: AN EARLY WARNING SYSTEM FOR CANCER REGISTRIES

J. W. BERG*[1] and Jack L. FINCH*[2]

Pathology, University of Colorado Health Sciences Center, School of Medicine[1] *and Data Analysis, Colorado Central Cancer Registry, Colorado Department of Health*[2]

New human carcinogens often make their presence known by increasing the incidence of previously rare or at least uncommon cancers. The rarer the cancer in the past, the bigger will be the change in its relative frequency by the accumulation of even a few extra cases.

We here discuss what we have learned about the design and operation of an automated surveillance system based on comparison of relative frequencies in a large standard population and a smaller study population.

Cancer epidemiology can be thought of as a science of comparisons. Causes are found by comparisons of individuals: cases *versus* controls or exposed *versus* non-exposed members of a cohort. Before one gets to this stage however, the problems most often are defined by comparisons of groups; cancer rates in different countries, cancer rates in different states or prefectures, or changes in cancer rates over time, all subjects in which Professor Mitsuo Segi was preeminent. The extension of these latter kinds of studies from common cancers to rarer ones has been profitable even while unsystematic. The present discussion concerns the conceptual problems encountered in efforts to systematize such comparisons.

We have created such a system for use in U.S. registries but since experience still is meager about moving it from one computer to another or one registry system to another, we prefer to use the space available to us to consider aspects important for any software program. The importance of the less common cancers is perhaps best known through the story of how asbestos was recognized as a carcinogen by studies of patients with mesotheliomas. Other well-known examples are Burkitt's lymphoma, the production of hepatic angiosarcomas by vinyl chloride, the vaginal adenocarcinomas produced by *in utero* stilbestrol exposure, while more recently there are the Kaposi's sarcomas associated with acquired immunodeficiency syndrome (AIDS), T-cell leukemias due to viral infections, and brain lymphomas in transplant patients. Perhaps most important, excepting viral tumors, the most newly recognized carcinogens are found to cause other cancers as well. All of these cancers had been so very rare that only a few cases were enough to suggest that a new carcinogen was active. Once the alert had been given, the cause usually was identified reasonably rapidly.

Cancer epidemiologists may take pride in the speed with which they helped track

---

*[1] B216, Denver, Co. 80262, U.S.A.

*[2] Denver, Co. 80220, U.S.A.

down the causal agents. There must be some chagrin, however, that it took others to discover the problems clinically while cancer registries, to which so much time and effort have been devoted, contributed little or nothing to the early work. We believe there are practical ways that cancer registry data can be used to warn us early of new kinds of cancer that signal (belatedly) the introduction of new carcinogens into the environment.

Cancer registries currently are collecting quite detailed information on cancer cases including the exact site of origin of the cancer (378 code numbers are given for cancer in the 1975 edition, ICD) and the histologic type (385 types of cancer are given different codes in the companion, ICD—Oncology). Theoretically, registries could and should report *incidence rates* on all site-type combinations and then determine which are changing with time and which seem to differ from one subpopulation to another or from one registry to another. Practically this could not be done because of limitations on resources, manpower above all, but also because of such mundane considerations as the size of publications. Rarer tumors must have lower priority than common ones for verification, a feature which would add to the delays in reporting incidence trends, delays which are already considerable because of the time it takes to make sure all cases diagnosed in a given year are collected and encoded correctly. Finally, there has been the problem of lack of specificity or at least variation in specificity. Just as registry data are weakened to the extent they must rely on death certificate diagnoses with their notorious imprecision, so more specific studies are weakened to the extent that pathologists use only non-specific diagnoses. Even terms like "adenocarcinoma" which are fairly specific when used to describe a lung cancer or cervical cancer are uniformative when applied without modifiers to stomach, thyroid, or breast cancers, for example.

This last problem is disappearing in developed countries as a quite precise and specific pathological "lingua franca" emerges. Staffing shortages are eased as computers take over the work of the tabulation. The problem of the delay in obtaining complete data on incidence has not been solved for most of us, and may not be for some time, but as suggested below it can be bypassed. Even when one does this though, other problems, only vaguely glimpsed before, remain. These and their partial solutions will be discussed following the outline of the proposed general solution.

The Practical Solution

It seems obvious that the fact of rarity itself can be taken advantage of when studying how rare cancers differ over time or among populations. Changes in importance for common cancers usually occur at most at a few percent per year. Therefore great effort must be expended to make sure that the most recent trend, alarming or reassuring, is not due to small artifacts, small errors in population estimates or small changes in medical or statistical practice. By contrast, the changes in rare tumors that have been important have been very large in *relative* terms. The first few mesotheliomas in Connecticut asbestos workers caused a 7-fold rise in their frequency in men (with a later rise in women). Changes of this magnitude can be seen even when case reporting is not complete. Thus, it is possible for cancer registries to have a truly early warning system. As soon as the bulk of a year's data is in, it can be screened to see if any changes have occurred large enough to merit immediate attention. The staffing costs of such monitoring should be reduced by computerization. When the quality of the basic data becomes good enough, rapid monitoring should be within the reach of most registries through the use of *comparative relative frequencies.* If a type of neoplasm that previously accounted for one cancer in every 20,000 among men or even 1 among 1,000 suddenly becomes 7 times as common, the relative increase can be recognized and proven significant even if only 80% of the year's cases have been registered. It is on this basis that we developed and tested a working early warning system.

Before such a system is designed, certain obvious problems must be addressed. The first of these is the *problem of too much specificity* or *"data dispersion."* One reason it was difficult for cancer registrars to see the rise in mesotheliomas when it first occurred was that these neoplams were assigned to multiple sites in different parts of the cancer classification system. The most common site is pleura, considered part of the respiratory system, and the second commonest site is the peritoneum, considered part of the digestive system. For each of these two basic sites of origin, there are several alternative codes that can be used. A mesothelioma arising from the pleural surface of the lung may grow into the lung and be coded to that organ. If a similar tumor grows outward destroying ribs and becomes a mass in the chest wall beneath the skin, the soft tissue of the trunk area is a defensible primary location. The visceral and soft tissue possibilities for origin of a peritoneal mesothelioma obviously are that much greater. Thus, too much specificity can be as big a problem as too little. There was little chance to spot the mesothelioma problem when the pleural majority were merged with all other cancers of the pleura, mediastinum, nose, nasal sinuses, and middle ear as "other respiratory cancers," but there would be as much of a problem if every site-type combination in the body were looked at separately.

The theoretical solution is simple enough; divide up cancers only enough to separate, in this case, etiologic entities. In other cases one would want to classify cancers by their responsiveness to a specific treatment, *etc.*.

The problem with this approach, however, is that it presupposes the answers we are searching for. Practically, we have found virtue in a 3-step approach. First, existing knowledge is used as much as possible to devise meaningful major categories such as cancer of the mouth or large bowel (colon *and* rectum). Breaking with tradition, anal cancers are separated from the latter group since they have a different epidemiology, one well enough known to justify separate analysis. On one hand, a major group need not be large, if it has its own distinctive epidemiology. On the other hand, cancers with features in common need to be brought together. Retroperitoneum clearly is a soft-tissue site, mediastinum probably is, and pleura and peritoneum can be included if, as in Europe, mesothelioma is considered a soft tissue tumor.

When terminology is variable and cases are quite rare, subgroups of cases should be formed at the beginning. It seems counterproductive for a first analysis to separate every sarcoma and lymphoma type for an organ like the thyroid where such cancers are rare. If there is a sudden significant increase in the category of "sarcomas of the thyroid," the few cases involved can be subclassified for a full review. (The capability for individual case review is a prime necessity for any kind of monitoring. A system can never anticipate exactly which groupings are optimal.)

Often beyond the groupings of very rare diagnoses that seem obvious, there are others that are useful as summary statements even though one does not want to lose sight of the basic data. When performing analyses of this kind from very basic type-by-site cross-tabulations, far too much time must be spent combining categories because there may be different names for the same entity with respect to etiology. Fortunately, a computer can be programmed to count items more than once. We found great value in having our itemized list of special sites and types followed by a few additional summary groupings such as "all adenocarcinomas" (=minor salivary gland cancers) for the lip and the oral cavity, and "all malignant Brenner tumors" of the ovary which, following Scully's definition, are *recalculated* as the total of a) squamous cell carcinomas, b) transitional cell carcinomas, c) adenosquamous carcinomas, and d) cases diagnosed specifically as Brenner-type cancers.

Finally, in direct response to the mesothelioma problem, we found it useful to follow the tabulations of subsite and histology within each major site with a tabulation of relative frequencies of specific histologies from *all* sites. Carcinomas were not included because any major affinity across sites had been used to define the original site groups. *i.e.*, "oral cavity," "pharynx excluding nasopharynx," and "large bowel" (colon plus rectum). Hence we limited our across-site tabulations to non-carcinomas (histologies above 857 in MOTNAC, SNOP, and ICD-O).

The *problem of false positives* is even a greater problem than the dispersion of data. It had a great deal to do with our choice of comparison standards and comparison methods and so consideration of these points was postponed until this section.

Our general plan was to compare frequencies in the newest data set with the frequencies seen in previous data that could serve as a standard. When there has been little change in the population over the time-period, there is correspondingly little need for adjustment for age, sex, or race. However, when one is comparing, say, the relative frequencies of specific cancers in blacks with those in the much larger white population, it seems much safer to make the comparisons separately for each sex and age subgroup, then sum the expectations and observations (indirect standardization). Problems arise whenever the standard population is not large so that many age- and sex-specific subgroups do not by chance have a case of the rare cancer in question. We are still using trial and error to determine when we gain and when we lose by various degrees of stratification.

When studying changes in relative frequencies over time, most of the commonest specific diagnoses will show increases. On inspection, these increases will be mainly due to greater precision of diagnosis, and decreased use of "wastebasket" categories such as "cancer," "carcinoma," or "mouth." Our solution to the problem has worked reasonably well. We include along with the comparison in overall relative frequencies, a comparison of *within-site* relative frequencies using only *specific diagnoses*. Thus, for esophageal locations we look at observed and standard relative frequencies in two ways: once as a fraction of all cancers in a) the data set and, b) within the organ. We evaluate the distribution past and present only of those cases which were assigned to a specific location, ignoring the cases coded to merely "esophagus." Similarly, we consider the within-site frequency of esophageal adenocarcinomas only in terms of the carcinomas of specified types, excluding those without such specification. (Because at most sites carcinomas predominate and can usually be separated from sarcomas, *etc.*, we used only specific types of *carcinomas* in the histology analysis.) This aspect of our work is still unfinished; we have not determined whether moving from a single definition of "specific carcinomas" and "specific sites" applied across all major groups is good enough or whether group-specific definitions would repay the extra programming that such specificity would require.

Adjusting for improved specificity, or other changes, is one way of reducing the number of changes in frequency that need to be explored in further detail. Another simplification is related to significance testing. The object of the whole surveillance system is to identify changes most likely to be important. In this regard, testing for "statistical significance" can be helpful even when not all criteria for statistical rigor are met.

Since the principal use we visualized for our system was the comparison of a *relatively small* set of new data against a *relatively large* standard set with at least a 1 to 10 ratio, we felt the requirements for a Poission test were approached, and that this test would be appropriate for the very small frequencies that made up the bulk of our data. The test also was attractive because of the relative ease of programming the Bailar-Ederer (1) method. After use we still recommend it but with a warning and a modification. First, the Poisson test is inappropriate and misleading when two data sets of comparable size are being studied. In that situation a stratified χ^2 (Mantel-Haenszel (3)) approach theoretically would be better, though we have not determined the storage- and time-requirements needed to apply it to every comparison. Secondly, we obtained many "significant" results because a diagnosis appeared in the new, but not in the standard data-set. Such events will be common if the diagnosis is rare, but the finding is of practical importance only if the "new" diagnosis occurs more than once or twice in the new data set. We now recommend against a significance test when the observed and expected frequencies are both less than 3, or even 5.

What sample sizes are necessary for a useful test? As described below, we obtained useful information when we compared the distribution of the 15,388 cancers in whites reported from Colorado during the Third National Cancer Survey (TNCS (2)) with the cancers in the remaining TNCS white population—147,331 cases or a 1:10 ratio. We also obtained good information on black-white differences by comparing 41,661 cancers in blacks (TNCS plus the first 5 years of SEER data (4)) with about 450,000 cancers in whites. We did not get much usable information from the same data set when our study groups consisted of about 4,000 Japanese-Americans, 2,200 Chinese-Americans or 4,300 Hispanics. For study populations of these sizes, almost all usable information resides in the actual incidence rates of more common cancers. We have not had enough experience with study groups in the 7,000–10,000 case-range to determine the usefulness of results. On the other hand, *negative* information may be useful from a group of any size, since it would mean that the group had no evidence of a sizable cancer problem.

At this point there will have been some winnowing of the "significant" increases in rare cancers, but it is almost sure that the number of "false" increases will greatly outnumber the true and important changes. The next step probably is to go over the list with knowledgeable pathologists. They should be able to identify some terms as representing novel occurrences, or entities that have probably been continuously present but unrecognized, *e.g.*, hairy cell leukemia. A second set of diagnoses will be characterized as not epidemiologically important, just newly fashionable because of advocacy by a particularly persuasive diagnostician. The shift of many brain tumors from the "glioblastoma" category to "astrocytoma" would be a case in point. Whatever the pathological and clinical justification for this particular shift, the result has been the loss of previously distinct epidemiological or at least demographic differences between the two diagnoses. Again, recently in the U.S.A. at least, "malignant fibrous histiocytoma" is now the most popular diagnosis for spindle-cell sarcomas, replacing principally "fibrosarcoma," just as 40 years ago "fibrosarcoma" displaced "neurosarcoma." Finally, the pathologist will note entities such as "medullary carcinoma of the colon" that are not standard but most

TABLE I.   Examples of Special Cancers Seen in Excess in Colorado 1969–1971

Site-type	Ratio observed to expected[a]	Number of cases
Eye–squamous cell ca.	2.7	10
Lip—women under 60	10.0	4
Larynx and pharynx—women under 55	1.7	31
Fallopian tube—1969–1971	2.6	8
1972–1974	2.3	12
1975–1978	1.8	19
Islet cell—1969–1971	2.2	13
1972–1974	4.9	8
1975–1978	Not increased	
Neurilemmal sarcomas all sites	2.0	7
Hepatic angiosarcomas	6.5	3
Bladder cancer—one community	4.8	12

[a] Expected rates from Third National Cancer Survey, 1969–1971; Colorado data also from survey. Later data came from incomplete coverage. Expected values for histologic types calculated from *within-site* TNCS distributions except for neurilemmal sarcomas.

likely represent the idiosyncratic use of language by certain pathologists. Tomorrow's discoveries may, however, be included in today's idiosyncrasies.)

The search for real geographic or occupational clustering would seem the last level of screening for the possible positive findings within the cancer registry. With this information in hand, hopefully some choice in priority can be made as to which of the "significant" increases are most likely to be real and which are more likely to be statistical fluctuations. At the level of actual investigations of apparent increases, we have been as limited by time and money as most other registries would be. In one investigation using questionnaire follow-back, we found causal explanations for some, but far from all, of the largest fluctuations in Colorado cancer rates from 1970 (Table I). Explanations included a) residence at high altitudes for cancers of the conjunctiva, b) early occupational exposure to the sun while farming (younger women with lip cancer), and c) high frequency of employment as cocktail waitresses and bartenders among younger women with pharyngeal and laryngeal cancer. Other high rates have persisted without obvious cause, including 2- to 4-fold increases for cancers of the fallopian tube and islet cell carcinomas of the pancreas. Other rates once high have since returned to normal, including high frequencies of neurilemmosarcomas, hepatic angiosarcomas, and high bladder cancer rates in one *community* that raised the rate for all the Denver area significantly above the national average.

In conclusion, while we do not minimize the efforts and difficulties still inherent in surveillance of populations for important increases in previously uncommon cancers, we believe that enough knowledge about epidemiology, pathology, and computers exists to make such surveillance both feasible and ultimately profitable in terms of early attention to new cancer risks.

Acknowledgment

The development and testing of this system was supported by Grants CA 17060-03 NCI and 5R18CA25254 from the National Cancer Institute to the Colorado Regional Cancer Center.

REFERENCES

1. Bailar, J. C. III and Ederer, F. Significance factors for the ratio of a Poisson variable to its expectation. *Biometrics*, **20**, 639–643 (1964).
2. Cutler, S. J. and Young, J. L., Jr. Third National Cancer Survey: Incidence data. *Natl. Cancer Inst. Monogr.*, **4**, 1–454 (1975).
3. Mantel, N. and Haenszel, W. Statistical aspects of the analysis of data from retrospective studies of disease. *J. Natl. Cancer Inst.*, **22**, 719–748 (1959).
4. Young, J. L., Jr., Percy, C. L., and Asire, A. J. Surveillance epidemiology and end results: Incidence and mortality data, 1973–77. *Natl. Cancer Inst. Monogr.*, **57**, 1–1082 (1981).

END RESULTS OF CANCER PATIENTS: FROM POPULATION-BASED CANCER REGISTRY DATA

Akira Takano and Yoshi Okuno

Miyagi Prefectural Cancer Registry*

Relative 5-year survival rates derived from data of population-based cancer registries could become a standard for evaluating the medical care of each hospital within a certain area. These could also become the indices of the present medical care system aiming at early detection and early treatment of cancer.

Five-year survival rates for cancer patients of selected sites diagnosed in 1978 and 1979 in Miyagi Prefecture were computed in the following groupings: all cases (including cases registered for which no information is available other than death certificates-DCO); reported cases (excluding DCO); surgically treated cases; and histologically confirmed cases.

Hospital cancer registries which conduct active follow-up yield different rates than those of the population-based cancer registries which depend upon passive follow-up by determining survival from death notifications only. Such notifications may sometimes yield higher survival rates than the actual rates. All the survivors in the file of the registry were followed as much as possible, and the rates were computed using the data corrected by the follow-up survey.

Allowing for a few differences, we are confident that the rates which were computed "according to records" can be used as a standard for the above-mentioned purposes.

It was in 1951 that the first population-based cancer survey in Japan was started by the late Professor Mitsuo Segi in Miyagi Prefecture. A quarter century has passed since the "survey" changed to "registration" in 1959.

Since 1962 cancer registration has been started in Osaka, Aichi, and some other prefectures and cities. The research group for these population-based cancer registries is organized under a grant of the Ministry of Health and Welfare of Japan.

In both 1975 and 1977 the authors made follow-up surveys on cancer patients for computing survival rates (7, 8). At that time they sensed that the reliability of the data including identification items was an essential problem needing further study not only regarding end results but also for computing survival rates. Also, they found that survival rates of cancer patients varied greatly according to the reliability of registration. Thus it was deemed necessary to find a way to decrease the fallibility of the registration figures.

Since then, we have gradually improved the reliability of registration. The average annual number of registrations and related data in the Miyagi Prefectural Cancer Registry

---

* 6-2-81 Kamisugi, Sendai 980, Japan (高野　昭，奥野ヨシ).

of recent years (1980–1982) are as follows: population, 2,032,320 (1980 census); number of incident cases, 4,700; number of deaths, 2,950; the proportion of incidence to death, 1.6 times; the proportion of cases registered for which no information is available other than death certificates, 14%; and the proportion of histologically confirmed cases to all incidence, 70%, and to reported cases, 81%. Information has been received for 79% of the deaths with mention of cancer somewhere on the death certificates (5). About 80% of the incident reports are actually abstracted from hospital records (active way), and the rest are voluntarily reported from hospitals and clinics within the area (passive way).

Using the above divisions, relative 5-year survival rates were computed by sex and site for cancer patients who were diagnosed in 1978 and 1979.

Relative 5-Year Survival Rates in Miyagi Prefecture

Relative 5-year survival rates were computed by the method introduced by Ederer et al. (1), which is used commonly in cancer registration. The survival rates given in the life tables for Japan in 1980 (6) are used for the computation of expected survival rates. The data have been collated with all the death certificates of the region up to December 31, 1984, and all the rest are treated as survivors in the file.

The focus of this study is the cancer patients diagnosed in 1978 and 1979. The incident year for cases diagnosed by death certificate only (DCO) is set at 1/2 of the "duration of illness" listed on the death certificates. However, if a date of surgical operation is listed, that is taken as the incident date. Only the first primary is considered, because the second or subsequent primary is liable to have been affected by the first one.

As shown in Table I, the rates have been calculated for the following groups: all cases (including DCO); reported cases (excluding DCO); surgically operated cases including both curative and non-curative operations; and histologically confirmed cases. The inclusion of the latter two groups was thought to be important for the results to more accurately comparable with hospital data.

Relative 5-year survival rates showed more favorable results for females (41.0%) than for males (31.0%) for all sites. Female rates were probably influenced by the favorable survival for cancer of the breast and the cervix; for other sites also generally higher survival was shown for females. However, it is of interest that female rates were lower than male rates for cancer of the stomach, liver and biliary passages, skin, and leukemia. Further study is needed of the sex differences by histological type and age distribution.

When observing the rates by group, we noticed that survival rates for the latter two groups, i.e., surgically treated (III) and histologically confirmed (IV), were higher than those for all (I), and reported (II) for all sites with the exception of cancer of the pancreas, and leukemia for which the diagnosis is considered to be difficult. This suggests that some doubtful cases might have been registered as cancer of the pancreas and leukemia.

Death Certificates Only (DCO)

DCO is defined as cases registered for which no information is available other than a statement on the death certificate that the deceased died from or with cancer (9).

The proportion of DCO for 1978 and 1979 in Miyagi Prefecture was 16.1% (1,325)

TABLE I. Relative 5-Year Survival Rates (%) of Selected Sites in Miyagi Prefecture (1978–1979)

Site (ICD-9th)		I All[a]				II Reported[b]				III Surgically treated				IV Histologically conf.			
		No.	OSR	RSR	SE	No.	OSR	RSR	SE	No.	OSR	RSR	SE	No.	OSR	RSR	SE
140–208 Malignant neoplasms, all sites	M	4,421	25.7	31.0	0.8	3,722	30.5	35.9	0.9	2,465	38.5	43.9	1.1	2,870	35.7	41.2	1.1
	F	3,797	36.3	41.0	0.9	3,173	43.4	47.7	1.0	2,193	50.3	54.0	1.1	2,506	48.9	52.8	1.1
140–149 Lip, oral cavity, and pharynx	M	67	22.4	26.4	6.4	61	24.6	28.7	6.7	33	27.3	31.5	9.3	52	23.1	26.6	7.1
	F	37	35.1	42.5	9.8	33	39.4	45.3	10.0	13	30.8	34.2	14.6	30	40.0	44.9	10.2
150 Oesophagus	M	276	8.0	9.8	2.2	229	9.6	11.6	2.5	124	13.7	15.6	3.7	190	10.5	12.4	2.8
	F	100	11.0	14.2	4.5	72	15.3	18.7	5.6	34	20.6	22.3	7.7	51	19.6	22.5	6.7
151 Stomach	M	1,694	35.3	42.0	1.4	1,447	41.3	47.9	1.5	1,215	44.9	50.5	1.6	1,224	45.6	51.8	1.6
	F	1,028	31.3	35.7	1.7	847	38.0	42.1	1.9	681	43.5	46.6	2.0	675	43.3	46.8	2.1
152, 153 Intestine, except rectum	M	187	33.7	41.3	4.4	168	37.5	45.0	4.6	149	40.3	47.5	4.8	138	41.3	48.4	5.0
	F	238	38.2	44.2	3.7	207	44.0	49.7	3.9	192	44.3	49.9	4.1	167	47.9	53.1	4.3
154 Rectum	M	188	35.6	42.5	4.3	171	39.2	45.9	4.5	159	41.5	47.9	4.6	141	46.1	53.5	4.9
	F	201	39.3	45.1	4.0	168	46.4	51.4	4.3	158	43.7	48.1	4.4	140	51.4	56.3	4.6
155, 156 Liver and biliary passages	M	342	4.1	5.1	1.5	244	5.7	6.8	1.9	115	8.7	10.0	3.2	152	7.2	8.4	2.6
	F	265	1.9	2.3	1.1	164	3.0	3.5	1.6	94	3.2	3.6	2.2	95	2.1	2.4	1.8
157 Pancreas	M	190	4.2	5.2	2.0	137	5.8	6.9	2.6	75	2.7	3.1	2.3	85	2.4	2.8	2.1
	F	133	6.0	7.1	2.6	92	8.7	10.1	3.6	49	10.2	11.7	5.3	57	7.0	8.0	4.1
161 Larynx	M	43	37.2	43.3	8.8	41	39.0	45.1	9.0	25	24.0	28.4	10.7	41	39.0	45.1	9.0
	F	8	37.5	44.1	20.1	6	50.0	58.5	23.5	3	33.3	40.6	34.5	6	50.0	58.5	23.5
162 Trachea, bronchus, and lung	M	592	8.4	10.6	1.6	499	10.0	12.3	1.8	136	27.9	31.8	4.5	223	15.7	18.3	3.0
	F	250	10.0	11.9	2.5	185	13.5	15.6	3.1	39	35.9	38.3	8.3	66	21.2	23.5	5.8
172, 173 Skin	M	47	72.3	90.1	5.4	46	73.9	90.5	5.3	27	70.4	89.9	7.4	42	76.2	92.8	4.9
	F	48	62.5	76.7	7.5	45	66.7	79.7	7.2	23	65.2	78.0	10.3	42	66.7	79.5	7.4
174 Breast	F	501	71.1	74.3	2.0	486	73.3	76.6	2.0	413	71.4	74.5	2.2	449	72.6	75.8	2.1
179–182 Uterus, all parts	F	368	61.4	66.3	2.7	341	66.3	70.9	2.6	185	78.9	81.4	2.9	292	67.8	72.0	2.8
185 Prostate	M	114	33.3	47.9	6.7	99	38.4	54.0	7.0	58	39.7	54.2	8.9	85	37.6	52.0	7.5
188 Bladder	M	132	46.2	58.2	5.4	114	53.5	65.1	5.4	103	54.4	65.6	5.6	106	54.7	65.7	5.5
191, 192 Brain and nervous system	M	46	39.1	47.6	9.0	40	45.0	52.1	9.1	28	50.0	57.1	10.7	37	48.6	56.1	9.4
	F	44	34.1	35.1	7.4	43	34.9	35.9	7.5	34	35.3	36.2	8.5	41	31.7	32.7	7.6
193 Thyroid	M	30	33.3	33.9	8.8	30	33.3	33.9	8.8	25	36.0	36.3	9.7	30	33.3	33.9	8.8
	F	28	57.1	64.7	10.5	26	61.5	69.8	10.2	19	78.9	83.9	9.0	24	66.7	72.8	9.9
204–208 Leukemia	M	110	11.8	13.0	3.5	83	15.7	16.7	4.4	—	—	—	—	56	7.1	7.7	3.8
	F	92	8.7	9.1	3.1	72	11.1	11.5	3.9	—	—	—	—	49	4.1	4.2	3.0

OSR, observed survival rates; RSR, relative survival rates; SE, standard error to RSR.
a Including cases of DCO.
b Excluding cases of DCO.

of the total cases (8,218), and surgical operations and even autopsy findings were often mentioned on these certificates. These are the cases which should be registered as cancer cases. We have not yet made further inquiry to the certifying physicians in these cases because of confidentiality, and because we intend to use this proportion of DCO as an index to evaluate the reliability of our registration. We believe that the DCO cases should be decreased as much as possible, however, this should be done by collecting more information on cancer patients during their lifetime. We fear that only the *apparent* reliability is improved by referring death certificates to certifying physicians, but that non-fatal cases would be overlooked.

In computing the incidence rate, the date of diagnosis for DCO cases has generally been assigned as the date of death (*10*). However, for this date we have gone back to half of the mentioned duration of illness on death certificates because "duration of illness" is often counted from the first symptom, and diagnosis is made during the course of the illness. This date of diagnosis is also used for computing survival rates, as we use the same file for all purposes.

Comparison of Survival Rates in Miyagi and Osaka

Five-year survival rates show more favorable results for Miyagi Prefecture than for Osaka Prefecture (*3*) (Table II).

In comparing the survival rates between the two prefectures, the difference in the observed period (1978–1979 for Miyagi and 1975–1977 for Osaka Prefectures) should be borne in mind. However, the most important factor with a marked difference between the rates in the two prefectures might be the proportion of DCO cases and the way of case collection, *i.e.*, by the active way in Miyagi Prefecture. Comparison of survival rates can be affected by variations in coverage and reporting of cases, by definitions of stage and treatment, and by methods used for patient follow-up (*2*).

Follow-up

Active and direct follow-up is generally limited to hospital cancer registries. On the other hand, population-based cancer registries usually undertake passive follow-up (based on death certificates or hospital notification of death) assuming survival in the absence of this information. They do not use direct follow-up, although they can refer to the active follow-up by hospitals (*4*).

The survival rates shown in Table I are based on the data from passive and indirect follow-up of the population-based cancer registry. Even if every precaution is taken under these limitations, survival analysis must still be considered unreliable (*4*).

To remove this apprehension, we conducted another survey to the extent that this population-based cancer registry allowed through related records such as resident ledgers, health insurance or social security register, *etc*. This survey is of all the patients who were diagnosed in 1978 and 1979 for whom no information of death has been received, *i.e.*, supposed survivors in the file. These data have been collated with all the death certificates through December 1984. All survivors except for residents of Sendai, which is about 1/3 of the total population of this Prefecture, were objects of the study.

TABLE II. Comparison of Relative 5-Year Survival Rates (%)
in Miyagi Prefecture and Osaka Prefecture

Site (ICD-9th)		Miyagi[a] (1978–1979)		Osaka[b] (1975–1977)	
		All[c]	Reported[d]	All[c]	Reported[d]
Oesophagus (150)	M	9.8	11.6	5.7	7.8
	F	14.2	18.7	7.7	11.2
Stomach (151)	M	42.0	47.9	24.2	30.9
	F	35.7	42.1	22.4	28.6
Intestine, except rectum (152, 153)	M	41.3	45.0	—	—
	F	44.2	49.7	—	—
Colon (153)	M	—	—	27.3	34.7
	F	—	—	25.6	34.6
Rectum (154)	M	42.5	45.9	24.6	31.7
	F	45.1	51.4	22.8	29.7
Pancreas (157)	M	5.2	6.9	1.5	5.2
	F	7.1	10.1	3.3	4.6
Larynx (161)	M	43.3	45.1	56.7	63.3
	F	44.1	58.5	50.9	57.6
Trachea, bronchus, and lung (162)	M	10.6	12.3	6.2	8.1
	F	11.9	15.6	6.9	9.1
Breast (174)	F	74.3	76.6	64.8	69.6
Uterus (179–182)	F	66.3	70.9	—	—
Cervix uteri (180)	F	71.4	73.0	56.1	62.5
Corpus uteri (182)	F	74.2	75.3	57.6	60.7
Ovary, adnexa (183)	F	27.1	29.5	18.2	24.2
Prostate (185)	M	47.9	54.0	32.8	38.8
Bladder (188)	M	58.2	65.1	46.0	54.5
	F	47.6	52.1	34.8	45.8

[a] Proportion of DCO: 15.8% for males; 16.4% for females.
[b] Proportion of DCO: 26.5% for males; 22.7% for females.
[c] Including cases of DCO.
[d] Excluding cases of DCO.

1. Follow-up based on resident ledgers

By the Resident Registration Act, Japanese are requested to register their names, dates of birth, addresses, *etc.* in public offices where they reside, and they must also register changes caused by their moving in and out. The first follow-up survey was based on resident ledgers kept in public offices of the relevant cities, towns, and villages. A separate inquiry was made for patients having more than one address.

Public health nurses were asked to complete or check the following categories: 1) surviving, 2) date of death, 3) date and place of moving, and 4) missing.

The number of cases checked in this way was 1,673 including some with carcinoma *in situ*, and some with tumors of uncertain behavior. We had responses from all the public offices. One pair of duplicate registrations, one mistake in relating sex, and one mistaken address were found from this survey.

Before the 2nd follow-up based on hospital medical records, the 'missing cases' reported as "new address unknown," "unidentified", and "legally missing" were checked by collating with telephone directories, residence maps, and available staff lists around their incident year. Their whereabouts during the incidence period were confirmed.

TABLE III. Results of Follow-up Survey on 1,673 Cases Diagnosed in 1978 and 1979

		1st follow-up by resident ledgers	2nd follow-up by hospital records
1)	Surviving	1,525	1,560
2)	Deceased	23	23
	Deceased, no death certificate	13	15
3)	Moved out of area	12	12
4)	Missing	100	63
	New address unknown	23	17
	Unidentified	75	45
	Legally missing[a]	2	1
	Total	1,673	1,673

[a] Their records have been deleted from the official ledgers.

TABLE IV. Comparison of 5-Year Survival Rates (%): Stomach, Rectum, Lung, and Breast in Miyagi Prefecture, Excluding Sendai-city

Site (ICD-9th)		Original				Revised				Difference	
		No.	OSR	RSR	SE	No.	OSR	RSR	SE	OSR	RSR
Stomach (151)	M	1,239	34.8	41.5	1.7	1,241[a,b]	33.6	40.0	1.7	1.2	1.5
	F	764	28.5	32.6	1.9	763[a]	27.8	31.8	1.9	0.7	0.8
Rectum (154)	M	135	34.8	41.6	5.1	135	34.4	41.1	5.1	0.4	0.5
	F	140	38.6	45.2	4.9	140	38.2	44.7	4.9	0.4	0.5
Trachea, bronchus, and	M	445	8.5	10.7	1.8	445	8.2	10.2	1.8	0.3	0.5
lung (162)	F	182	9.9	11.9	2.9	182	9.1	10.9	2.8	0.8	1.0
Breast (174)	F	310	68.1	71.6	2.7	310	66.9	70.3	2.7	1.2	1.3

[a] Mistaken sex.
[b] Change of address.

2. Follow-up based on hospital records

Out of the 100 cases reported as "missing" in the first follow-up survey, 35 surviving and 2 deceased were newly confirmed by the 2nd follow-up.

As shown in Table III, from both parts of this survey 1,560 cases (93.2%) were found to be surviving and 38 cases (2.3%) were deceased. Among the latter, we discovered 23 cases which should have been linked with death certificates. They resulted from mistaken sex, disagreement in identification of data such as name, date of birth, etc. and clerical mistakes inside and outside of the Registry. The 15 other deaths, however, could not be collated with the death lists which we used. They might be cases who died after moving away. From among all the follow-up cases, 63 (3.8%) were untraceable after their last hospital discharge.

The following are some of the complex details related to the 37 cases which were cleared up by our 2nd follow-up.

Surviving but moved because of work transfer or divorce

Deceased after moving

No detailed address such as c/o

Surviving, but no resident registration

Survival Rates after Follow-up

The data were corrected according to the new results, and differences between the former rates were scrutinized for some selected sites. Table IV shows revised relative 5-year survival rates based on the data obtained in the follow-up. Cancer of the stomach, rectum, lung, and breast only were selected for observation in this paper. The differences within the range of standard error were noted.

Accordingly, if present reliability is maintained with regard to our registration or proportion of DCO, proportion of histologically confirmed cases, and proportion of incidence to death, *etc.*, then relative survival rates by passive follow-up can be used as a standard for evaluating the medical care provided by various hospitals.

Acknowledgments

The authors wish to express their sincere thanks to the Miyagi Prefectural Cancer Registry Committee and the Miyagi Cancer Society for their generous support to the follow-up survey program. The authors are especially grateful to the public health nurses and medical-records personnel of the hospitals for their kind cooperation, and to Ms. Kishi Fujishima for her thoughtful arrangements.

REFERENCES

1. Ederer, P., Axtell, L. M., and Cutler, S. J. The relative survival rate: Statistical methodology. *Natl. Cancer Inst. Monogr.*, **6**, 101–121 (1961).
2. Haenszel, W. Contribution of end results data to cancer epidemiology. *Natl. Cancer Inst. Monogr.*, **15**, 21–33 (1964).
3. Hanai, A. and Fujimoto, I. Survival rate as an index in evaluating cancer control. *In* "The Role of the Registry in Cancer Control," eds. D. M. Parkin, G. Wagner, and C. Muir, IARC Scientific Publications, No. 66, pp. 87–107 (1985). IARC Lyon.
4. Maclennan, M., Muir, C., Steinitz, R., and Winkler, A. "Cancer Registration and Its Techniques," IARC Scientific Publications, No. 21 (1983). IARC, Lyon.
5. Okuno, Y. and Takano, A. The assessment of the reliability of cancer registration. Unpublished data.
6. Statistics and Information Department, Minister's Secretariat, Ministry of Health and Welfare, The 15th Life Tables (1983). Kosei-Tokei-Kyokai, Tokyo.
7. Takano, A. and Okuno, Y. Survivors in the file of population-based cancer registry. Annual Report, Research Group for Population-based Cancer Registries 1975, pp. 79–86 (1976) (in Japanese).
8. Takano, A., Okuno, Y., Otomo, Y., and Aihara, S. Survival rates of cancer patients in Miyagi Prefecture. Annual Report, Research Group for Population-based Cancer Registries, 1977, pp. 112–118 (1978) (in Japanese).
9. Waterhouse, J., Muir, C., Shanmugaratnam, K., and Powell, J. (eds.) "Cancer Incidence in Five Continents," Vol. IV, IARC Scientific Publication, No. 42 (1982). IARC Lyon.
10. Young, J. L., Percy, C. L., Asire, A. J., Berg, J. W., Cusano, M. M., Gloeckler, L. A., Horm, J. W., Lourie, W. I., Pollack, E. S., and Shambaugh, E. M. Cancer incidence and mortality in the United States, 1973–77. *Natl. Cancer Inst. Monogr.*, **57**, 1–9 (1981).

THE IMPACT OF THE COMPUTER ON THE CANCER REGISTRY

R. G. SKEET

The Thames Cancer Registry*

The development of cancer registries is described against the background of the growth of the computer industry, beginning with the precomputer days of mechanical punched card systems, through the era of magnetic tape based batch systems to the present time of online, disk based procedures. During this time more and more of the manual work of the Registry has been taken over by the computer and the whole operation has greatly increased in sophistication. The growth of information systems in the health industry now creates opportunities to generate cancer registration data as a spin-off from routine hospital systems, but growing public concern over the confidentiality of information, especially that held on computer files, has given rise to a serious threat to many population-based registries. A further danger is identified, the temptation to use sophisticated techniques which are very easy to carry out on "friendly" computers without full understanding of the underlying statistical validity of the method.

> *"Man is a tool-using animal . . . . . .*
> *Without tools he is nothing, with tools he is all"*

Carlyle

The latter half of the twentieth century has been characterised by the explosion of what might be called the "information industry." In many areas of human activity the development of the "tools of the trade" leads to development of the trade itself, and this in turn puts pressure on the toolmakers to introduce further improvements, resulting in a seemingly endless cycle of development. This phenomenon is nowhere better demonstrated than in the relationship between the growth of the computer industry and information science. As quickly as the engineer develops a computer processor which runs twice as fast as his previous model or a storage device which holds five times as much data as before, so the computer user requires even better and faster hardware to satisfy his demands for more and more information.

It is against this technological background that epidemiology in general, and Cancer Registration in particular, has developed in recent decades. The earliest cancer registries were children of their time, born into a world of mechanical punched card equipment, which then seemed amazingly fast and sophisticated, but which are viewed by today's young information scientists as quaint relics of former days.

A modern cancer registry is very different from that of 30 or 40 years ago—indeed they are hardly recognisable as functionally the same. Almost all of the changes which have taken place over recent years have been due to the introduction and development

---

* Surrey, SM2 5PY, U.K.

of electronic data processing. In parallel with the ongoing evolution of the long-standing registries there has also been a very significant increase in the number of new registries which have come into operation, particularly new hospital tumour registries. In the U.S.A. this seems to have given rise to a whole new light industry with an Association of Tumor Registrars boasting more than 1,100 members. Much of this expansion must be due to the opportunities afforded by the development of the microcomputer which brings powerful and relatively cheap information processing into all but the smallest hospital.

In this chapter we trace in outline how the development of the computer has influenced the evolution of the cancer registry, both in its internal working and its external relationships. We will also consider some of the possibly adverse effects that a high degree of computerisation can produce. Finally, and cautiously, we will look a little way into the future to see where technology might lead us.

Infancy

Cancer registration predates the age of the modern computer by a generation, the basic principles of operation being established within the limitations of punched card technology. Today it is easy to underestimate the sophistication of the equipment of 30 or 40 years ago. Despite their primitive appearance, these machines could sort, count, tabulate, collate, and print and, indeed, when the first attempts at computerisation took place, it was sometimes less easy for registries to extract statistics from their data. Their punched card equipment was usually housed within the registry and controlled by it, while the computer generally was not. It usually belonged to someone else and the registry was only one of a number of users—and not among the top priorities of the installation.

Punched card equipment was quite adequate for enabling registries to calculate incidence and survival rates and produce simple tabulations which demonstrated that such information systems could be made to work and produce worthwhile data.

By the time computers began to replace punched card equipment, the large population-based registries were already becoming embarrassed by the very large volume of cards they had accumulated. Punch cards have a limited lifespan, repeated passes through the machines rapidly aging them until the point when reproduction becomes essential. There is a practical limit as to how often a large database can be read and some registries were reaching this limit in the 1960's when computers came to their rescue.

The first problem was to convert data from the old punched cards to magnetic tape. This depended upon being able to find a suitable computer connected to the right sort of card reader, and some registries showed considerable ingenuity in solving the practical difficulties with which they were presented. The commercial world made a very rapid transition from cards to computers and soon the old-fashioned equipment became obsolete and some registries ran the very real risk of losing all their historical data because the machinery for transferring it to computer tape no longer existed.

The advent of computers solved the problem of data storage once and for all, but it did much more than that.

The logical power of even the earliest available computers far exceeded that of punched card equipment, and it became possible to perform a much more sophisticated type of data validation. Codes could be checked for legality, and cross-validation between data items became feasible. From now on considerable progress could be made to improve the quality of the data—the first validity checks on converted punched card data was sometimes a salutary experience!

The case-record could also be expanded considerably. The limit of 80 columns (or 65 plus interstage positions) per card no longer restricted the length of the record as a much longer computer record could be created. On punched card equipment a long record had to be split over two or more cards and it was very inconvenient if two items of data on different cards had to be processed together. Using the computer a "master record" could be set up which could then be updated and "filled out" from data on as many cards as required. The role of the punched card changed but was certainly not eliminated. From being the permanent storage medium it became a purely transitory device, the means by which data could be supplied to the computer. Once a card had served its single purpose it was destroyed.

One of the features of the early computer systems was that each registry developed its own suite of programmes. Despite a dearth of programmers and the high cost of development a large number of systems were written with little reference to others—although there was much borrowing of basic ideas. This introduced a lack of standardisation which has continued ever since, though it has to be admitted that it is not only Cancer Registries which have been guilty of re-inventing the wheel many times over. Very few registries owned their own computer. Almost all used those of Health or Government authorities or a university, and often these were situated some distance from the registry. Data was transmitted by car or van, usually at great inconvenience to everyone concerned.

Youth

Perhaps it was this very lack of standardisation which promoted the development of the sophisticated computer systems of the 1970's. Magnetic tape continued to be the most frequently used storage medium for the basic data set. It was cheap, relatively fast, and trouble-free. The system philosophy was simple. Data were generally stored as fixed format records in numerical order along the tape. When a tape was full, a continuation reel was used which enabled the registry database to expand indefinitely. It was also possible to use standard utility programs to tabulate data or produce lists of cases meeting certain criteria. The main "update" programs, however, were usually developed as a one-off system for each registry. A diversity of software developed quickly but once a system was introduced it was unlikely to be changed for quite a long time. Alterations to the structure of the database are an anathema to a cancer registry. Minor changes were made, however. Disks became used for sorting small volumes of data, including amendment and print files, which greatly facilitated the update cycle.

Even with relatively advanced systems there was much manual work to be done. Each registry held a large alphabetic index which was used to check each incoming registration. New cases were identified as such and multiple notifications of the same tumour were linked through this index. This process was entirely manual and was far from straightforward. The misspellings of names and the use of nicknames created many problems and considerable experience was necessary to avoid duplicate registrations or erroneous linkages, and there was little incentive to depart from time-honoured procedures.

The coding of various data items was also carried out manually. While some items could be coded very easily using simple lists of terms, others, such as the diagnostic variables of site, histology, and stage, required much expertise and experience to maintain the accuracy of the data.

This period of development gave rise to automated follow-up systems. The computer could produce pre-printed follow-up forms addressed to the appropriate hospital or general practitioner. Full identification details were printed on the form which was printed at the appropriate time intervals until death information was supplied. The registry could be given an early indication of any cases with overdue follow-up, but for most patients the routine was simple and efficient. Much credit is due to these systems for the marked success in the completeness of the follow-up in many registries.

By this time many registries had seen the advantages of pooling data relating to tumours of specific types. A number of collaborative studies had been set up which involved the processing of the data from several registries at one installation. The economic and practical advantages of this were obvious, but, although computer manufacturers had developed so-called "Industry Compatible Magnetic Tape," in practice there were often great difficulties in transferring data files between computers of different types.

At the same time as cancer registries were developing, largely as a result of new information technology, so information systems were being set up in other health applications, Government departments and in industry. Epidemiologists saw the opportunities which this presented for very efficient studies. Hundreds of hours had been spent in the past by researchers sorting through lists of factory employees, for example, in an attempt to discover registered cancers. If both cancer file and employee data were computerised it became possible to perform this task in a matter of minutes or, at most, hours, provided some form of linkage could be made between the files. In some countries where a unique personal identity number was used the linkage was often easy; in others where linkage could only be made using the patient's name and, perhaps, date of birth, there were more problems but these could usually be overcome by the use of phonetic linkages and other devices.

By the end of the 1970's it began to look as if endless opportunities for linkage studies were opening up.

During this time computers were still expensive pieces of equipment, often requiring much space and special accommodation with false floors and air conditioning. Only the largest registries found it economically worthwhile to have their own machine. Most registries were one of many users of large mainframe computers having access to them by means of terminals connected by telephone wires. In some respects, registries had the best of both worlds—ready access to a large computer without the responsibility of heavy maintenance costs and for the security and physical conditions necessary in computer installations. Few registries, though, were regarded as high priority users of these large machines. Their work often represented only a small fraction of the processing carried out and in many cases the service suffered as a result. Furthermore, when machines were upgraded, replaced, or moved, the registry was unlikely to be meaningfully consulted, and certainly its views would not weigh heavily with the managers of major installations. This gave rise to much instability for many registries which had come to depend more and more upon the computer for their everyday work. Small wonder, when computer costs began to fall in the late 1970's and early 1980's, that many registries began to consider acquiring their own machines in order to gain their independence and became, for the first time in many years, in this respect at least, masters of their own destiny.

Maturity

Until the 1980's, computers in cancer registries were used primarily to store data in a convenient form for analysis, to perform validation checks and to carry out the analysis itself. The present decade has seen the development of computer systems which carry out much of the clerical work necessary to organise data before storage. This is a fundamental change, bringing the computer into the data creation phase of the operation for the first time.

As we have seen, the first process necessary to place a record on a population-based cancer register is to determine whether the patient is already registered and, if so, whether the new report relates to the primary tumour already registered or to an entirely new tumour. A record linkage task such as this is by no means confined to cancer registries; it is a common component of many computer systems and it is not surprising that this was one of the first of the "data-creation" functions to be transferred to the computer. Where there is a large data set, the procedure is usually to link registrations at the earliest opportunity, as with manual linkage using alphabetic index cards. Where the data set is small, it is often more economical to merge completed registrations, rejecting the duplicates at a later stage. In countries where each member of the population has a National Identity Number, which uniquely identifies the patient on different computer systems, it has been the custom for many years to link certain types of records, given the necessary safeguards for protecting confidentiality. In such cases the linkage is a comparatively simple one. The type of linkage which is now being developed in some cancer registries is more complex. Usually only the name and date of birth are available for linkage, and errors in spelling and discrepancies in dates are not uncommon. The computer programs to achieve accurate and efficient linkage are sophisticated, requiring the use of random access files and online mass storage.

The second area in which the computer is beginning to have a new and significant impact is that of data coding. In computer systems, data are coded primarily in order to provide an organisation of data capable of analysis and retrieval, and a saving of storage space is now often of secondary importance. A number of registries now have systems which allow data to be entered in textual form. This may represent a very large saving in clerical resources and almost certainly, in well written systems, there will be improvements in accuracy. The coding process is carried out using disk-based dictionaries which are also used in an inverted form to decode the data on output, so that the whole process of coding and decoding is transparent to the user. Thus the input and output components of a system can be logically interlinked.

The advent of inexpensive mini- and micro-computers has resulted in the establishment of many new tumour registries and at the same time the quite spectacular increase in the use of computers in hospitals has resulted in other information systems which have a strong relevance to cancer registration, although not organised as such. These systems often hold much, or even all, of the data required for cancer registration and the challenge of the next decade will be to feed the larger population based registries from these local sources. In some cases this may mean that the central registry has less control over the quality of its data than has obtained in the past and the role of the registry may well change as a result of these developments. Many population based registries have provided a "cancer information" service to the hospitals from which their cases are registered and this has helped to provide support among clinicians, ensuring the continuity of funding on which registries depend. There is a danger that, as local schemes are developed, attitudes within hospitals may become more parochial and conflicts of interest between a local "mini-registry" and the larger population-based registry may emerge. Health Authorities may question whether a "two-tier" system of cancer registration is necessary and funding difficulties may arise. Thus the advent of the mini- and micro-computer in the hospital may cause population-based registries to re-examine their role and perhaps a return to the small-data-set, epidemiologically-orientated registry will occur. If data are supplied from other systems, this might result in relatively inexpensive registries with a major proportion of their costs being directed towards output and research rather than data creation. The growth of computing thus holds both threats and promises for population-based registries.

The greatest threat to cancer registration in the closing years of the century, however, comes as a direct result of the growth of the information industry in general. The computerisation of personal data has brought with it a growing concern for maintaining the confidentiality of such material. In many countries this has resulted in legislation which restricts access to personal data of all kinds. It is vital that health research is not impeded by the necessity to safeguard personal privacy from the activities of less altruistic consumers of data, but in some countries legislation has, perhaps unintentionally, made cancer registration virtually unworkable.

Thus, in its most recent phase of development, the computer has given cancer registration its greatest opportunity of increasing in efficiency, and the exploitation of its data has presented its greatest challenge. Potentially, in an indirect way, the computer has brought about the greatest threat to registries since they began.

CONCLUSION

On anything more than a very small scale, cancer registration without a computer is rather like microbiology with only a magnifying glass or surgery without anaesthetics. It is difficult to imagine how the early enthusiasm for cancer registration could have been maintained in the face of the problem of processing ever-expanding data mechanically. The writer has attempted to show how the growth of electronic data processing has led to the advancement of cancer information science.

Information systems depend fundamentally on the establishment and following of rules. In manual systems it is possible to operate with vague and incomplete rules, since arbitary decisions can be taken when required and, furthermore, such decisions need not necessarily be consistent. Because the computer has no intelligence of its own, the rules it is to follow must be complete and unambiguous. Once established, of course, the rules are followed without deviation. Thus the computerisation of cancer registration must concentrate the mind of those who have the responsibility for the design of such systems. It has often been remarked that cancer registration is not an exact science and, while it has to be accepted that the data will always be less than perfect, the use of computers should have done much to eliminate other sources of variability.

The general development of computing has resulted in the obvious threat with regard to confidentiality, but there is also another, more subtle, danger. The computer now makes it very easy to perform complex analyses which, until recently, would only be attempted by expert statisticians. In some areas technology has overtaken information science and because certain procedures *can* be done, they *will* be done, without a proper evaluation of the validity of the techniques with respect to the data being processed. Computers now put sharp statistical tools into both expert and inexpert hands; the perils are obvious.

While the computer has made the cancer registry what it is today, like so much of technology it has brought with it problems of its own which must not be ignored. As Thomas Carlyle also wrote: "The tools to him that can handle them."

MIGRANT STUDY

CANCER AMONG JAPANESE-AMERICANS
IN HAWAII

Grant N. Stemmermann,[*1] Abraham M. Y. Nomura,[*1]
and Laurence N. Kolonel[*2]

*The Japan-Hawaii Cancer Study, Kuakini Medical Center[*1]
and the Cancer Research Center of Hawaii[*2]*

The migration of Japanese to Hawaii has been followed by a change in the frequency of different cancers among them. Cancers of the esophagus, stomach, bile duct, and uterine cervix have decreased relative to the native Japanese experience; while cancers of the colon, rectum, breast, endometrium, ovary, urinary bladder, and reticuloendothelial system have increased. The incidence of some tumors in Hawaii Japanese is intermediate between U.S. white and native Japanese rates, while the incidence of others now exceeds U.S. white rates (colon, rectum, leukemia). Hawaii Tumor Registry data indicate that over the past 20 years different tumors have followed different trends, with colon cancer in men showing the greatest increase, and gastric cancer the greatest decrease. This report gives the details of these changes and highlights the results of some recent epidemiologic studies that the Japanese migration to Hawaii has generated.

Migration of the Japanese to Hawaii has been followed by changes in their cancer risks. The extent of these changes has been recorded in "Cancer in Five Continents" (*32*), as shown in Table I. In comparing the Japanese in Hawaii with their counterparts in Japan, cancers of the esophagus, stomach, and biliary tree have decreased in incidence in Hawaii, while cancers of the large bowel, liver, lung, breast, uterine corpus, prostate, urinary bladder, and reticuloendothelial system have increased in incidence. For many tumors (*viz.*, stomach, breast), the Hawaii Japanese risk is intermediate between the risk experienced by U.S. whites and Japanese in Japan. In contrast, the Hawaii Japanese risk of developing liver and colorectal cancer exceeds that of the U.S. white.

The sources of data for the comparisons in Table I are the Miyagi and Hawaii Cancer Registries. Since the Hawaii data are population-based and obtained from a single geographic area where both whites and Japanese receive their medical care from the same institutions, it is believed that their cancer rates represent an unbiased picture of the differences in cancer risk between these ethnic groups. Although comparisons between Miyagi and Hawaii are based on the unproven assumption that the two population groups are similar in the completeness of cancer surveillance, in the criteria used to determine malignancy and in medical care practices, it is unlikely that procedural variations could account for the 3-fold differences in rates that have been observed for esophageal, stomach, and colon cancer.

[*1] Honolulu, Hawaii 96817, U.S.A.
[*2] Honolulu, Hawaii 96813, U.S.A.

TABLE I. Post Migrational Changes in Japanese Cancer Incidence

Cancer site	Age-adjusted[a] rates									
	Male					Female				
	JJ[b]	HJ[b]	HW[b]	HJ: JJ	HJ: HW	JJ	HJ	HW	HJ: JJ	HJ: HW
Esophagus	13.8	4.5	2.4	0.32	1.8	3.2	0.6	1.9	0.18	0.3
Stomach	88.0	34.0	12.2	0.38	2.8	42.0	15.1	5.0	0.34	3.0
Colon	8.3	27.5	25.3	3.3	1.1	7.3	18.8	17.8	2.6	1.1
Rectum	9.2	21.4	14.1	2.3	1.5	6.5	8.8	8.9	1.35	1.0
Liver	2.5	5.7	2.7	2.2	2.1	0.9	2.2	1.4	2.4	1.6
Pancreas	7.4	8.6	8.6	1.2	1.0	4.2	4.5	6.5	1.1	0.7
Biliary tree	5.9	4.3	2.1	0.7	2.0	5.5	3.9	2.2	0.7	1.8
Lung	25.5	38.3	64.2	1.5	0.6	7.5	11.5	23.2	1.5	0.5
Breast	0.1	0.5	1.0	5.0	0.5	17.5	47.5	85.6	2.7	0.6
Uterine cervix	—	—	—	—	—	12.1	6.4	9.3	0.5	0.7
Uterine corpus	—	—	—	—	—	2.0	19.4	34.8	9.7	0.6
Ovary	—	—	—	—	—	3.4	7.0	9.4	2.1	0.7
Testes	0.8	1.0	5.0	1.25	0.2	—	—	—	—	—
Prostate	4.9	35.9	59.7	7.3	0.6	—	—	—	—	—
Urinary bladder	5.3	9.9	23.5	1.9	0.4	1.6	3.4	3.9	2.1	0.9
Hodgkin's	0.5	1.3	2.0	2.6	0.5	0.2	1.0	2.5	5.0	0.2
Lymphosarcoma[c]	2.8	5.7	6.3	2.0	0.9	1.5	5.1	7.5	3.4	0.7
Myeloma	1.1	1.3	2.0	1.2	0.7	0.7	1.0	2.5	1.4	0.4
Granulocytic leukemia	2.6	5.0	4.3	1.9	1.2	1.9	2.8	2.9	1.5	1.0

[a] Age-adjusted to world population.
[b] JJ, Japanese in Miyagi, Japan; HJ, Japanese in Hawaii; HW, whites in Hawaii.
[c] Combined lymphosarcoma and lymphocytic leukemia.

The assumption is also made that the Hawaii Japanese would have experienced the prevailing rates in Miyagi Prefecture if they had lived in Japan. Since the Japanese in Hawaii migrated primarily from seven different prefectures in Japan, an earlier study was done which took into account the prefecture-of-origin of the migrant Japanese in comparing their site-specific cancer mortality rates with people in Japan (27). One of the observations from the study is that the comparison of the 1960–1964 cancer incidence rates between Miyagi and Hawaii reflected reasonably well the comparison of the 1960 cancer mortality rates between the Japanese in Hawaii and Japan after standardizing for the prefecture-of-origin of the Hawaii Japanese.

This report will summarize recent trends (1962–1981) of major cancers in the Hawaii Japanese population. The Hawaii Cancer Registry began in 1960. As a consequence, it is possible that there was some under ascertainment of cancer cases during the early years of the Registry. In this regard, the 1962–1965 rates in this report may be lower than they should be. However, by 1967 case ascertainment throughout the state was almost entirely complete (14). Since then, few cases (less than 1%) are identified only by death certificate and more than 94% of cases overall are histologically confirmed. On this basis, time trend patterns from 1966 to 1981 should be more reliable than the earlier period. In addition to the trends, this report will present, in capsule form, a summary of the epidemiologic data that are pertinent to the Hawaii Japanese cancer experience.

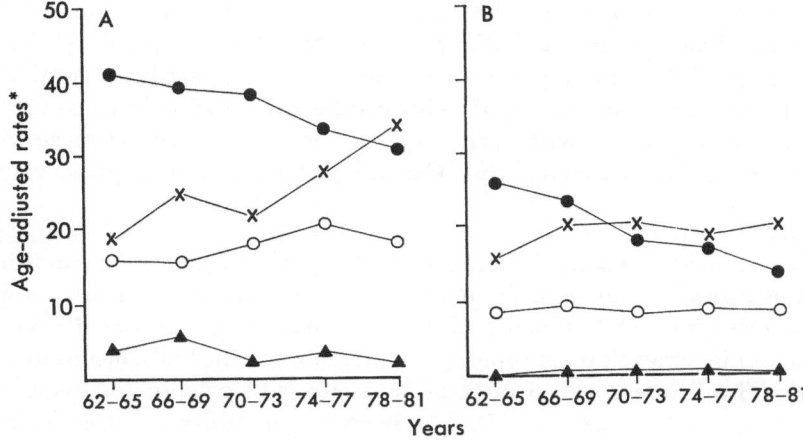

Fig. 1. Trends, gastrointestinal cancer, Hawaii Japanese, 1962–1981
A: male. B: female. ● stomach; × colon; ○ rectum; ▲ esophagus. * age adjusted
to Hawaii population, all races.

Gastrointestinal Tract

1. Trends, 1962–1981

The recent trends in cancer risk in the esophagus, stomach, colon, and rectum are shown in Fig. 1. The steady decline in gastric cancer has affected both sexes in equal degree. A rise in colon cancer has also been noted for both sexes, but this rise is steeper for men. Age specific trends indicate that the increase in male colon cancer is greatest among men over 60 years of age, whereas the increase in female risk is confined to women over 70 years of age. Recent trends for rectal cancer have been fairly stable for both sexes. Esophageal cancer continues to decline among Hawaii Japanese men, and is almost nonexistent among Hawaii Japanese women.

2. Epidemiology
1) Esophagus

Cigarette smoking and heavy alcohol use have been associated with esophageal cancer in the U.S.A. (2, 13, 28, 34). There is indirect evidence that this holds true for Hawaii since the races with the highest use of cigarettes and alcohol (Hawaiians and Caucasians) have the highest rates of this tumor (13). A prospective study of two age matched cohorts of men in Hiroshima and Honolulu (the NiHonSan study) indicates that Hawaii Japanese men consume less alcohol than native Japanese men (12). There is also a smaller proportion of current cigarette smokers among the men in Hawaii, although more of them are heavy smokers (more than one pack a day).

2) Stomach

Diets high in the intake of pickled vegetables and dried/salted fish, and low in the intake of raw vegetables have been linked to increased risk of gastric cancer (6). A similar diet favors development of atrophic gastritis and intestinal metaplasia of the pyloric antrum (4, 25). The high pH of the stomach that accompanies atrophic gastritis also favors nitrosation of dietary amines, producing endogenous mutagens (19) that resemble nitroso compounds known to be carcinogenic in the experimental animal (*18*). The 5-year relative survival rates in the SEER program range from a low of 7% for American Indians to a high of 27% for Japanese (*35*); and, in Hawaii, Japanese survival with this tumor is twice that of Caucasians (*33*). This can be attributed only in part to the larger percent of Japanese patients with early stage tumors (*13*), since Japanese with stage 1 and 2 cancers show better survival than Caucasians with cancers at these stages (*35*).

3) *Large bowel*

Colonic and rectal cancers differ in respect to epidemiologic associations in prospective studies of Hawaii Japanese. Colonic tumors are associated with a low fat intake (*30*), low serum cholesterol (*31*), but increased weight gain after age 25 (*23*). Rectal tumors are associated with higher levels of fat intake (*30*) and increased alcohol consumption, especially beer (*26*). The 5-year survival rates of Japanese with colonic and rectal cancer are higher than those of U.S. whites (*35*). The basis for the difference has not been established.

Tumors of the Liver, Pancreas and Extrahepatic Biliary Tree

1. *Trends*

The age adjusted mean incidence rates of cancers at these sites for the years 1962–1981 are shown in Fig. 2. The stability of the rates of pancreatic cancer in this population suggests that Hawaii Japanese do not share in the reported increase in frequency of this cancer among U.S. whites. Biliary tract cancer appears to be decreasing in both sexes, while hepatoma rates are fairly stable.

2. *Epidemiology*
1) *Liver*

Prospective studies show that hepatitis B infection is strongly tied to the development of hepatoma among Hawaii Japanese (*24*) as it is among Taiwanese (*3*).

2) *Pancreas*

There is no direct or indirect evidence that links any epidemiologic variable with

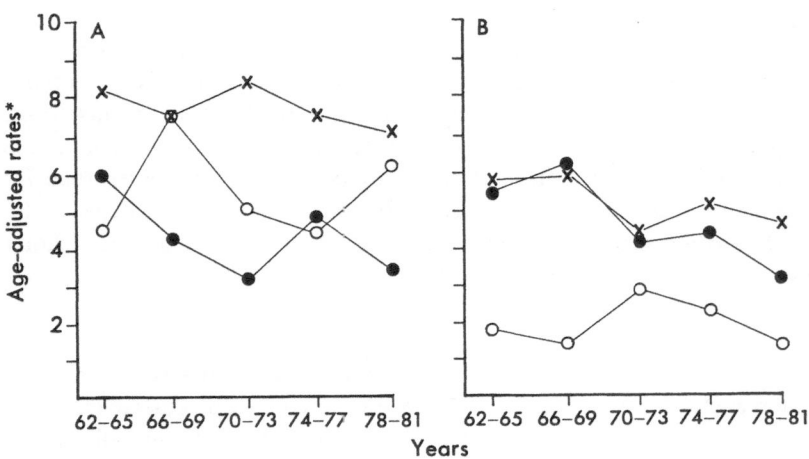

FIG. 2. Trends, cancer of the liver, biliary tree and pancreas, 1962–1981
A: male. B: female. ● biliary tree; × pancreas; ○ liver.

pancreatic cancer in the Hawaii Japanese. Studies regarding this cancer are being planned in the future.

3) Biliary tract cancer

Although tumors of the extrahepatic biliary tree are decreasing in frequency among Hawaii Japanese, their risk for this tumor is still much higher than it is for other races in Hawaii. As in other races, women predominate over men for gallbladder cancer, while bile duct cancer is more frequently found in males, especially elderly males. Although gallstones are a more common cause of hospitalization for other ethnic groups than the Japanese in Hawaii, the Hawaii Japanese experience a higher rate of cancer of the gall-bladder (5, 11).

Cancer of the Lung

1. Trends

Lung cancer rates have increased more in Japanese men than in women in Hawaii between the years 1962–1981, but in the last 4 years the rates have stabilized in both sexes (Fig. 3).

2. Epidemiology

Japanese women experience the lowest lung cancer rates among any of the races in Hawaii, while Japanese men rank third in this category, after Caucasians and Hawaiians (7). A state survey of cigarette use failed to show a correspondence with the rank order of lung cancer in the different races in Hawaii (13). This suggests that other factors might affect lung cancer risk. The results of four studies support this hypothesis. The rank order of alcohol use corresponds with the lung cancer incidence among Hawaiians, Caucasians, and Japanese (13), and a prospective study of Japanese men indicates that alcohol intake may be related to lung cancer risk (26). A study of women in Hawaii indicates that Japanese and Chinese women are more likely to be nonsmokers than other races, and are more liekly to develop adenocarcinoma of the lung than epidermoid or small cell carcinoma (8). A case-control study of lung cancer among Japanese and other ethnic groups in Hawaii showed an inverse relationship to vitamin A, particularly ca-

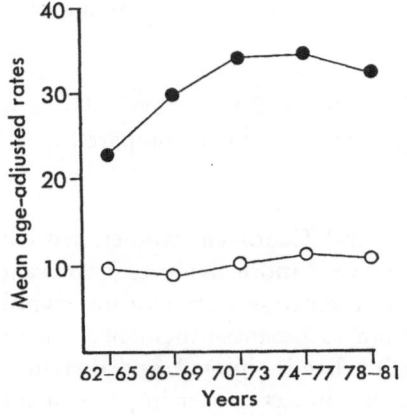

FIG. 3.   Lung cancer trends, Hawaii Japanese.
● male; ○ female.

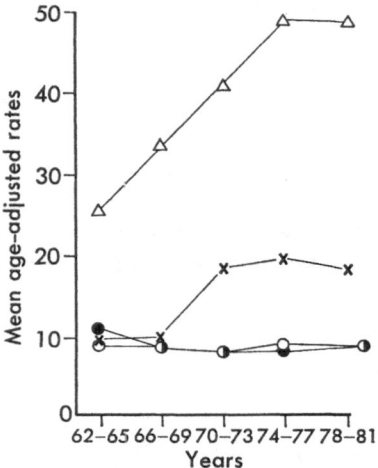

FIG. 4.   Time trends, breast, uterus, ovary cancer, Hawaii Japanese
△ breast; × uterine corpus; ○ ovary; ● uterine cervix.

rotene consumption (10). Lastly, the serum β-carotene level in Hawaii Japanese men is inversely related to lung cancer risk at every level of cigarette consumption (22). It remains to be determined whether β-carotene is protective against lung cancer or whether cigarette consumption actually lowers the serum level of this substance.

Cancer of the Breast and Female Reproductive System

1.   Recent trends

There has been a steep rise in the frequency of breast cancer in the 20 years from 1962 through 1981 (Fig. 4). During the same period cancer of the endometrum has shown a moderate increase, ovarian cancer has been fairly stable and cancer of the uterine cervix has shown a small decrease. In the case of breast cancer, all age groups above age 29 have participated in the increase although the sharpest rise has been noted in the age groups between 50 and 69 (Fig. 5A). The increase in the risk of endometrial cancer appears to have been limited to the ages between 50 and 69 (Fig. 5B).

2.   Epidemiology

A wide disparity in the relative 5-year survival has been demonstrated between Japanese in the U.S.A. (85% survivors) when compared to all other races (whites, 73%; blacks, 61%) (35).

1)   Breast

Comparison of Japanese and Caucasian women with breast cancer in Hawaii indicates that Japanese women were more likely to have cancer at an earlier stage than Caucasian women (9). This difference was statistically significant only after age 55. The age specific ratios of Caucasian to Japanese incidence rates were least for *in situ* cancer and successively greater for localized, regional, and distant breast cancer. These results were interpreted to indicate that breast cancer in post-menopausal Japanese women had slower growth rates than in Caucasian women. Pathology studies of breast cancer in the two races indicate that Japanese women are more likely to show increased lymphocytic

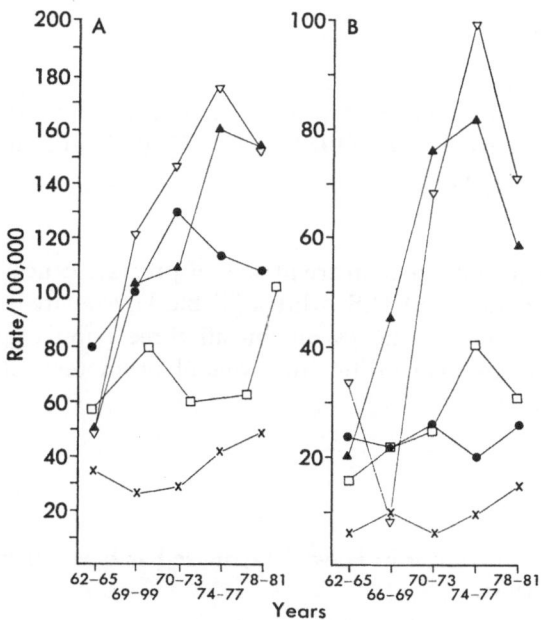

FIG. 5. Age specific cancer trends, Hawaii Japanese
× 30–39; ● 40–49; ▲ 50–59; △ 60–69; □ 70+.
A: breast. B: endometrium.

infiltration of mammary tumors, more extensive sinus histiocytosis and less frequent lymph node metastasis (29). Comparative survival studies of Caucasian and Japanese women in Hawaii at 5 years (16) and 10 years (17) indicate that the survival advantage of Japanese over Caucasian women is not retained after adjustment for stage at diagnosis. Second generation Japanese women had better survival than Issei women, even after adjusting for stage. This suggests that westernization and genetic constitution do not explain the overall or stage adjusted breast survival patterns.

2) *Carcinoma, uterine corpus* (endometrium)

Hawaii Japanese women rank fourth in their risk of endometrial cancer, after Caucasians, Hawaiians, and Chinese (7), but experience the same survival rates with this cancer as U.S. whites (35). No epidemiologic studies of this cancer have yet been conducted among the Hawaii Japanese.

3) *Carcinoma of the ovary*

A comparison of the histologic types of ovarian cancer among Japanese and Caucasian women in Hawaii indicates a similar distribution of subtypes in each race, with epithelial carcinomas constituting over 90% of the tumors in each race (20). This differs from the distribution of histologic subtypes of ovarian cancers in Miyagi, Japan, where 79% of these tumors are epithelial in type (27). In contrast, germ cell tumors constitute only 3.5% of Hawaii cases but 19% of the Miyagi cases. Because the incidence rates of ovarian cancer are higher among the Japanese in Hawaii than in Miyagi, it would appear, then, that the post migration increase in the frequency of ovarian tumors among Hawaii Japanese women is due to an increase in the frequency of epithelial tumors. Although the numbers are small, there may have been a post migrational decrease in the frequency of germ cell malignancies among the Japanese in Hawaii.

Tumors of the Prostate

1. Recent Trends

Comparison of the frequency of prostate cancer prior to autopsy among Hawaii Japanese between the periods 1968–1972 and 1973–1977 indicates that this tumor is fairly stable in this population (*7*).

2. Epidemiology

In spite of the great difference in frequency of prostate cancer as a clinical problem in Japan, Hawaiian Japanese and U.S. whites (Table I), the latent form of this tumor is found with about the same frequency among all three populations (*1*). This suggests that these populations experience different levels of promoters rather than initiators of this tumor.

Urinary Bladder

1. Recent trends

The frequency of this tumor in Hawaii Japanese has been fairly stable for both sexes over the period 1962–1981.

2. Epidemiology

Japanese men rank second among the five major races in Hawaii in the incidence of urothelial cancer, but Japanese women rank fifth for this tumor (*13*). A preliminary report of a case-control study being conducted in Hawaii weakly suggests that urothelial cancer cases consume less vitamin A than their controls (*15*).

Reticuloendothelial System

1. Recent trends

The frequency of tumors of this system has been stable over the period 1962–1981 for Hawaii Japanese. There are too few cases of the subtypes of tumors in this category to assess trends for lymphosarcoma, Hodgkin's disease, myeloma, and leukemia individually.

2. Epidemiology

There are no studies that explain the increased frequency of each of the tumors of the reticuloendothelial system among Hawaii Japanese as compared to native Japanese.

Acknowledgment

This work was supported by Grants Nos. R01 CA33644 and 1-P01 CA33619, and Contract Nos. N01 CN55424 and N01 CA15655, awarded by the National Cancer Institute, DHHS.

REFERENCES

1. Akazaki, K. and Stemmermann, G. N. Comparative study of latent carcinoma of the prostate among Japanese in Japan and Hawaii. *J. Natl. Cancer Inst.*, **50**, 1137–1144 (1973).
2. Auerbach, O., Stout, A. P., Hammond, C., and Garfinkel, L. Histologic changes in esophagus in relation to smoking habits. *Arch. Environ. Health*, **11**, 4–15 (1965).

3. Beasley, R., Lin, C.-C., Wang, L.S.Y., and Chien, C.-S. Hepatocellular carcinoma and hepatitis B virus—a prospective study of 22,707 men in Taiwan. *Lancet*, **ii**, 1129–1132 (1981).

4. Correa, P., Cuello, C., Fajardo, F., Haenszel, W., Bolanos, O., and de Ramirez, B. Diet and gastric cancer. Nutrition survey in a high risk area. *J. Natl. Cancer Inst.*, **70**, 673–678 (1983).

5. Glober, G. and Stemmermann, G. Hawaii ethnic groups. *In* "Western Diseases: Their Emergence and Prevention," eds. H. C. Trowell and D. P. Burkitt, pp. 319–333 (1981). Edward Arnold, London.

6. Haenszel, W., Kurihara, M., Segi, M., and Lee, R.K.C. Stomach cancer among Japanese in Hawaii. *J. Natl. Cancer Inst.*, **49**, 969–988 (1972).

7. Hinds, M. W., Kolonel, L. N., Nomura, A.M.Y., Burch, T., and Rellahan, W. 1973–77 Cancer incidence in Hawaii with special reference to trends since 1968–72 for certain sites. *Haw. Med. J.*, **40**, 7–11 (1981).

8. Hinds, M. W., Stemmermann, G. N., Yang, H. Y., Kolonel, L., Lee, J., and Wegner, E. Differences in lung cancer risk from smoking among Japanese, Chinese and Hawaiian women in Hawaii. *Int. J. Cancer*, **27**, 297–302 (1981).

9. Hinds, M. W., Kolonel, L., Nomura, A.M.Y., and Lee, J. Stage specific breast cancer incidence. *Br. J. Cancer*, **45**, 118–123 (1982).

10. Hinds, M. W., Kolonel, L. N., Hankin, J. H., and Lee, J. Dietary vitamin A, carotene, vitamin C, and risk of lung cancer in Hawaii. *Am. J. Epidemiol.*, **119**, 227–236 (1984).

11. Inouye, A. and Whelan, T. J., Jr. Carcinoma of the extra hepatic bile ducts. *Ann. J. Surg.*, **136**, 90–94 (1978).

12. Kagan, A., Harris, B. R., Winkelstein, W., Johnson, K., Kato, H., Syme, S. L., Rhoads, G. G., Gay, M. L., Nichaman, M. Z., Hamilton, H. B., and Tillotson, J. Epidemiologic studies of coronary heart disease and stroke in Japanese men living in Japan, Hawaii and California: demographic, dietary and biochemical characteristics. *J. Chron. Dis.*, **7**, 345–364 (1974).

13. Kolonel, L. Smoking and drinking patterns among different ethnic groups in Hawaii. *Natl. Cancer Inst. Monogr.*, **53**, 81–87 (1979).

14. Kolonel, L. N. Cancer patterns of four ethnic groups in Hawaii. *J. Natl. Cancer Inst.*, **65**, 1127–1139 (1980).

15. Kolonel, L. N., Nomura, A.M.Y., Hinds, M. W., Hirohata, T., Hankin, J. H., and Lee, J. Role of diet in cancer incidence in Hawaii. *Cancer Res.*, **43**, 2397s–2402s (1983).

16. LeMarchand, L., Kolonel, L. N., and Nomura, A. Relationship of ethnicity and other prognostic factors to breast cancer survival patterns in Hawaii. *J. Natl. Cancer Inst.*, **73** 1259–1265 (1984).

17. LeMarchand, L., Kolonel, L. N., and Nomura, A. Breast cancer survival among Japanese and Caucasian women. *Am. J. Epidemiol.*, **122**, 571–578 (1985).

18. Matsukura, N., Kawachi, T., Sugimura, T., Nakadate, M., and Hirota, T. Induction of intestinal metaplasia and carcinoma in the glandular stomach of rats by N-alkyl-N'-nitro-nitrosamine. *Gann*, **70**, 181–185 (1979).

19. Mirvish, S. S. The etiology of gastric cancer. *J. Natl. Cancer Inst.*, **71**, 631–647 (1983).

20. Nathan, P., Navin, J., Stemmermann, G., and Rellahan, W. Ovarian cancer in Japanese women in Hawaii. *In* "An International Survey of Distributions of Histologic Types of Tumours of the Testis and Ovary," ed. H. Stalsberg, pp. 243–246 (1983). UICC Technical Report Series 75, Geneva.

21. Nomura, A. and Hirohata, T. Cancer mortality among Japanese in Hawaii. *Haw. Med. J.*, **35**, 293–297 (1976).

22. Nomura, A.M.Y. Serum vitamin levels and the risk of cancer of specific sites in men of Japanese ancestry in Hawaii. *Cancer Res.*, **45**, 2369–2372 (1985).

23. Nomura, A.M.Y., Heilbrun, L. K., and Stemmermann, G. N. Body mass index as a predictor of cancer in men. *J. Natl. Cancer Inst.*, **74**, 319–323 (1985).

24. Nomura, A., Stemmermann, G. N., and Wasnich, R. D. Presence of hepatitis B surface antigen before primary hepatocellular carcinoma. *JAMA*, **247**, 2247–2249 (1982).

25. Nomura, A., Yamakawa, H., Ishidate, T., Kamiyama, S., Masuda, H., Stemmermann, G., Heilbrun, L. K., and Hankin, J. Intestinal metaplasia in Japan: association with diet. *J. Natl. Cancer Inst.*, **68**, 401–405 (1982).

26. Pollack, E., Nomura, A., Heilbrun, L., and Stemmermann, G. Prospective study of alcohol consumption and cancer. *N. Engl. J. Med.*, **310**, 617–621 (1984).

27. Sasano, N., Tateno, H., Takano, A., and Okuno, Y. Ovarian cancers in Miyagi Prefecture, Japan. *In* "An International Survey of Distributions of Histologic Types of Tumours of the Testis and Ovary," ed. H. Stalsberg, pp. 193–198 (1983). UICC Technical Report Series 75, Geneva.

28. Schoenberg, B. C., Bailor, J. C., and Fraumeni, J. F. Certain mortality patterns of esophageal cancer in the United States. 1930–1967. *J. Natl. Cancer Inst.*, **46**, 63–73 (1970).

29. Stemmermann, G., Catts, A., Fukunaga, F., Horie, A., and Nomura, A.M.Y. Breast cancer in women of Japanese and Caucasian ancestry in Hawaii. *Cancer*, **56**, 206–209 (1985).

30. Stemmermann, G. N., Nomura, A.M.Y., and Heilbrun, L. K. Dietary fat and the risk of colorectal cancer. *Cancer Res.*, **44**, 4633–4637 (1984).

31. Stemmermann, G. N., Nomura, A.M.Y., Heilbrun, L. K., Pollack, E. S., and Kagan, A. Serum cholesterol and colon cancer incidence in Hawaii Japanese men. *J. Natl. Cancer Inst.*, **67**, 1179–1182 (1981).

32. Waterhouse, J., Muir, C., Shanmugaratnam, K., and Powell, J. Cancer in Five Continents, Vol. IV (1982). IARC, Lyon.

33. Wronkowski, Z., Stemmermann, G., and Rellahan, W. Stomach carcinoma among Caucasians and Hawaiians in Hawaii. *Cancer*, **39**, 2310–2316 (1977).

34. Wynder, E. L. and Brosa, I. J. A study of etiologic factors in cancer of the esophagus. *Cancer*, **14**, 389–913 (1961).

35. Young, J. L., Ries, L. G., and Pollack, E. Cancer patient survival among ethnic groups in the United States. *J. Natl. Cancer Inst.*, **73**, 341–352 (1984).

Gann Monograph on Cancer Research 33, 1987

CANCER MORTALITY AMONG POLISH MIGRANTS

Jerzy Staszewski

*Institute of Oncology**

The results of studies of cancer mortality among Polish-born migrants to the United States, Australia, and England and Wales, and in their countries of birth and of adoption are discussed and compared with similar studies of migrants from other European countries and Japan to the United States. Polish migrants offer unusually attractive opportunities for epidemiologic studies as Poland has distinctive cancer patterns (*e.g.*, high stomach and low intestinal tract, breast and prostate cancer risk). Among the 12 major white foreign-born groups in the United States, the Polish-born displayed the highest mortality from cancers of the esophagus, stomach, larynx, and lung, but also fairly high mortality from cancers of the intestinal tract, breast, and prostate. Direction and timing of the shifts in migrants' site-specific cancer risks may shed new light on cancer etiopathogenesis.

In comparison with other countries (*10, 11, 13*), Poland is characterized by a low, but increasing risk of cancer of the intestinal tract, breast, corpus uteri, ovary, and prostate. The risk of cancer of the stomach and of the uterine cervix in Poland is high, and only in recent years has shown some decline. (Similarity of cancer occurrence in Poland and Japan is noticeable—surprising in view of great differences between the two countries in so many respects).

The contrasts in risks between the United States and Poland have been more marked than those provided by other European countries. Further, Polish migrants have constituted one of the largest migrant groups in the United States. They also displayed the highest mortality from cancer at all sites, and from cancers of the esophagus, stomach, larynx, and lung among the 12 major white foreign-born groups in the United States in 1950 (*4*). To exploit those adventages, studies have been initiated to explore the site-specific displacements in cancer risks from those recorded in home and host countries.

Cancer mortality among the Polish-born in the United States in 1950 and in 1959–1961 has been compared with the experience reported for Poland and United States natives (*12–14*). Similar studies have been carried out for Polish-born migrants in Australia, 1962–1966 (*13, 15*), and in England and Wales, 1970–1972 (*1*).

The results of these studies will be compared with the mortality among migrants to the United States from six other European countries, 1950 (*4*), and from Japan, 1959–1962 (*7*). For the latter, data have been presented both for Japanese-born Issei and for second generation of migrants, Nisei.

More detailed data, such as age-specific rates, can be found in references given above, particularly in ref. *13*, while the basic data for the Polish-born and the native (for the United States) and total (for Australia, England and Wales) populations of the three

---

* 44-100 Gliwice, Poland.

TABLE I. Age-standarized Mortality Rates for Selected Cancer Sites in the United States, 1950 and 1959–1961, Australia, 1962–1966, and England and Wales, 1970–1972, and in Polish-born Migrants, Expressed as Ratios of the Rates for Poland in the Similar Period Taken as 100.0

ICD, 1955 rev.	Site	Sex	U.S.A., 1950 Polish-born	U.S.A., 1959–1961[a]		Australia, 1962–1966[b,c]		England and Wales 1970–1972[b,d]	
				Native white Americans	Polish-born	All	Polish-born	All	Polish-born
150	Esophagus	M	255 (131)	74	145 (332)	—	— (5)	101	132 (31)
151	Stomach	M	95 (413)	26	59 (1,085)	31	58 (54)	53	64 (125)
		F	90 (176)	27	67 (634)	32	96 (21)	55	57 (27)
152–154	Intestinal tract	M	490 (284)	376	482 (1,344)	222	124 (19)	213	140 (66)
		F	551 (216)	420	529 (1,078)	207	205 (17)	212	175 (38)
161	Larynx	M	212 (48)	118	171 (161)	—	— (2)	—	— (5)
162–163	Lung	M	212 (434)	183	241 (1,909)	127	104 (65)	185	114 (232)
		F	145 (54)	133	209 (252)	—	— (9)	250	209 (32)
170	Breast	F	320 (167)	368	331 (655)	153	153 (28)	225	218 (66)
177	Prostate	M	312 (125)	397	329 (648)	—	— (7)	122	92 (29)

Standard—"world" population (3). Number of deaths in parenthesis: rates not given when number of deaths of Polish-born is below 10.

a Mortality rates for Poland in 1959–1961 were taken as 100.0.

b Rates truncated for ages 40–79.

c Mortality rates for Poland, 1964–1965, were taken as 100.0.

d Mortality rates for Poland, 1971, were taken as 100.0.

host countries are presented in Table I as ratios of age-adjusted cancer mortality rates by site and sex. (Ratios for U.S. native whites are not shown for 1950 because they were not available when this paper was prepared). These ratios were calculated in the following manner: age-standardized mortality rates were calculated using Segi's "world" population as modified by Doll and Cook (3) as the standard; only for migrants in Australia was indirect standardization used (15). (For Australia and England and Wales [all and Polish-born] and the corresponding rates for Poland, age groups below 40, and 80 and over were omitted: the first contained almost no cancer deaths in migrants, and the last was prone to frequent underreporting). Then, the rates for Poland were taken as 100.0 and the rates for the Polish-born and their host countries for the same sex and similar time period were expressed as ratios thereof. (For the Polish-born in the United States for 1950, the rates for Poland in 1959–1961 instead of 1950 were used, because site-specific cancer mortality rates are not available for Poland for the years before 1959).

Comparative interpretation of the data presented is difficult because they cover different time periods while cancer risks change with time. But even when comparisons of cancer risks among migrants with the risks in their country of birth and their country of adoption are limited to the same time period, the problem remains that the risks are not uniform among three compared populations, and that migrants are not a random sample of the population of their country of birth. The selective factors of economic, political, and other influences that determine the composition of migrants are difficult to define, and their effects are difficult to quantify. But knowing them is of great significance. For instance, in studies of cancer mortality among foreign-born whites in the United States, the relatively low stomach cancer mortality among migrants from Italy may be related to a high proportion of them coming from the southern part of Italy where the stomach cancer risk is distinctly lower than in northern Italy. The origin from the rural areas of Poland of most of the Polish migrants to the United States probably has some bearing on their extremeely high mortality from cancer of the lung, larynx and esophagus.

Composition of migrant populations may vary with time as well as with host country. For example, the just mentioned preponderance of migrants from rural areas, which moved mainly for economic motives, pertains only to the so called "old migration" from Poland to the United States before about 1924. The "new migration," which left Poland mainly because of the Second World War, is quite different. These migrants of the United States, and also to England and Australia (where, in contrast to the United States, the largest majority of Polish migrants), are more often from the urban areas of Poland, better educated and from higher socio-economic classes. That indicates that analyses of time trends in cancer risks among migrants may be further complicated by changes in their composition, and by changes in their origin. But not only comparisons of migrants with perople who remained in their country of birth may be difficult. Also, the area of the country of adoption, and the population stratum in which these migrants settle, may display distinctive cancer risks. For example, mortality rates for cancer of the intestinal tract were higher by some 20% for Polish-born Americans than for native Americans. But the rates for the natives are higher in the northeastern states than in the other regions of the United States, and the increased mortality among Polish migrants can be attributed to their concentration in these high risk states.

The following discussion of the selected major cancer sites follows the ICD (International Classification of Disease—Seventh Revision 1955, WHO) order but for esophageal cancer which is considered next to cancers of the larynx and lung because of some common features.

Stomach

Poland belongs to the countries with a high risk of stomach cancer, and the decrease in that risk first started in Poland probably after 1960. On the other hand, the risk in the United States has been decreasing since before 1930, and now is among the lowest in the world. In 1950, Polish-born migrants to the United States experienced about the same stomach cancer mortality as in Poland, and much higher than the mortality among native white Americans. Ten years later, mortality from stomach cancer among the U.S. native whites decreased some 30%, as it did among Polish migrants (slightly more for males). Also, among Polish migrants to Australia, another country with a low risk of stomach cancer, mortality from that cancer was intermediate, and for females much closer to the high rate reported for Poland than to the low mortality among the natives of Australia. The Australian study pertained to the period 1962–1966. On the other hand, stomach cancer mortality rates among Polish migrants to England and Wales in 1970–1972 appear to be closer to the rates in the host country than was observed in Australia and the United States, particularly in 1950. This may be due, at least partly, to the higher incidence of this cancer in England and Wales than in the other two host countries. Selective factors probably also have some bearing, migrants to the U.S. being more from the higher-risk groups (low socio-economic, rural). In all the three host countries the transition to their lower stomach cancer mortality rates was increasingly more pronounced with increasing age of the migrants.

Polish migrants to the U.S. demonstrate most clearly the pattern noticeable also in migrants to the U.S. from six other European countries for which data have been available (4), as well as from Japan (7) and in migrants within Colombia (2), suggesting that early exposures are critical in the etiology of stomach cancer. This has been subsequently corroborated by findings of the studies conducted in Colombia (2) that in high-risk populations the prevalence of chronic atrophic gastritis and intestinal metaplasia, believed to be precursors of stomach cancer, is also determined by events well before the age of 20.

Intestinal Tract

To decrease chance variation as well as the effects of possible differences in classification of borderline lesions (recto-sigmoid junction), no subdivision to more detailed sites has been made. This is also justified by the fact that for cancer of both colon and rectum Poland ranks low when compared with other countries (10, 11, 13); the colon/rectum ratio was 1.4: 1 in 1959–1961.

Epidemiology of this cancer differs from the epidemiology of stomach cancer. The risk of intestinal-tract cancer is low but increasing in Poland, and high in the United States. Mortality from intestinal-tract cancer among Polish-born Americans was much higher than in Poland, and even higher than among the U.S. native whites, both in 1950 and around 1960. It was similar to the mortality of the native in the Northeast and East North Central States, where mortality from intestinal-tract cancer is above the U.S. average, and where Polish migrants are concentrated. Intestinal-tract cancer mortality rates for Polish female migrants to Australia and to England and Wales also approached the high levels experienced by the native populations of these two countries, whereas for males the rates were intermediate between the high rates in these two host countries and the low rates in Poland. As the migrants to the United States originated more from rural areas of Poland, where the risk of intestinal-tract cancer was the lowest, one would expect their transition to the high risk to be, if anything, slower than for migrants to England and Wales and Australia, derived from higher risk groups. The incomplete transition observed for male migrants to these two countries is hard to explain; it may be partly an artefact due to chance variation, the male rate for migrants to Australia, for example, being based on only 19 deaths.

In the study of cancer mortality among foreign-born Americans in 1950 (4), out of the six other European countries of birth for which data are available, only Norway might confidently be said to experience substantially lower intestinal tract cancer mortality than the United States, even if not as low as in Poland. The findings for Polish and Norwegian migrants reinforce each other in demonstrating that rates for persons moving from low-risk areas tend to rise to the level prevailing at the new place of residence. Furthermore, a study of persons migrating within the United States demonstrated that intestinal tract cancer mortality conforms to the rates characteristic of the most recent residence and not of the place of birth (6).

The experience of Japanese migrants to the United States (7) seems consistent with other migrant populations, although quantitatively the Issei, and even Nisei, have not made as complete a transition from the low risk of intestinal tract cancer in their country of birth to the high risk in the United States, as did migrants from Norway and Poland within one generation.

The shifts in risk of stomach cancer, and of intestinal tract cancer, as observed in the same population of migrants, are going in opposite directions and are not synchronous. For intestinal tract cancer, the shift from the low risk prevailing in the country or region of birth to the high risk characteristic for the host population is completed usually in one generation, and apparently in a relatively short time. Recent events appear to be the important ones in the etiology of intestinal tract cancer, whereas the risk of stomach cancer is probably determined early in life.

Incidentally, Polish migrants display an exception to the general rule of a negative correlation of the risk of cancers of the stomach and of the intestinal tract. The risks of both these cancers are high among Polish-born Americans.

Adenomatous polyps are suspected to be the precursors of intestinal tract cancer. These polyps tend to appear later in life, at ages over 40 (5). This indirectly supports the conclusion from the migrant studies that relatively recent events determine the risk of intestinal tract cancer, whereas exposures early in life are important in the epidemiology of stomach cancer, for which the precursor lesion can appear as early as age 15.

Esophagus

Still another pattern of displacements in mortality for migrants, from the levels recorded in home and host countries, is observed for cancer of the esophagus. Mortality from this cancer among male migrants is frequently higher than in the country of birth as well as higher than in the host country. This has been more pronounced for Polish migrants to the United States than for migrants from the six other European countries (4). The difference in esophageal cancer mortality between U.S. native whites and native

Poles was not remarkable for either sex, whereas among Polish male migrants in 1950 the rates were about three times higher than in both of the two native population, and were about double 10 years later. During both periods, the excess mortality among polish migrants increased with age. The female migrants did not deviate from the mortality among natives.

The experience of Japanese migrants is similar (7). Among Issei males, mortality from cancer of the esophagus was higher than in either home and host population. Nisei rates were lower than the Issei rates and similar to mortality among U.S. native whites.

Larynx

Laryngeal cancer mortality among male Polish-born Americans followed the pattern described for esophageal cancer : it was much higher than among the natives of the United States and of Poland. The preponderance of Polish-born Americans was most marked for the age groups over 60, for laryngeal as well as for esophageal cancer. For other migrant groups, I could find no comparable data related to cancer of the larynx.

Lung

A similar patterns is seen for cancer of the lung in males, but only among some migrant groups, whereas the typical pattern for lung cancer among males, as observed in migrants of other European countries to the United States (4), is a displacement of mortality rates upward or downward to a position intermediate to the home and host countries. Polish male migrants ranked first among all ethnic groups in the United States in lung cancer mortality, as they did in esophageal and laryngeal cancer mortality. Their lung cancer mortality was much higher than in Poland, and was almost twice as high as among the native white Americans in 1950, and over 30% higher in 1959–1961. In this second period, the prepondernace of the migrant rates was limited to the older age groups, 65 and over. Likewise, only in the oldest age groups was the lung cancer mortality higher among Polish migrants to Australia and perhaps also to England and Wales, than among natives of these host countries. Also, among Japanese Americans (7) mortality from lung cancer was higher among Issei, especially age 65 and over, than among native white Americans. In the younger age groups it decreased with time, as among Polish migrants.

It is interesting to note that an increased risk of lung cancer, independent of smoking history, in migrants from rural farming to urban areas, has been described for the U.S. native whites (8, 9). As mentioned, most of the migrants who left Poland before the Second World War were born in rural farming areas and settled, particularly in the United States, in urban areas. Also, most of the Issei were born in rural farming areas of Japan and settled in American cities. Reduction in Nisei rates might represent the absence of special hazards to migrants from rural farming areas in that country.

The increased lung cancer risk in migrants from rural farming areas to the cities has recently been corroborated in another setting, in Poland. In a study of cancer incidence in Zabrze, an industrial city in the Katowice District, incidence of lung cancer among immigrants born in villages was higher than among immigrants born in towns, and similar to that of the natives of Zabrze City (16). The natives of that city have a very heavy and lifelong exposure to air pollutants originating from coal mines, foundries, cockeries, and other heavy industry.

Breast and Prostate

Mortality from cancer of the breast as well as of the prostate is low but increasing in Poland. In the 1950s it was almost as low as in Japan, amounting to about one-quarter of the rates for native white Americans. The increase in breast cancer mortality among polish migrants to the higher levels of the three host countries was virtually complete up to the age of about 55, but not quite as high in the older age groups. A similar incomplete transition in older groups was observed only among Italian and Japanese migrants but not among migrants from the other five European countries (England and Wales, Ireland, Norway, Sweden, and Germany). A similar shift in risk was noted for prostatic cancer, but comparisons are based on smaller numbers and less reliable data, as this cancer occurs mainly at an age when reliability of comparison of cancer statistics is at its lowest.

Final Remarks

There is an old, but still frequently recalled hypothesis that cancer incidence is the same in all populations, so that an increase in risk of one form of cancer in a population is compensated by a decrease in risk of some other cancer. The results of the study of Polish-born Americans are not compatible with that hypothesis: their great increase in risk of cancer of the lung and of the intestinal tract was not compensated by a decrease in risk of other cancers.

Review of cancer mortality among Polish migrants has revealed distinctive site-specific patterns (particularly in regard to direction and timing) of displacement in risk which are helpful in formulating and checking hypotheses on cancer etiopathogenesis.

REFERENCES

1. Adelstein, A. M., Staszewski, J., and Muir, C. S. Cancer mortality in 1970–1972 among Polish-born migrants to England and Wales. *Br. J. Cancer*, **40**, 464–475 (1979).
2. Correa, P., Haenszel, W., and Tannenbaum, S. Epidemiology of gastric carcinoma: review and future prospects. *Natl. Cancer Inst. Monogr.*, **62**, 129–134 (1982).
3. Doll, R. and Cook, P. Summarizing indices for comparison of cancer incidence data. *Int. J. Cancer*, **2**, 269 (1967).
4. Haenszel, W. Cancer mortality among the foreign-born in the United States. *J. Natl. Cancer Inst.*, **26**, 37–132 (1961).
5. Haenszel, W. and Correa, P. Cancer of the colon and rectum and adenomatous polyps. A review of epidemiologic findings. *Cancer*, **28**, 14–24 (1971).
6. Haenszel, W. and Dawson, E. A. A note on mortality from cancer of the colon and rectum in the United States. *Cancer*, **18**, 265–272 (1965).
7. Haenszel, W. and Kurihara, M. Studies of Japanese migrants. I. Mortality from cancer and other diseases among Japanese in the United States. *J. Natl. Cancer Inst.*, **40**, 43–68 (1968).
8. Haenszel, W., Loveland, D. B., and Sirken, M. G. Lung cancer mortality as related to

residence and smoking histories. I. White males. *J. Natl. Cancer Inst.*, **28**, 947–1001 (1962).

9. Haenszel, W. and Taeuber, K. E. Lung cancer mortality as related to residence and smoking histories. II. White females. *J. Natl. Cancer Inst.*, **32**, 803–838 (1964).

10. Segi, M. and Kurihara, M. "Cancer Mortality for Selected Sites in 24 Countries," No. 4 (1962–1963) (1966). Department of Public Health, Tohoku University School of Medicine, Sendai.

11. Segi, M., Kurihara, M., and Matsuyama, T. "Cancer Mortality for Selected Sites in 24 Countries," No. 5 (1964–1965) (1970). Department of Public Health, Tohoku University School of Medicine, Sendai.

12. Staszewski, J. Cancer of the upper alimentary tract and larynx in Poland and in Polish-born Americans. *Br. J. Cancer*, **29**, 389–399 (1974).

13. Staszewski, J. "Epidemiology of Cancer of Selected Sites in Poland and Polish Migrants" (1976). Ballinger Pub. Co., Cambridge.

14. Staszewski, J. and Haenszel, W. Cancer mortality among the Polish-born in the United States. *J. Natl. Cancer Inst.*, **35**, 291–297 (1965).

15. Staszewski, J., McCall, M., and Stenhous, N. S. Cancer mortality in 1962–1966 among Polish migrants to Australia. *Br. J. Cancer*, **25**, 599–610 (1971).

16. Zemla, B. Pulmonary carcinoma in a population of immigrants. *Pol. Tyg. Lak.*, **XXXV**, 17, 597–600 (1981) (in Polish).

CANCER PATTERNS AMONG KOREANS IN JAPAN

Akira Oshima,[*1] Takashi Ubukata,[*2]
and Isaburo Fujimoto[*3]

*Section of Cancer Epidemiology, Research Institute of the Center for Adult Diseases,[*1] Department of Epidemiology and Mass Examination for Stomach Cancer,[*2] and Department of Field Research, Center for Adult Diseases[*3]*

Cancer patterns among Koreans living in Japan were analyzed using cancer mortality and/or incidence data for Osaka and Japan. The following points were elucidated: 1) compared with Japanese males, Korean males had significantly higher mortality rates from cancers of the esophagus, liver, and lung. In Korean females liver cancer was more frequent and breast cancer was less frequent than in Japanese females; 2) among Korean males, stomach cancer mortality rate seems to have been decreasing more rapidly than it has in Japanese males; 3) the most prominent feature in cancer patterns for Koreans in Japan is the much higher rate of liver cancer. Hepatitis B virus and alcohol were suggested to be involved in this Korean-Japanese difference.

According to the 1980 census of Japan, about 600,000 Koreans who retain their Korean nationality live in Japan. In all almost all cases, they themselves, their parents or their grandparents migrated to Japan before or during World War II. In the background of their migration there is the unhappy history that Korea had been annexed to Japan during the 1910–1945 period.

In 1965 Hirayama *et al.* analyzed various demographic data for foreigners in Japan and showed that stomach cancer mortality rates were higher among Koreans in Japan than those among Japanese during the 1955–1963 period (*1*). In 1981 Song showed that mortality rates from liver cirrhosis and liver cancer were much higher among Koreans in Osaka, Japan than those among Japanese (*10*).

In 1982 Oshima *et al.* calculates systematically age-specific and age-adjusted cancer mortality rates of selected sites among Koreans in Osaka during 1968–1977, using data from the Osaka Cancer Registry (*7*). The following points were elucidated: 1) among Koreans in Osaka, the mortality rate for liver cancer was about twice that among Japanese; 2) among Koreans in Osaka, the mortality rate of stomach cancer has been declining more rapidly than it has among Japanese. Recently Ubukata *et al.* have analyzed cancer mortality rates of Koreans in Japan during the 1963–1980 period and confirmed the findings described above (*11*). Ubukata *et al.* also analyzed cancer mortality rates of Koreans and Japanese in Osaka during the 1973–1982 period and discussed the factors involved in the differences between Korean and Japanese cancer patterns.

In this paper the previous information is updated and summarized, and some com-

---

[*1]–[*3] Nakamichi 1-3-3, Higashinari-ku, Osaka 537, Japan (大島　明，生方享司，藤本伊三郎).

parisons between cancer patterns among Koreans in Japan and among Koreans in Korea are shown.

Cancer Mortality Patterns among Koreans in Osaka, Japan

Table I shows the age-adjusted cancer mortality rates of selected sites among Koreans and Japanese in Osaka Prefecture during 1973–1982. The population at risk by nationality was estimated from the 1970, 1975, and 1980 census. As of 1980, the Korean population was 158,079 and the Japanese population was 8,295,801. The number of deaths in Osaka was obtained from death certificate files with permission from the authorities concerned.

The number of deaths during this 10-year period was 7,844 from all causes and 1,859 (23.7%) from cancer for Korean residents, and was 425,331 and 98,783 (23.2%) respectively for Japanese residents in Osaka.

As shown in Table I, cancer of the liver was the commonest among Korean males, followed by stomach, lung, and esophagus cancer. Among Korean females stomach cancer was the most frequent malignant neoplasm, followed by uterine, liver, and lung cancer. Compared with Japanese males, Korean males had significantly higher mortality rates from cancers of the esophagus (the Korean-Japanese rate ratio was 1.5), liver (2.9), and lung (1.5). In Korean females liver cancer was significantly higher than in Japanese females (1.9). Among Koreans the mortality rates from stomach cancer were significantly lower in both sexes (0.8 and 0.7) and breast cancer in females (0.6).

Figure 1 shows the age-specific mortality rates from liver cancer among Koreans and among Japanese in Osaka. The mortality rate among Koreans were 1.9 to 2.9 times

TABLE I. Age-adjusted Mortality Rates[a] for Selected Cancer Sites among
Koreans and Japanese in Osaka Prefecture, 1973–1982

Site (ICD-8[b] Code)	Males			Females		
	Koreans	Japanese	Ratio	Koreans	Japanese	Ratio
Cancer—all sites (140–209)	215.4	165.0	1.3**	86.7	93.4	0.9
Mouth and pharynx (140–149)	2.3	2.1	1.1	0.3	0.7	0.4
Esophagus (150)	10.6	7.2	1.5*	1.0	1.8	0.6
Stomach (151)	43.6	56.4	0.8**	18.1	27.6	0.7**
Colon (153)	6.9	6.1	1.1	3.8	4.7	0.8
Rectum (154)	6.4	6.2	1.0	2.9	3.6	0.8
Liver (155, 1978)	65.7	22.3	2.9**	12.2	6.4	1.9**
Gallbladder and bile duct (156)	4.3	3.3	1.3	3.0	3.2	0.9
Pancreas (157)	7.1	6.1	1.2	3.0	3.6	0.8
Larynx (161)	1.7	1.7	1.0	0.0	0.3	0.0
Lung and trachea (162)	42.3	27.6	1.5**	10.6	7.8	1.4
Breast (174)	0.0	0.0	—	3.6	6.0	0.6**
Uterus (180–182)	—	—	—	12.5	10.3	1.2
Prostate (185)	1.2	1.3	1.0	—	—	—
Bladder (188)	2.3	2.9	0.8	0.5	0.9	0.6
Leukemia (204–207)	2.8	4.2	0.7	2.2	2.9	0.8

* p<0.05   ** p<0.01.
[a] per 100,000 population, standard population: UICC's world population.
[b] International Classification of Diseases, 8th revision.

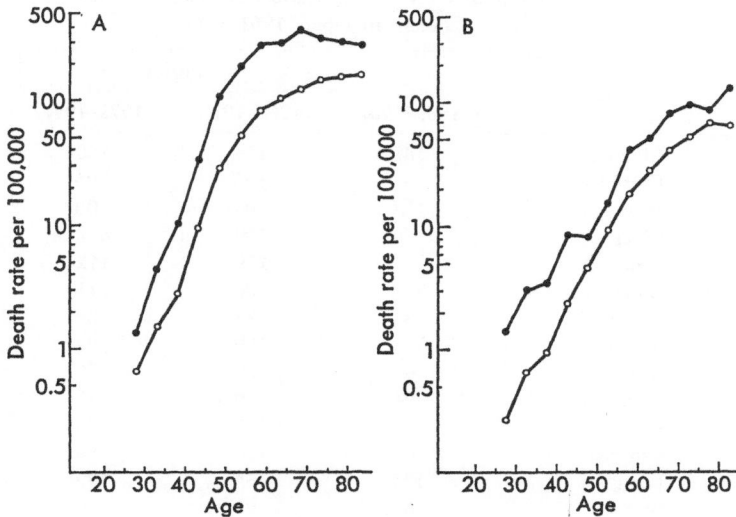

FIG. 1.   Age-specific mortality rate of liver cancer for Koreans (●) and Japanese in Osaka, Japan (○), 1973–1982
A: male. B: female.

higher than those among Japanese and exceeded in all age groups. A similar patterns was also observed in liver cirrhosis mortality rates.

Trends in Cancer Mortality Rates among Koreans in Japan

The Annual Report of Vital Statistics published by the Ministry of Health and Welfare of Japan provides the total number of deaths according to major cause for foreigners in Japan by sex and nationality, but it is not described by age-group. The age-adjusted cancer mortality rates, therefore, cannot be calculated by the direct method. Instead, we calculated the standardized mortality ratios (SMR's) of selected cancer sites for Koreans in Japan by 5-year periods during 1963–1982 with the age-specific rates for Japanese in the same periods as standards (Table II). Although the SMR's for Koreans were generally similar to the Korean-Japanese ratios in Table I, some discrepancies were observed. It should, however, be taken into consideration that Koreans living in Osaka came mainly from Cheju Island remote from the mainland of Korea and that the cancer patterns among them might be somewhat different from those among all Koreans in Japan. It should also be taken into consideration that there is a larger Korean population in western Japan including Osaka where liver cancer is more prevalent than in eastern Japan.

Figure 2 shows the trends of estimated age-adjusted cancer mortality rates for Koreans in Japan. We estimated these rates by applying the SMR's for Koreans to the age-adjusted rates for Japanese of the same period. From Table II and Fig. 2, the trends for Koreans can be considered to be similar to those for Japanese except in stomach cancer mortality rate. This rate for Korean males seems to have been decreasing more rapidly than it has for Japanese males.

TABLE II. Standardized Mortality Ratios[a] of Selected Cancer
Sites for Koreans in Japan, 1963–1982

Sex	Site	Period			
		1963–1967	1968–1972	1973–1977	1978–1982
Males	All sites	181	154	160	166
	Esophagus	—	196	204	152
	Stomach	137	108	100	96
	Liver[b]	—	409	418	476
	Pancreas	—	119	112	139
	Lung	253	206	211	181
	Leukemia	84	75	89	77
Females	All sites	113	100	97	118
	Esophagus	—	89	59	78
	Stomach	94	80	73	93
	Liver[b]	—	165	178	252
	Pancreas	—	126	89	116
	Lung	136	154	172	189
	Breast	63	91	60	65
	Uterus	150	135	151	154
	Leukemia	104	63	65	90

[a] Calculated on the basis of sex- and age-specific cancer mortality rates for Japanese in the same period.
[b] ICD-8: 155, 1977, 1978.

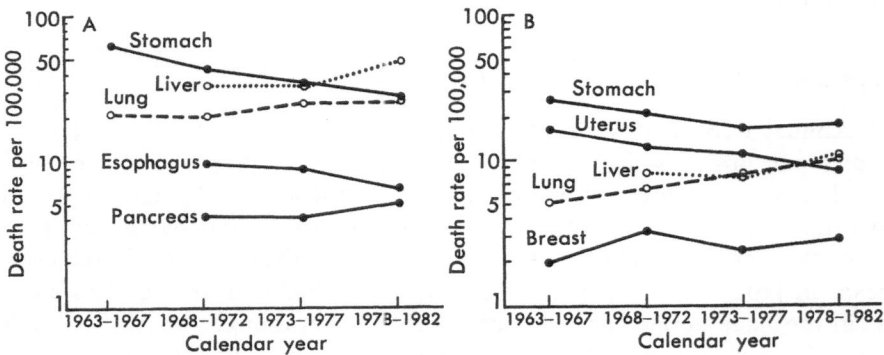

FIG. 2. Trends of age-adjusted cancer mortality rates of selected sites for Koreans
in Japan, 1963–1982. A: male. B: female.

Factors Involved in the Korean-Japanese Difference of Liver Cancer

The most prominent feature in cancer patterns for Koreans in Japan is the much higher rate of liver cancer. The mortality rate from liver cirrhosis is also much higher among them. These high mortality rates for chronic liver diseases among Koreans in Japan can be explained by the high prevalence rate of hepatitis B surface antigen (HBs-Ag) positives among them. The prevalence rate of HBs-Ag positives among Korean male and female blood donors in Osaka was 7.6% and 3.2%, and this was 3.5 and 1.9 times higher than that among Japanese males and females, respectively (8).

Another etiologic factor of chronic liver disease, i.e., alcohol, was discussed by

TABLE III. Distribution of Cancer Incidences of Selected Cancer Sites
for Koreans in Korea[a] and for Koreans in Osaka[b]

Sex	Site	Incidences among Koreans in Korea, July 1980–June 1984			Incidences among Koreans in Osaka, 1973–1982		
		Observed	Expected[c]	SPIR[d]	Observed	Expected[c]	SPIR[d]
Males	All sites	41,318	41,318.0	100	358	358.0	100
	Esophagus	1,132	1,264.4	90	19	14.9	147
	Stomach	12,169	14,456.5	84	77	129.4	60
	Colon	1,038	1,759.5	59	13	15.4	84
	Rectum	1,406	1,834.6	77	12	15.6	77
	Liver	6,468	4,699.8	138	102	40.4	252
	Pancreas	781	556.6	140	12	10.1	119
	Lung	5,036	4,726.3	107	52	50.1	104
Females	All sites	36,468	36,468.0	100	247	247.0	100
	Esophagus	537	369.3	49	2	3.0	67
	Stomach	6,430	8,174.6	79	52	59.1	88
	Colon	839	1,357.2	62	13	10.4	130
	Rectum	1,299	1,203.0	108	10	8.7	115
	Liver	1,669	1,087.4	156	18	9.4	191
	Pancreas	518	602.5	86	2	5.2	39
	Lung	1,394	1,594.8	87	13	13.8	94
	Breast	3,357	5,580.8	60	21	32.0	66
	Uterus	11,461	8,505.5	135	62	51.1	121

[a] From the Korean Cancer Registry.
[b] From the Osaka Cancer Registry; restricted to those cases whose residence was in Ikuno-ku or Higashi-nari-ku where Koreans live very densely.
[c] Expected numbers were calculated on a sex- and age-specific distribution of cancer incidences among Japanese in Osaka, 1980–1983.
[d] Standardized proportional incidence ratio, calculated as Observed/Expected × 100.

Ubukata *et al.* (*12*). They suggested that heavy drinkers are more frequent among Korean males in Japan than among Japanese males.

Comparison of Cancer Patterns among Koreans in Japan with Those among Koreans in Korea

Any study of cancer patterns in a migrant population should be conducted by comparing their cancer mortality or incidence patterns with those of the home and the host countries. Therefore, the findings presented so far should be said to be incomplete because there were no comparisons made for cancer patterns among Koreans in Japan with those among Koreans in Korea.

In Korea there is a complete system for population census and a rather complete death registration system. Many Koreans, however, have died without physician care. Kim reported that the proportion of deaths certified by physicians was 28% in 1965 and 57.3% in 1974 (*2*). Therefore, it is difficult to obtain age-specific cancer mortality rates for Koreans in Korea.

Although there was no population-based cancer registry system before 1982 in Korea, some information on relative frequencies of cancer can be obtained from hospital-based cancer registries (*4, 9*). Since 1980 the Korean Cancer Registry has been in operation and it covers about fifty teaching hospitals in Korea. Table III shows the distribution of cancer incidences of selected sites for Koreans in Korea and for Koreans in Osaka. Data for Koreans in Korea came from the Korean Cancer Registry (5, 6). Data for Koreans in Osaka were obtained from the Osaka Cancer Registry. Because nationality is not included as an item on the registration form of the Osaka Cancer Registry, it is necessary to check each card for whether the case's surname is Korean or not. Due to the large load of this work, this step was restricted to those cases whose residence was in Ikuno-ku or Higashinari-ku which has the largest Korean population in Osaka.

In Table III, standardized proportional incidence ratios (SPIR's) of selected cancer sites for Koreans in Korea and for Koreans in Osaka are also shown. We calculated the SPIR's with the sex- and age-specific distribution of cancer incidences among Japanese in Osaka as a standard. From the two series of SPIR's in Table III, it seems that stomach cancer is less prevalent and liver cancer is more frequent among Koreans in Osaka than among Koreans in Korea. However, the limitations of proportional methodologies and the representativeness or comparability of the subjects should be taken into consideration.

Ongoing study

A comparative study of cancer risk among Koreans in Japan, Koreans in Korea and Japanese is now being carried out. Much information can be obtained from the further analysis of data from the Korean Cancer Registry (5, 6) and the accumulation of data from the population-based Kangwha Cancer Registry (3). A survey on the lifestyle factors, such as smoking, drinking, diet and so on for Koreans in Japan, Koreans in Korea and Japanese is also being conducted.

In 1984 a Japan-Korea cooperative study of comparative cancer epidemiology began with a research grant from the Ministry of Education, Science and Culture of Japan (Chief researcher: Professor S. Kamiyama, Department of Hygiene, Akita University School of Medicine, and his Korean counterpart: Professor Kim Jin-Pok, Department of Surgery, Seoul National University College of Medicine). Under this project a comparative study has been initiated, and it is expected that some important clues on the etiologic factors of cancer will be obtained in the near future.

REFERENCES

1. Hirayama, T., Fukasawa, T., and Kimura, M. Demographic studies among a foreign population in Japan. *Kosei-no-shiyo*, **12**, 8–14 (1965) (in Japanese).
2. Kim, I. S. Comparative study of mortality patterns between Korea and Japan—An overview. *Korean J. Epidemiol.*, **1**, 47–54 (1970).
3. Kim, I. S., Kim, H. J., Oh, H. C., Kim, B. S., and Lee, Y. The cancer registry program in Kangwha County—The first report (July 1982–June 1984). *Korean J. Epidemiol.*, **6**, 100–111 (1984) (in Korean).
4. Korean Cancer Society. Cancer registry report for 1975. *J. Korean Med. Assoc.*, **19**, 673–681 (1976) (in Korean).
5. Ministry of Health and Social Affairs. Three year report for cancer register programme in the Republic of Korea, July 1, 1980–June 30, 1983. *J. Korean Cancer Res. Assoc.*, **16**, 73–228 (1984).
6. Ministry of Health and Social Affairs. One year report for cancer register programme in the Republic of Korea, July 1, 1983–June 30, 1984. *J. Korean Cancer Res. Assoc.*, **17**, 109–191 (1985).

7. Oshima, A., Hanai, A., Fujimoto, I., and Song, K. Cancer mortality among Koreans in Osaka, Japan. *Natl. Cancer Inst. Monogr.*, **62**, 13–16 (1982).

8. Oshima, A. Hiyama, T., Fujimoto, I., Song, K., Yamano, H., and Tanaka, M. The epidemiology of liver cancer. *Jpn. J. Cancer Clin.*, **28**, 962–971 (1982).

9. Seel, D. J. Observed cancer incidence in Southwest Korea. *Cancer*, **46**, 852–858 (1980).

10. Song, K. Epidemiology of liver cancer and liver cirrhosis for Koreans living in Japan. *Med. J. Osaka Univ.*, **32**, 357–373 (1981).

11. Ubukata, T., Oshima, A., and Fujimoto, I. Comparison of the causes of death between Koreans in Japan and Japanese. 2. Death from cancer. *Jpn. J. Public Health*, **31**, 71–77 (1984) (in Japanese).

12. Ubukata, T., Oshima, A., and Fujimoto, I. Mortality among Koreans living in Osaka, Japan during 1973–1982. *Int. J. Epidemiol.*, **15**, 218–225 (1986).

TOPICS IN CANCER
EPIDEMIOLOGY

PASSIVE SMOKING AND CANCER: AN EPIDEMIOLOGICAL REVIEW

Takeshi HIRAYAMA

Institute of Preventive Oncology

There is sufficient evidence that tobacco smoke is carcinogenic to humans. Epidemiological evidence supporting this statement was reviewed. An elevated, mostly dose-dependent, risk for lung cancer was observed in non-smoking wives with smoking husbands in five or more epidemiological, both cohort and case-control, studies in Japan, Greece, and the U.S.A. The results are compatible with much higher concentrations of carcinogens in sidestream smoke and other laboratory evidence such as elevated cotinine level in urines, impaired lung function, and demonstration of mutagens in urines in persons passively exposed to tobacco smoke. A significant association was also found with nasal sinus cancer and brain tumors in a large scale cohort study in Japan, probably reflecting the carcinogenic hazard of continued inhalation of sidestream smoke. Solid action to minimize the victims is urgently required.

Most constituents in tobacco smoke occur in markedly higher concentration in sidestream smoke than in mainstream smoke (*3, 4*). If inhaled at a close distance, or when ventilation of space is poor or there are many smokers in the room, polluted air could create a carcinogenic potentials and cause adverse health effects such as pulmonary dysfunction in people exposed to such air (*30*). Bos *et al.* (*2*) demonstrated excretion of mutagens in human urine after passive smoking. Eight nonsmokers were experimentally exposed to cigarette smoke by being in a poorly ventilated room together with heavy smokers for 6 hr. Inhalation of the contaminated air by the passive-smokers resulted in an increase in the urinary excretion of products mutagenic in the *Salmonella*/microsome assay. If such conditions last for a long time it is possible the risk of cancer fo selected sites could go up. Such speculation was supported by reports of epidemiological studies from Japan, Greece, and the U.S.A. which demonstrated an elevated risk of lung cancer in non-smoking women with smoking husbands.

Passive Smoking and Cancer: Epidemiologic Evidence

1. Prospective studies
1) Study in Japan

A prospective study was conducted of the mortality of 91,540 non-smoking wives in Japan in relation to the husbands' smoking habit (*12–15*).

A total of 265,118 adults, 122,261 men and 142,857 women, aged 40 years and above, 95% of the census population in 29 Health Center Districts in Japan, were in-

---

* 1-2 Ichigaya-Sadoharacho, Shinjuku-ku, Tokyo 162, Japan (平山　雄).

terviewed from October 1 to December 31, 1965 and were followed up by establishing a record linkage system between the risk factor records and death certificates.

a) *Lung cancer*

A total of 429 deaths from lung cancer in women was recorded during the 16 year follow-up (1966–1981). Samples of these showed that 74% of them were adenocarcinomas. Out of these 429 lung cancers, 303 were nonsmokers and 200 occurred among 91,450 non-smoking married women whose husband's smoking habits were known. The standardized mortality ratio of lung cancer in non-smoking women was 1.00, 1,36. 1.42, 1.58, and 1.91 when husbands were nonsmokers, ex-smokers, daily smokers of 1–14, 15–19, and 20 or more cigarettes per day, respectively (*p*: 0.00178) (Table I, Fig. 1). A Similar significant dose-response relationship was observed by age and by occupation of husbands, by age of wives, and in each time period of observation (internal consistency of association) (*13*). No other characteristics of husbands or wives themselves were found to elevate the risk of lung cancer in their non-smoking partners (specificity of association) (*13*). Non-smoking husband with smoking wife also showed an elevated risk of lung cancer, standardized mortality ratio being 1.00, 2.14, and 2.31 in non-somking husbands with non-smkoking wives, with wives smoking 1–19, and with wives smoking 20 or more cigarettes daily, respectively (*p*: 0.0177) (*15*). Based on this large scale cohort study it was estimated 1,029 non-smoking women annually die from lung cancer in Japan due to their husband's smoking.

b) *Nasal sinus cancer and brain tumor*

A significant risk elevation of cancer of paranasal sinuses and brain tumor in non-smoking wives was also observed according to the amount of a husband's smoking, relative risk for nasal sinus cancer being 1.00, 1.67, 2.03, 2.55 and for brain tumor being, 1.00, 3.03, 6.25, 4.32 when husbands were nonsmokers, smokers of 1–14, 15–19, and 20 or more cigarettes daily (*15*) (Table I). No other risk factors studied were identified to significantly alter the risk of nasal sinus cancer in women. The finding thus strengthens the plausibility of carcinogenic hazards of sidestream smoke inhalation through the nose. For brain tumor, a significant risk elevation by passive smoking was reported for child-hood brain tumor (*24*). It is of importance that a similar risk elevation by passive smoking was observed also for adult brain tumor. Other causes of death in non-smoking wives which showed significant association with husbands smoking habit were ischemic heart disease and suicide. All causes of death also showed significant association (Table I).

2) *Study in the U.S.A.*

A large scale prospective study was conducted by the American Cancer Society for 176,739 non-smoking women from 1960 through 1972 for whom smoking habits of the husbands were known (*7*). Of these, 47% or 375,000 non-smoking women were studied. Of 153 cases of lung cancer among non-smoking females, 88 were married to smokers. The lung cancer mortality ratio was 1.00, 1.27, and 1.10 for women married to men who never smoked, currently smoked less than 20 cigarettes per day, and currently smoked 20 or more cigarettes per day, repectively. When matched on the basis of wife's 5-year age group, husband's occupational exposure, highest educational level of husband and wife, race, urban-rural residence and absence of serious disease at the start of the study, the mortality ratio became 1.00, 1.37, and 1.04, respectively. The mortality ratio in non-smoking women with a smoking husband was above 1.00 throughout the study, although not statistically significant.

TABLE I. Spouse Smoking and Major Causes of Death: Dose-response Relationship

	(Number of deaths)	Mantel-extension chi	One-tail p value
Cancer of all sites	(2,705)	2.659	0.00392[a]
Cancer			
Mouth and pharynx	(22)	−0.829	0.20355
Esophagus	(58)	0.246	0.40284
Stomach	(854)	−0.270	0.39358
Colon	(142)	0.463	0.32168
Rectum	(112)	−0.007	0.49721
Bile duct and gallbladder	(91)	0.972	0.16553
Liver	(226)	0.696	0.24321
Pancreas	(127)	−0.860	0.12500
Nasal sinus	(28)	1.963	0.02482[a]
Lung	(200)	2.915	0.00178[a]
Breast	(115)	1.320	0.09342
Cervix	(273)	1.156	0.12384
Ovary	(54)	0.394	0.34679
Urinary organs	(49)	0.125	0.45026
Skin	(23)	1.445	0.07423
Bone tumor	(17)	0.358	0.36017
Brain tumor	(34)	2.673	0.00376[a]
Malignant lymphoma	(85)	1.134	0.12840
Leukemia	(51)	1.389	0.08242
Tuberculosis	(100)	0.608	0.27159
Diabetes	(227)	0.800	0.21186
Subarachnoid haemorrhage	(126)	1.622	0.05240
Cerebrovascular disease	(2,609)	1.604	0.05436
Ischemic heart disease	(494)	1.979	0.02391[a]
Other heart disease	(680)	1.254	0.10492
Hypertensive heart disease	(226)	0.927	0.17696
Ulcer	(57)	0.772	0.22006
Cirrhosis	(180)	−0.808	0.20955
Emphysema/bronchitis	(106)	0.940	0.17361
Suicide	(200)	1.859	0.03151
All causes	(9,106)	4.351	0.00001[a]

Husbands smoking[b]		Non	Ex	1–14	15–19	20–
Rate ratio	Ca. all sites	1.00	1.16	1.13	1.04	1.20
in non-smoking	Ca. lung	1.00	1.36	1.42	1.58	1.91
wives	Ca. nasal sinus	1.00	—	1.57	2.02	2.55
	Brain tumor	1.00	—	3.05	6.25	4.32
Rate ratio	All causes	1.00	1.26	1.16	1.06	1.19
in non-smoking	Ischemic heart disease	1.00	1.03	1.17	1.06	1.30
wives	Suicide	1.00	0.94	1.52	0.85	1.60

[a] Significant at 2.5% level (based on one-tail p).
[b] non, nonsmoker; ex, ex-smoker; 1–14, 15–19, 20–, daily number of cigarettes smoked.

3) Study in Scotland

Sixteen thousand one hundred seventy-one individuals from a health survey in Scotland (1972–1976) were followed up until December 1982 (9). Eight thousand one

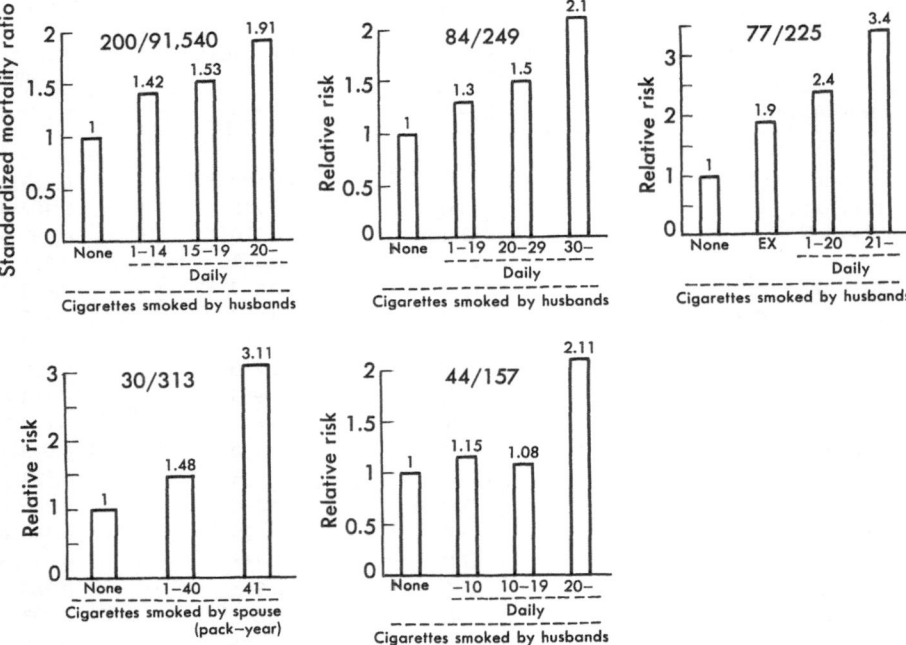

FIG. 1.   Lung cancer risk in non-smoking wives by number of cigarettes smoked by husbands
A: cohort study (Japan) (*13*). B: case control study (Japan) (*1*). C: case control study (Greece) (*28*). D: case control study (U.S.A.) (*6*). E: case control study (U.S.A.) (*8*).

hundred twenty-eight of these were couples and could be paired according to smoking habits. The lung cancer mortality expressed as the annual age-standardized rate per 10,000 males was 4 in nonsmokers not exposed to passive smoking, 13 among nonsmokers exposed to passive smoking, 22 among smokers, and 24 among smokers exposed to external passive smoking. The clear dose-response relationship with lung cancer observed in males exposed to passive smoking supports observations from other studies reported.

2.   Retrospective studies
1)   Study in Japan

A case-control study on passive smoking and lung cancer was conducted in Hiroshima and Nagasaki (*1*). Four hundred twenty-eight out of 525 newly diagnosed cases of primary lung cancer ascertained from the Hiroshima and Nagasaki Tumor and Tissue Registries, and 957 age-sex matched controls, 2 for each lung cancer case in Hiroshima, and 3 for each case in Nagasaki, were interviewed. Among 84 female nonsmokers, those with husbands smoking 1–19, 20–29, and 30 or more cigarettes daily showed odds ratios of 1.3, 1.5, and 2.1, respectively (p for trend$=0.06$) (Fig. 1), and those not exposed and exposed within the last 10 years showed odds ratios of 1.3 and 1.8, respectively (p for trend$=0.05$). When subclassified by occupation of subjects, odds ratios became more apparent in white and blue collar workers, p for trend being 0.03.

2)   Study in Greece

A case-control study on passive smoking and lung cancer was conducted in Greece

(1978–1982) (*27, 28*). Study subjects were non-smoking female residents of Athens. For a total of 77 cases and 225 controls, the risk ratio (RR) of lung cancer, other than adeno-carcinoma or terminal bronchiolar carcinoma for never-married women or those with husbands who were nonsmokers or ex-smokers for 5 to 20 years was 1.0, for wives of men who were ex-smokers for less than 5 years, RR was 1.9; for wives of men currently smoking 1 to 20 cigarettes daily, RR was 2.4; and for wives of men currently smoking 20 or more cigarettes daily, RR was 3.4 (Fig. 1). The dose-response relationship was highly statistically significant.

3)   *Study in Louisiana, U.S.A.*

A case-control study was conducted in Louisiana, U.S.A. on the smoking habits of parents and spouses involving 1,338 lung cancer patients and 1,393 comparison sub-jects (*6*). The exposure to passive smoking was calculated as total lifetime pack/years smoked by the spouses at the time of the interview. Nonsmokers married to heavy smokers had an increased risk of lung cancer, the relative risk being 1.00, 1.48, and 3.11 when spouses smoked none, 1–40 and 40 or more pack-years in the past (Fig. 1). In the non-smoking women, 54% of the cases were adenocarcinomas but the trends with regard to passive smoking exposure remained if these cases were excluded. The association with maternal smoking was significant (RR: 1.66) and statistical significance persisted after controlling for variables indicative of active smoking.

4)   *Study in New York, U.S.A.*

A case-control study was conducted in New York between 1971 and 1980 (*16*). One hundred thirty-four cases of lung cancer in nonsmokers were compared with an equal number of age-, sex-, race-, and hospital-matched non-smoking controls. Preliminary data on exposure to passive inhalation of tobacco smoke for a subset of cases and con-trols showed more frequent exposure among male cases (18 of 25 cases) than among controls (11 out of 25 cases) to sidestream tobacco smoke at work, the relative risk being 3.27 ($p < 0.045$). No extra risk was found for those exposed to smoke at home only.

5)   *Study in New Jersey and Ohio, U.S.A.*

A case-control study was conducted in three hospitals in New Jersey and one hos-pital in Ohio from 1971–1981 (*8*). One hundred thirty-four cases of lung cancer and 402 controls of colon-rectum cancer in non-smoking women were identified. All cases and controls were confirmed by histologic review of slides, and non-smoking status and exposures were verified by interview. The odds ratio increased with increasing number of cigarettes smoked by the husband, particularly for cigarettes smoked at home (Fig. 1). The odds ratio for women whose husbands smoked 20 or more cigarettes at home was 2.11 (95% confidence limits 1.13, 3.95). A logistic regression analysis showed a significant positive trend of increasing risk with increased exposure to husband's smoking at home when age, hospital, socioeconomic class, and year of diagnosis were controlled.

6)   *Study in North Carolina, U.S.A.*

A case-control study was conducted in North Carolina on passive smoking and can-cer utilizing a hospital based tumor registry (*25, 26*).

Information on smoking by the spouse was obtained for 518 cancer cases and 518 noncancer controls, identified from the hospital-based tumor registry. Cancer risk among individuals ever married to smokers was 1.6 times that of those never married to smokers ($p < 0.01$). Elevated risks were seen for several specific cancer sites such as cervix, breast, and endocrine organs and were not limited to lung cancer or other "smoking-related" tumors. Then, cancer risk from cumulative household exposure to cigarette smoke was evaluated. Over an individual's lifetime, overall cancer risk rose steadily and significantly with each additional household member who smoked. Cancer risk was also greater for individuals with exposures during both childhood and adulthood than for individuals with exposures during only one period. Trends were observed for both smoking-related and other sites. Odds ratios varied with extent of exposure from 1.4 to 2.7. Risk rose by 60% for those exposed during childhood and by 50% for those exposed during adulthood only, reaching 2.7 of those exposed during both periods.

7)   *Study in Hong Kong*

A case-control study was conducted on passive smoking and lung cancer in Hong Kong (*5*). Out of 189 female lung cancer patients, 84 were non-smoking married women. Out of these, 40.5% lived with a smoking husband, whereas of the 139 control patients, 47.5% lived with a smoking husband.

Later, another case-control study was conducted in Hong Kong (*18, 19*) in which 200 female lung cancer patients and 200 healthy district controls were interviewed. Compared with individuals claiming no exposure either passive or active, nonsmokers who were exposed to passive smoke at home, work or both had lung cancer risks (RRs) of 1.22, 0.91, and 1.59, respectively. Further, 120 female lung cancer patients were compared with the same number of healthy controls matched for age, socioeconomic status, and residential district (*20*). Among those who had never smoked, patients had an average excess of 3.8 years ($p \leq 0.123$) of passive exposure compared with control subjects. Passively exposed patients had predominantly adenocarcinoma or large cell carcinoma.

8)   *Study in West Germany*

Out of 59 female bronchogenic carcinomas in the region of Mannheim-Ludwig-shafen-Heidelberg, 39 appeared in non-smoking patients; 61.5% of these had lived in a domestic community with smokers. This is nearly 3-fold the number expected on the basis of smoking behavior of men in respective groups of the same age (*17*).

Evaluation of Currently Available Data

1.   *Lung cancer and passive smoking*

As shown in Fig. 1, there are several reports showing a consistent dose-dependent elevated risk of lung cancer in nonsmokers whose spouses have a smoking habit, and no essential statistical difference exists among the major reported results (*11*). Obviously, exposure to spouse smoking is only a part of the total exposure to passive smoking. These results thus strongly indicate the carcinogenic potential of continued inhalation of sidestream smoke. It is likely that passive smoking is more closely related to adenocarcinoma of the lung, common in women, than active smoking, reflecting the different histological responses to the two routes of inhalation: side stream smoke is inhaled mainly through the nose while mainstream smoke is inhaled solely through the mouth.

2.   *Cancer other than lung and passive smoking*

Since sidestream smoke is usually inhaled through the nose, it is of importance to study the influence of passive smoking on cancers other than lung. A large scale prospective study in Japan showed a statistically significant elevated risk of cancer of the nasal sinus and brain tumor in non-smoking women with smoking husbands. Association of childhood brain tumors with passive smoking was shown in a case-control study conducted in California (*24*). These results confirm the carcinogenic potential of inhaled side-stream smoke over a long time. Thus cancers observed to be significantly influenced by household passive smoking (lung cancer, nasal sinus cancer, and brain tumor) mostly statisfy each of the necessary postulates of causality: the consistency, the strength, the specificity, the temporal relationship of the association and, above all, the biological plausibility.

3. Radioactivity and cigarette smoke

One aspect which might be of importance in interpreting the carcinogenic mechanisms of passive smoking is the radioactivity of cigarette smoke. The passive smoker was reported to be exposed to the same radioactive elements in the tobacco as the smoker: moreover, 50–70% of the ^{210}Po appears in sidestream smoke, far more than in mainstream smoke (31). Increased exposure to radon daughters through passive smoking would be expected to increase the risk of lung cancer in passive smokers. In Little and O'Toole's study (21), four out of eight "nonsmokers" had significant ^{210}Po at the bifurcations, demonstrating exposure to airborne ^{210}Po or ^{210}Pb α-radiation, in line with the increased incidence of lung cancer seen in passive smokers.

4. Urinary cotinine in passive smokers

Urinary cotinine, a metabolite of nicotine with a longer half-life, was demonstrated in persons exposed to passive smoking (23, 29). The cotinine levels among heavy passive smokers in Japan (23) were about one-seventh the levels in average smokers, in contrast to about one-fiftieth in Wald's study in Britain (29), possibly reflecting higher exposure to passive smoking due to the closer physical proximity of spouses at home in Japan. In both studies, the urinary levels increased in proportion to estimated passive smoking exposure. The cotinine concentrations among Japanese nonsmokers living with 2-pack-a-day smokers were roughly equivalent to the cotinine levels of smokers of less than 3 cigarettes per day.

5. Parental smoking

The effect of parental smoking on the risk of lung cancer in family members must also seriously be considered as shown in the Louisiana (6) and North Carolina studies (26), and as suggested by studies which demonstrated elevated levels of cotinine in saliva, serum and urine from infants exposed to passive smoking (10, 22, 32).

6. Passive smoking in the workplace

As shown in Kabat and Wynder's study (16) and the Hiroshima-Nagasaki study (1) some suggestive evidence exists for the carcinogenic influence of passive smoking in the workplace. In view of the practical and social considerations, the issue is an important item for future research.

REFERENCES

1. Akiba, S., Kato, H., and Blot, W. J. Passive smoking and lung cancer among Japanese women. *Cancer Res.*, **46**, 4804–4807 (1986).
2. Bos, R. P., Theuws, J.K.G., and Henderson, P. Excretion of mutagens in human urine after passive smoking. *Cancer Lett.*, **19**, 85–90 (1983).
3. Brunnemann, K. D., Adams, J. D., and Ho, D.P.S. The influence of tobacco smoke on indoor atmospheres. II. Volatile and tobacco specific nitrosamines in main and sidestream

smoke and their contribution to indoor pollution. *In* "Proceedings of the 4th Joint Conference on the Sensing of Environmental Pollutants. New Orleans 1977," pp. 876–880 (1978). American Chemical Society, Washington.

4. Brunnemann, K. D. and Hoffmann, D. Chemical studies on tobacco smoke LIX. Analysis of volatile nitrosamines in tobacco smoke and polluted indoor environments. *In* "Environmental Aspects of N-nitroso Compounds," eds. E. A. Walter, L. Griciute, and M. Gastegnaro, pp. 343–356 (1978). IARC Scientific Publications No. 19, WHO, Lyon.

5. Chan, W. C. and Fund, S. C. Lung cancer in non-smokers in Hong Kong. *In* "Cancer Campaign 6, Cancer Epidemiology," ed. E. Grundmann, pp. 199–202 (1982). Gustav Fischer Verlag, Stuttgart and New York.

6. Correa, P., Pickle, L. W., Fontham, E., Lin, Y., and Haenszel, W. Passive smoking and lung cancer. *Lancet*, **ii**, 595–597 (1983).

7. Garfinkel, L. Time trends in lung cancer mortality among non-smokers and a note on passive smoking. *J. Natl. Cancer Inst.*, **66**, 1061–1066 (1981).

8. Garfinkel, L., Auerbach, O., and Joupert, L. Involuntary smoking and lung cancer; a case-control study. *J. Natl. Cancer Inst.*, **75**, 463–469 (1985).

9. Gillis, C. R., Hoke, D. J., Hawthorne, V. M., and Boyle, P. The effect of environmental tobacco smoke in two urban communities in the West of Scotland. *Eur. J. Resp. Dis.* (Suppl. 133), 199–124 (1983).

10. Greenburg, R., Etzel, R., and Haley, N. Exposure of the fetus, neonate, and nursed infant to nicotine and cotinine from maternal smoking. *N. Engl. J. Med.*, **310**, 1075–1078 (1984).

11. Health or Smoking?—Follow-up Report of the Royal College of Physicians (1983). Pitman Publish. Ltd., London.

12. Hirayama, T. Non-smoking wives of heavy smokers have a higher risk of lung cancer; a study from Japan. *Br. Med. J.*, **282**, 183–185 (1981).

13. Hirayama, T. Passive smoking and lung cancer; consistency of association. *Lancet*, **ii**, 1425–1426 (1983).

14. Hirayama, T. Lung cancer in Japan. Effects of nutrition and passive smoking. *In* "Lung Cancer, Causes and Prevention," eds. M. Mizell and P. Correa, pp. 175–195 (1984). Verlag Chemie International Inc., New York.

15. Hirayama, T. Cancer mortality in nonsmoking women with smoking husbands based on a large-scale cohort study in Japan. *Prevent. Med.*, **13**, 680–690 (1984).

16. Kabat, G. C., and Wynder, E. L. Lung cancer in nonsmokers. *Cancer*, **53**, 1214–1221 (1984).

17. Knoth, A. Bohn, H., and Schmidt, F. Passivrauchen als Lungenkrebsursache bei Nichtraucherinnen. *Med. Klin.*, **78**, 66–69 (Nr. 2) (1983).

18. Koo, L. C., Ho, J.H.-C., and Saw, D. Active and passive smoking among female lung cancer patients and controls in Hong Kong. *J. Exp. Clin. Cancer Res.*, **4**, 367–375 (1983).

19. Koo, L. C., Ho, J.H.-C., and Saw, D. Is passive smoking an added risk factor for lung cancer in Chinese women? *J. Exp. Clin. Cancer Res.*, **3**, 277–283 (1984).

20. Koo, L. C., Ho, J.H.-C., and Lee, N. An analysis of some risk factors for lung cancer in Hong Kong. *Int. J. Cancer.*, **35**(2), 149–155 (1985).

21. Little, J. B. and O'Toole, W. F. Respiratory tract tumors in hamsters induced by benzo[a]pyrene and ^{210}Po radiation. *Cancer Res.*, **34**, 3026–3039 (1974).

22. Luck, W. and Nau, H. Exposure of the fetus, neonate, and nursed infant to nicotine and cotinine from maternal smoking. *N. Engl. J. Med.*, **311**, 672 (1984).

23. Matsukura, S., Taminato, T., Kitano, N., Seino, Y., Hamada, H., Uchihashi, M., Nakajima, H., and Hirata, Y. Effects of environmental tobacco smoke on urinary cotinine excretion in nonsmokers; Evidence for passive smoking. *N. Engl. J. Med.*, **311**, 828–832 (1984).

24. Preston-Martin, S., Yu, M. C., Benton, B., and Henderson, B. E. N-nitroso compounds and childhood brain tumors; a case-control study. *Cancer Res.*, **42**, 5240–5245 (1982).

25. Sandler, D. P., Everson, R. B., and Wilcox, A. J. Passive smoking in adulthood and cancer risk. *Am. J. Epidemiol.*, **121**, 37–48 (1985).

26. Sandler, D. P., Wilcox, A. J., and Everson, R. B. Cumulative effects of lifetime passive smoking on cancer risk. *Lancet*, **i**, 312–314 (1985).

27. Trichopoulos, D., Kalandidi, A., Sparros, L., and MacMahon, B. Lung cancer and passive smoking. *Int. J. Cancer*, **27**, 1–40 (1981).

28. Trichopoulos, D., Kalandidi, A., and Sparros, L. Lung cancer and passive smoking; conclusion of Greek study. *Lancet*, **ii**, 677–678 (1983).

29. Wald, N. J., Boreham, J., Bailey, A., Ritchie, C., Haddow, J., and Knight, G. Urinary cotinine as marker of breathing other people's tobacco smoke. *Lancet*, **i**, 230–231 (1984).

30. White, R. J. and Froeb, F. H. Small-airways dysfunction in non-smokers chronically exposed to tobacco smoke. *N. Engl. J. Med.*, **302**, 720–723 (1980).

31. Winters, T. H. and Difranza, J. R. Radioactivity and cigarette smoke. *In* "Lung Cancer: Causes and Prevention," eds. M. Miell and P. Correa, pp. 263–271 (1984). Verlag Chemie International Inc., New York.

32. Woodward, A., Miles, H., and Grgurinovich, N. Cotinine in urine of smokers' infants. *Lancet*, **ii**, 935 (1984).

EXOGENOUS HORMONES AND THE RISK OF CANCER

Brian E. Henderson, Ronald K. Ross, and Leslie Bernstein

Department of Preventive Medicine,
*University of Southern California School of Medicine**

Epidemiologic, clinical, and experimental data suggest that endogenous levels of estrogen and progesterone alter risk of cancers of the endometrium and breast. Risk of these cancers is similarly affected when these hormones are administered for therapeutic purposes, in the form of oral contraceptives, estrogen replacement therapy and for the prevention of habitual abortion. Estrogen replacement therapy and sequential oral contraceptives (unopposed hormone followed by an estrogen/progestogen in combination) both increase risk of endometrial cancer, whereas combination oral contraceptives (estrogen/progestogen in combination in each pill) lower risk. While there is no evidence that oral contraceptives alter risk of breast cancer when taken during most of reproductive life, these drugs may increase risk of breast cancer when taken at an early age (especially for those women taking pills with a high progestogen potency) and when taken during the perimenopausal period. Estrogen replacement therapy appears to increase risk of breast cancer when taken in high doses for long periods. There is a slight but consistent increase in risk of breast cancer in women given diethylstilbestrol during pregnancy. Male offspring of such women appear to have elevated risks of testis cancer.

We have published previously a review of the evidence that endogenous levels of certain steroid and polypeptide hormones are causally related to a group of human cancers including those of the breast, endometrium, prostate, ovary, and testis (25). Taken together, these sites currently account for 19% of all newly diagnosed male and 42% of all newly diagnosed female cancers in the U.S.

Because of this evidence and the importance of these cancers, there is reason for concern about the effects on cancer risk if the same or closely related hormones are administered for therapeutic purposes, e.g., as oral contraceptives, hormone replacement therapy in the menopause or for the prevention of abortion. We attempt to briefly review here the vast amount of epidemiological information on this subject, much of which has accumulated during the past ten years.

Oral Contraceptives

Oral contraceptives have been widely used since the early 1960s. By 1978 the WHO estimated that more than 80 million women throughout the world had been exposed to these drugs. There is now a substantial body of literature on the relationship between

---

* Los Angeles, California 90033, U.S.A.

oral contraceptive (OC) use and risk of cancers of the breast, endometrium, ovary, and cervix. Recently there have also been reports of a relationship between OC use and cancer of the liver.

1. Breast cancer

Numerous epidemiologic studies have examined the relationship between OCs and risk of breast cancer. The majority of these were summarized by Kelsey and Hildreth (40). Although results have now been published for seven cohort studies and 17 case-control studies, the possible relationship between OC use and breast cancer continues to be a major source of controversy (15, 46, 68).

As a group, these studies provide no strong evidence that OCs either increase or decrease breast cancer risk when used during the middle reproductive years. However, use at two particular times during the reproductive years, the post-menarcheal period and the perimenopausal period, may substantially increase risk. Five studies have reported an elevated risk of breast cancer with use of OCs around the time of menopause (7, 35, 43, 62, 74), although the range of risk estimates is wide (Table I). A probable explanation of this increased risk is that OCs produce a hormonal state approximating that of a normally menstruating woman, masking the onset of menopause by artificially prolonging menstrual life. The net effect of such use would be greater hormonal exposure to estrogens and progestogens than would have occurred naturally during the perimenopausal period.

A second group of OC users who may be at increased risk of breast cancer are those who use OCs for long periods of time early in menstrual life, particularly before first full-term pregnancy. Paffenbarger et al. (51) reported a relative risk of 2.7 for such use in a series of breast cancer cases and controls who were less than 50 years old. This effect was independent of age at childbirth. In a subsequent case-control study of women under age 33, Pike et al. (54) reported that the risk of breast cancer increased with increasing duration of OC use before the first full-term pregnancy; a relative risk of 3.5 was reached for 8 or more years of use compared with non-use. Data from a case-control drug surveillance program study indicate a significantly increased risk of breast cancer among women aged 30–39 who had more than 5 years of OC use which started or ended many years prior to diagnosis (59). The estimated relative risk for such use beginning at least 15

TABLE I.   Breast Cancer Risk and Oral Contraceptive Use during the Perimenopausal Period

First author	Reference	Relative risk of current users compared to non-users Age at diagnosis[a]	
		40–44	45–49
Vessey	74	0.7	1.5
Jick	35	0.8	4.0
RCGP[b]	62	1.1	1.7
Brinton	7	1.1	1.3
Lipnick[c]	43	1.8	1.7

[a] For Vessey's study, age groups are 41–45, 46–50.
[b] RCGP study presents data for upper age group as 45+.
[c] Risk estimates presented for women who were current users in 1976.

years earlier was 2.6; the estimated relative risk for use ending at least 10 years earlier was 5.0.

Recently, Pike et al. (55) updated their ongoing case-control study to include 317 breast cancer cases under 37 years of age. Cases used OCs for an average of 49 months compared to 39 months for the controls and a large part (60%) of this difference in average duration of use was for use before age 23. For OC use before age 25, the relative risk was 2.5 for 4 or more years of use and the trend of increasing risk with increasing duration of use was highly significant ($p < 0.0001$). Swedish investigators (49) subsequently reported a significant trend of increasing breast cancer risk with decreasing age at first use. The estimated relative risk for first OC use before age 20 was 11.5; for first use between ages 20 and 24, it was 3.3. Further evidence that early long-term OC use may increase breast cancer risk is provided by a recent report from Oxford which shows significantly increased breast cancer risk for more than 4 years use prior to first full-term pregnancy (47). Two other major studies, however, provide no support for these observations. Both the Cancer and Steroid Hormone Study, a large case-control study of OC use and risk of breast, endometrial and ovarian cancer in women aged 20 to 54 years (9, 69), and the first phase of a case-control study of young married women in Britain (78), found little or no evidence of an increased breast cancer risk with OC use before full-term pregnancy or before age 25.

Early studies of OC use and breast cancer risk generally were unable to adequately test the hypothesis that *early long-term OC use* increases breast cancer risk because OC use before first pregnancy was uncommon in the 1960s when these compounds first became widely available. Thus, in these studies, few women had histories of long-term exposures during the post-pubertal years. Many early studies considered only married women whose major reason for taking OCs was family spacing. Furthermore, a period of 10–20 years after such exposure may be necessary before exposure-related increases in breast cancer risk are detectable.

Because both timing of menarche and timing of first full-term pregnancy are critical risk factors for breast cancer, exposures during the years between these two events may also be critical for establishing breast cancer risk. The period immediately after onset of menses is characterized by frequent anovulartory cycles (79), and even when ovulatory cycles occur in adolescent girls they are characterized by significantly lower levels of estrogen and progesterone than are those of adult fertile women (2). For both reasons, OC use during the post-menarcheal years may expose young women to higher levels of estrogens and progestogens than would have occurred naturally, altering their subsequent risk of breast cancer. Logically, this would occur if a woman's average breast tissue mitotic activity when on OCs is greater than her average "normal" mitotic activity and could be due to either the estrogen or the progestogen component of the compound. Using a similar line of reasoning (in other words, measuring the effect of OC use relative to the woman's "normal" hormonal state), one might expect that the more recently introduced "low-dose" OCs may protect against breast cancer in regularly ovulating women (for example, those who are post-first full-term pregnancy and/or between the ages of 25 and 35).

2. Endometrial cancer

Following the establishment of the association between prolonged use of estrogen

TABLE II.   Case-control Studies of Combination Oral Contraceptives and Endometrial Cancer

First author	Reference	Relative risk	Number of cases using OCs
Kaufman	38	0.5	16
Weiss	80	0.5	17
Kelsey	41	0.6	6
Hulka	34	0.4	5
CDC	11	0.6	70
Henderson	22	0.5	43

TABLE III.   Case-control Studies of Oral Contraceptives and Epithelial Carcinoma of the Ovary

First author	Reference	Relative risk	Number of cases using OCs
Newhouse	48	0.6	19
McGowan	45	0.7	Unk
Casagrande	8	0.8	41
Hildreth	30	0.5	3
Willett	81	0.8	13
Francheschi	17	0.7	17
Rosenberg	60	0.6	29
Risch	57	0.9[a]	23
CDC	10	0.6	90
Cramer	13	0.4	34
La Vecchia	42	0.6	18

[a] Estimated.

replacement therapy and endometrial cancer, case series were reported suggesting a similar association between sequential OCs and endometrial cancer (64). Sequential OCs administer a constant, relatively high dose of estrogen without progestogen for 3 weeks, followed by 5 to 6 days of estrogen with progestogen. This results in a menstrual cycle with a normal or perhaps hyperplastic proliferation phase followed by a short secretory phase. Three of the four case-control studies that have data on sequential OCs (removed from sale in the U.S. in 1976) show a 2-fold increased risk for ever-use (11, 22, 80). The one negative study had only two cases who ever used sequential OCs (38).

In contrast, use of combination OCs in which an estrogen and progestogen are combined in each pill has been consistently reported in case-control studies to decrease the risk of endometrial cancer by about 50% (Table II). One prospective study observed a similar decrease in risk (56). The protective effect of combination OCs is biologically plausible since the presence of the progestogen reduces endometrial mitotic activity and causes differentiation of the endometrial cells to a secretory state.

In the largest study to date (11), there was no apparent difference in risk for use of OCs for short periods (<5 years) compared to longer use. However, we observed a clear decrease in risk with duration of use (relative risk for 5 or more years of use was 0.1) (22). Such protection was not evident for certain subgroups of women, including those who were obese and those of high parity.

3.   *Ovarian cancer*

At least 11 case-control studies have examined the association between prior use of

OCs and ovarian cancer (Table III). All the studies show a decrease in risk among OC users, averaging about 40% across all studies. The risk clearly decreases with increasing duration of use (8, 10) and appears to be longlasting. In the Centers for Disease Control study (10) the risk of ovarian cancer for women who had first used OCs 10 or more years earlier was about half that of non-users.

The risk of ovarian cancer is also decreased by pregnancy whether complete or incomplete (8). We combined periods of pregnancy and OC use into a single measure which we called "protected time." The risk of ovarian cancer was clearly decreased by increasing protected time. We hypothesized that this protection resulted from suppression of ovulation.

4. Cervix cancer

There has been no consistent evidence that longterm use of OCs alters the risk of squamous cell carcinoma of the cervix (4, 12, 71, 72, 73, 82). However, two case-control studies have shown an increased risk with increasing duration of OC use (20, 50). Stern et al. (70) demonstrated higher rates of progression from cervical dysplasia to carcinoma in situ among OC users in a large cohort study in Los Angeles. In a recent report from the Oxford-Family Planning Association Contraceptive Study there was an increasing trend of risk with duration of OC use (76, 77), Finally, an increasing incidence of adenocarcinoma of the cervix has been reported among women under 35 years of age in Los Angeles County (53). It was hypothesized that use of OCs during the teenage years might account for this trend.

5. Liver tumors

A causal association between the use of oral contraceptives and benign liver tumors, variously described as adenomas or focal nodular hyperplasia, is well documented (16, 58). Experimental animal studies have shown that OCs can cause hepatocellular carcinomas in mice and are effective promoters of hepatocarcinogenesis in diethyl-nitrosamine-primed rats (83). At least 10 case reports of hepatocellular carcinoma arising in women taking oral contraceptives have been published. Recently, we reported 11 further cases of malignant liver tumors in young women (23). Ten of the cases had used oral contraceptives for periods ranging from 6 to 168 months. The other patient had received multiple "hormone" shots of undetermined type for regulation of men-strual periods during the 9 months preceding diagnosis. Six of the 11 patients were taking hormones at the time of diagnosis. The average duration of use in the 11 cases was 65 months compared to 27 months in age-matched neighborhood controls—a difference which is highly significant statistically (1-sided $p<0.005$, test for trend retaining the matching triplets).

Hormone Replacement Therapy

There are currently over 30 million postmenopausal women in the U.S. The advisability of long-term use of estrogen replacement therapy for such women remains controversial. Nonetheless, by the mid 1970's, over 28 million prescriptions of non-contraceptive estrogens were being filled annually in the U.S. However, concerns about the carcinogenic potential of estrogen replacement therapy on the breast and endometrium led to a 50% decline in the number of estrogen prescriptions by 1980.

TABLE IV. Estrogen Replacement Therapy and Risk of Breast Cancer

First author	Reference	Relative risk	
		Ever use	Long-term use
Hoover	32	1.3	2.0
Ross	61	1.1	1.9
Jick	36	1.1	—
Brinton	6	1.2	1.3
Hoover	31	1.4	1.8
Hiatt	29	0.7	1.8

The decline in cervical cancer occurrence in the past few decades and the increase in endometrial cancer rates during the 1960s and early 1970s has made endometrial cancer the most common gynecologic malignancy in the U.S.. Case reports of this neoplasm occurring in women following use of estrogens have appeared in the medical literature for over 30 years, but only since 1975 have there been serious controlled efforts to study this relationship. Over 20 studies have now been published on this association. Nearly all of these studies demonstrated a strong association between estrogen use and disease risk that was related to both dose and duration of use (1, 44, 65, 84).

Most early studies of the possible effects of estrogen replacement on risk of breast cancer were uncontrolled follow-up studies. The most credible cohort study was done by Hoover et al. (32). Although they reported only a 25% excess of breast cancer in their cohort of menopausal estrogen users compared to the number expected based on general population rates (49 observed versus 39 expected), they did report a more substantial excess among women using high doses for a long time.

Early case-control studies which reported findings on menopausal estrogens and breast cancer were often limited by small numbers, by insufficient data on dose and duration of use, and by the definite possibility of bias. A new round of carefully conducted case-control studies using healthy population controls has recently been published (6, 29, 31, 36, 61) (Table IV). All of these studies with a sufficient number of longterm users found small increases in risk of breast cancer (relative risks of 1.3 to 1.9) after such use.

Two other recently reported studies which used hospital controls as their comparison group found no evidence to suggest that breast cancer risk was increased either overall or with long duration of use (37, 39). One possible explanation for this is that hospital controls have more contact with the health care system and are therefore more likely to use elective drugs than the population as a whole.

The continued controversy surrounding the advisability of long-term use of estrogen replacement therapy among postmenopausal women centers around three issues: the potential benefits to be derived from such therapy compared with the potential risks, the most favorable dose to maximize the benefit to risk ratio, and the benefits and risks to be derived by adding a progestogen to the estrogen regimen.

There is substantial epidemiologic and clinical evidence that estrogens prevent osteoporosis and its most serious medical consequence, hip fracture. Women using estrogens for 5 years in the postmenopausal period approximately halve their risk of sustaining a non-traumatic osteoporotic fracture (52). Recent case-control studies have provided compelling evidence that estrogens lower risk of coronary heart disease (24). This effect is most likely mediated through raised high density and reduced low density lipoprotein

TABLE V.   Relative Risks for Hormone Use during Pregnancy of Mothers of
Testis Cancer Cases and Controls from Three Case-control Studies

Reference		No. used/total		Relative risk
		Case	Control	
Schottenfeld	(63)	11/190	3/141	2.8
Henderson	(21)	5/78	1/78	5.3
Depue	(14)	9/107	2/108	4.9

cholesterol levels in estrogen users. Since death rates from coronary heart disease among U.S. women are four times those of breast and endometrial cancer combined, this benefit alone could far outweigh any carcinogenic potential.

Hormones during Pregnancy

Diethylstilbestrol (DES), a non-steroidal estrogen, was promoted during the 1940's as a useful drug for the treatment of habitual abortion and threatened abortion (66, 67). During the next twenty years it has been estimated that two to three million women were given DES during pregnancy. In 1971, Herbst et al. (28) reported a strong association between such maternal exposure and the occurrence of adenocarcinoma of the vagina in their offspring. The peak incidence occurred during the late teenage years with declining risk once these young women reached their 20's (26, 27). Interestingly, the highest risk occurred among the offspring of mothers initially exposed to DES during the first trimester.

Until recently there has been little information available on the cancer risk of male offspring exposed in utero to DES. Three case-control studies have demonstrated an increased risk of testis cancer in the male offspring of women exposed to DES, estrogen or the estrogen-progestogen combination used in pregnancy tests (14, 21, 63). The relative risks for such hormone exposure initiated during the first trimester ranged from 2.8 to 5.3 (Table V).

The effect of DES exposure during pregnancy on the risk of cancer in the mother, herself, has been the subject of several recent studies (3, 5, 18, 19, 33, 75). Three of these reports are based on long-term follow-up of women who were entered in randomized clinical trials (3, 5, 75). Taken together these reports demonstrated a 30% excess of breast cancer cases (48 in the treated compared to 37 in the placebo control). Although this excess is not statistically significant it is consistent with the magnitude of risk that might be expected for exposure to an estrogenic drug over a relatively short duration.

REFERENCES

1. Antunes, C.M.F., Stolley, P. D., Rosenshein, N. B., Davies, J. L., Tonascia, J. A., Brown, C., Burnett, L., Rutledge, A., Pokempner, M., and Garcia, R. Endometrial cancer and estrogen use. N. Engl. J. Med., 300, 9–13 (1979).
2. Apter, D., Raisanen, I., Ylostalo, P., and Vihko, R. Ultrasonographic and hormonal patterns of adolescent menstrual cycles. Paper presented at the XV Acta Endocrinologica Congress in Helsinki, Finland (1985).
3. Beral, V. and Cowell, L. Randomized trial of high doses of stilboestrol and thisterone in pregnancy: long-term follow-up of mothers. Br. Med. J., 281, 1098–1101 (1980).

4. Boyce, J. G., Lu, T., Nelson, J. H., and Fruchter, R. G. Oral contraceptives and cervical carcinoma. *Am. J. Obstet. Gynecol.*, **128**, 761–764 (1977).

5. Brian, D. D., Tilley, B. C., Labarthe, D. R., O'Fallon, W. M., Noller, K. L., and Kurland, L. T. Breast cancer in DES-exposed mothers. Absence of association. *Mayo Clin. Proc.*, **55**, 89–93 (1980).

6. Brinton, L. A., Hoover, R. N., Szklo, M., and Fraumeni, J. F. Menopausal estrogen use and risk of breast cancer. *Cancer*, **47**, 2517–2522 (1981).

7. Brinton, L. A., Hoover, R., Szklo, M., and Fraumeni, J. F. Oral contraceptives and breast cancer. *Int. J. Epidemiol.*, **11**, 316–322 (1982).

8. Casagrande, J. T., Louie, E. W., Pike, M. C., Roy, S., Ross, R. K., and Henderson, B. E. "Incessant ovulation" and ovarian cancer. *Lancet*, **ii**, 170–173 (1979).

9. Center for Disease Control. Long-term oral contraceptive use and the risk of breast cancer. *JAMA*, **249**, 1591–1595 (1983).

10. Centers for Disease Control. Oral contraceptive use and the risk of ovarian cancer. *JAMA*, **249**, 1596–1599 (1983).

11. Centers for Disease Control. Oral contraceptive use and the risk of endometrial cancer. *JAMA*, **249**, 1600–1604 (1983).

12. Clarke, E. A., Hatcher, J., McKeown-Eyssen, G. E., and Lickrish, G. M. Cervical dysplasia: association with sexual behavior, smoking and oral contraceptive use? *Am. J. Obstet. Gynecol.*, **151**, 612–616 (1985).

13. Cramer, D. W., Hutchinson, G. B., Welch, W. R., Scully, R. E., and Knapp, R. C. Factors affecting the association of oral contraceptives and ovarian cancer. *N. Engl. J. Med.*, **307**, 1047–1051 (1982).

14. Depue, R. H., Pike, M. C. and Henderson, B. E. Estrogen exposure during gestation and risk of testicular cancer. *J. Natl. Cancer Inst.*, **71**, 1151–1155 (1983).

15. Editorial. Another look at the pill and breast cancer. *Lancet*, **ii**, 985–987 (1985).

16. Edmondson, H. A., Henderson, B., and Benton, B. Liver cell adenomas associated with use of oral contraceptives. *N. Engl. J. Med.*, **294**, 470–472 (1976).

17. Franceschi, S., La Vecchia, C., Helmrich, S. P., Mangioni, C., and Tognoni, G. Risk factors for epithelial ovarian cancer in Italy. *Am. J. Epidemiol.*, **115**, 714–719 (1982).

18. Greenberg, E. R., Barnes, A. B., Reseguie, L., Barnett, J. A., Burnside, S., Lanza, I. L., Neff, R. K., Stevens, M., Young, R. H., and Colton, T. Breast cancer in mothers given diethylstilbestrol in pregnancy. *N. Engl. J. Med.*, **311**, 1393–1398 (1984).

19. Hadjimichael, O. C., Meigs, J. W., Falcier, F. W., Thompson, W. D., and Flannery, J. T. Cancer risk among women exposed to exogenous estrogens during pregnancy. *J. Natl. Cancer Inst.*, **73**, 831–834 (1984).

20. Harris, R.W.C., Brinton, L. A., Cowdell, R. H., Skegg, D.C.G., Smith, P. G., Vessey, M. P., and Doll, R. Characteristics of women with dysplasia or carcinoma-*in situ* of the cervix uteri. *Br. J. Cancer*, **42**, 359–369 (1980).

21. Henderson, B. E., Benton, B., Jing, J., Yu, M. C., and Pike, M. C. Risk factors for cancer of the testis in young men. *Int. J. Cancer*, **23**, 598–602 (1979).

22. Henderson, B. E., Casagrande, J. T., Pike, M. C., Mack, T., Rosario, I., and Duke, A. The epidemiology of endometrial cancer in young women. *Br. J. Cancer*, **47**, 749–754 (1983).

23. Henderson, B. E., Preston-Martin, S., Edmondson, H. A., Peters, R. L., and Pike, M. C. Hepatocellular carcinoma and oral contraceptives. *Br. J. Cancer*, **48**, 437–440 (1983).

24. Henderson, B. E., Ross, R. K., Paganini-Hill, A., and Mack, T. M. Estrogen use and cardiovascular disease. *Am. J. Obstet. Gynecol.*, **154**, 1181–1186 (1986).

25. Henderson, B. E., Ross, R. K., Pike, M. C., and Casagrande, J. T. Endogenous hormones as a major factor in human cancer. *Cancer Res.*, **42**, 3232–3239 (1982).

26. Herbst, A. L. The epidemiology of vaginal and cervical clear cell adenocarcinoma. *In*

"Developmental Effects of Diethylstilbestrol (DES) in Pregnancy," eds. A. L. Herbst and H. A. Bern, pp. 63–70 (1981). Thieme Stratton, New York.

27. Herbst, A. L., Cole, P., Norusis, M. J., Welch, W. R., and Scully, R. E. Epidemiologic aspects and factors related to survival in 384 registry cases of clear cell adenocarcinoma of the vagina and cervix. *Am. J. Obstet. Gynecol.*, **135**, 876–886 (1979).

28. Herbst, A. L., Ulfelder, H., and Poskanzer, D. C. Adenocarcinoma of the vagina. Association of maternal stilbestrol therapy with tumor appearance in young women. *N. Engl. J. Med.*, **248**, 878–881 (1971).

29. Hiatt, R. A., Bawal, R., Friedman, G. W., and Hoover, R. Exogenous estrogens and breast cancer after oophorectomy. *Cancer*, **54**, 139–144 (1984).

30. Hildreth, N. G., Kelsey, J. L., Li Volsi, V. A., Fischer, D. B., Holford, T. R., Mostow, E. D., Schwartz, P. E., and White, C. An epidemiological study of epithelial carcinoma of the ovary. *Am. J. Epidemiol.*, **114**, 398–405 (1981).

31. Hoover, R., Glass, A., Finkle, W. D., Azevedo, D., and Milne, K. Conjugated estrogens and breast cancer risk in women. *J. Natl. Cancer Inst.*, **67**, 815–820 (1981).

32. Hoover, R., Gray, L. A., Cole, P., and MacMahon, B. Menopausal estrogens and breast cancer *N. Engl. J. Med.*, **295**, 401–405 (1976).

33. Hubby, M. M., Haenszel, W. M., and Herbst, A. L. Effects on the mother following exposure to diethylstilbestrol in pregnancy. *In* "Developmental Effects of Diethylstilbestrol (DES) in Pregnancy," eds. A. L. Herbst and H. A. Bern, pp. 120–128 (1981). Thieme Stratton Inc., New York.

34. Hulka, B. S., Chambless, L. E., Kaufman, D. G., Fowler, W. C., and Greenberg, B. G. Protection against endometrial carcinoma by combination-product oral contraceptives. *JAMA*, **247**, 475–477 (1982).

35. Jick, H., Walker, A. M., Watkins, R. N., D'Ewart, D. C., Hunter, J. R., Danford, A., Madsen, S., Dinan, B. J., and Rothman, K. J. Oral contraceptives and breast cancer. *Am. J. Epidemiol.*, **112**, 577–585 (1980).

36. Jick, H., Walker, A. M., Watkins, R. N., D'Wart, D. C., Hunter, J. R., Danford, A., Madsen, S., Dinan. B. J., and Rothman, K. J. Replacement estrogens and breast cancer. *Am. J. Epidemiol.*, **112**, 586–594 (1980).

37. Kaufman, D. W., Miller, D. R., Rosenberg, L., Helmrich, S. P., Stolley, P., Schottenfeld, D., and Shapiro, S. Noncontraceptive estrogen use and risk of breast cancer. *JAMA*, **252**, 63–67 (1984).

38. Kaufman, D. W., Shapiro, S., Slone, D., Rosenberg, L., Miettinen, O. S., Stolley, P. D., Knapp, R. C., Leavitt, T., Watring, W. G., Rosenshein, N. B., Lewis, J. L., Schottenfeld, M. D., and Engle, R. I. Decreased risk of endometrial cancer among oral contraceptive users. *N. Engl. J. Med.*, **303**, 1045–1047 (1980).

39. Kelsey, J. L., Fischer, D. B., Holford, J. R., Livolsi, V. A., Mostow, E. D., Goldeberg, I. S., and White, C. Exogenous estrogens and other factors in the epidemiology of breast cancer. *J. Natl. Cancer Inst.*, **67**, 327–333 (1981).

40. Kelsey, J. L. and Hildreth, N. G. "Breast and Gynecologic Cancer Epidemiology," pp. 5–10 (1983). CRC Press, Inc., Boca Raton, Fla.

41. Kelsey, J. L., Li Volsi, V. A., Holford, T. R., Fischer, D. B., Mostow, E. D., Schwartz, P. E., O'Connor, T., and White, C. A case-control study of cancer of the endometrium. *Am. J. Epidemiol.*, **116**, 333–342 (1982).

42. La Vecchia, C., Franceschi, S., and Decarli, A. Oral contraceptive use and the risk of epithelial ovarian cancer. *Br. J. Cancer*, **50**, 31–34 (1984).

43. Lipnick, R. J., Buring, J. E., Hennekens, C. H., Rosner, B., Willett, W., Bain, C., Stampfer, M. J., Colditz, G. A., Oeto, R., and Speizer, F. E. Oral contraceptives and breast cancer: a prospective cohort study. *JAMA*, **255**, 58–61 (1986).

44. Mack, T. M., Pike, M. C., Henderson, B. E., Pfeffer, R. I., Gerkins, V. R., Arthur, M.,

and Brown, S. E. Estrogens and endometrial cancer in a retirement community. *N. Engl. J. Med.*, **294**, 1256–1258 (1976).

45. McGowan, L., Parent, L., Ledner, W., and Norris, H. J. The woman at risk for developing ovarian cancer. *Gynecol. Oncol.*, **7**, 325–344 (1979).

46. McPherson, K. and Coope, P. A. Early oral contraceptive use and breast cancer risk (letter). *Lancet*, **i**, 685–686 (1986).

47. McPherson, K., Neil, A., Vessey, M. P., and Doll, R. Oral contraceptives and breast cancer (letter). *Lancet*, **ii**, 1414–1415 (1983).

48. Newhouse, M. L., Pearson, R. M., Fullerton, J. M., Boesen, E.A.M., and Shannon, H. S. A case control study of carcinoma of the ovary. *Br. J. Prev. Soc. Med.*, **31**, 148–153 (1977).

49. Olsson, H., Landin-Olsson, M., Möller, T. R., Ranstam, J., and Holm, P. Oral contraceptive use and breast cancer in young women in Sweden (letter). *Lancet*, **i**, 748–749 (1985).

50. Ory, H. W., Conger, S. B., Naib, Z., Tyler, C. W., and Hatcher, R. A. Preliminary analysis of oral contraceptive use and risk of developing premalignant lesions of the uterine cervix. *In* "Pharmacology of Steroid Contraceptive Drugs," eds. S. Garratini and H. W. Berendes, pp. 211–224 (1977). Raven Press, New York.

51. Paffenbarger, R. S., Kampert, J. B., and Chang, H. Oral contraceptives and breast cancer risk. *INSERM*, **83**, 93–114 (1979).

52. Paganini-Hill, A., Ross, R. K., Gerkins, V. R., Henderson, B. E., Arthur, M., and Mack, T. M. Menopausal estrogen therapy and hip fractures. *Ann. Intern. Med.*, **95**, 28–31 (1981).

53. Peters, R. K., Chao, A., Mack, T. M., Thomas, D., Bernstein, L., and Henderson, B. E. Increased frequency of adenocarcinomas of the uterine cervix in young women in Los Angeles County. *J. Natl. Cancer Inst.*, **76**, 423–428 (1986).

54. Pike, M. C., Henderson, B. E., Casagrande, J. T. Rosario, I., and Gray, G. E. Oral contraceptive use and early abortion as risk factors for breast cancer in young women. *Br. J. Cancer*, **43**, 72–76 (1981).

55. Pike, M. C., Henderson, B. E., Krailo, M. D., Duke, A., and Roy, S. Breast cancer in young women and use of oral contraceptives: possible modifying effect of formulation and age at use. *Lancet*, **ii**, 926–930 (1983).

56. Ramcharan, S., Pellegrin, F. A., Ray, R., and Hsu, J-P. A prospective study of the side effects of oral contraceptives. *In* "The Walnut Creek Contraceptive Drug Study," NIH Publ. 81-564, Vol. 3 (1981). U.S. Dept. of Health and Human Services, Natl. Population Research, Bethesda.

57. Risch, H. A., Weiss, N. S., Lyone, J. L., Dailing, J. R., and Liff, J. M. Events of reproductive life and the incidence of epithelial ovarian cancer. *Am. J. Epidemiol.*, **117**, 128–139 (1983).

58. Rooks, J. B., Ory, H. W., Ishak, K. G., Strauss, L. T., Greenspan, J. R., Paganini-Hill, A., and Tyler, C. W. Epidemiology of hepatocellular adenoma. The role of oral contraceptive use. *JAMA*, **242**, 644–648 (1979).

59. Rosenberg, L., Miller, D. R., Kaufman, D. W., Helmrich, S. P., Stolley, P. D., Schottenfeld, D., and Shapiro, S. Breast cancer and oral contraceptive use. *Am. J. Epidemiol.*, **119**, 167–176 (1984).

60. Rosenberg, L., Shapiro, S., Slone, D., Kaufman, D. W., Helmrich, S. P., Miettinen, O. S., Stolley, P. D., Rosenshin, N. B., Schottenfeld, D., and Engl, R. L. Epithelial ovarian cancer and combination oral contraceptives. *JAMA*, **247**, 3210–3212 (1982).

61. Ross, R. K., Paganini-Hill, A., Gerkins, V. R., Mack, T. M., Pfeffer, R., Arthur, M., and Henderson, B. E. A case-control study of menopausal estrogen therapy and breast cancer. *JAMA*, **243**, 1635–1639 (1980).

62. Royal College of General Practitioners. Breast cancer and oral contraceptives: findings

in Royal College of General Practitioner's study. *Br. Med. J.*, **282**, 2089–2094 (1981).

63. Schottenfeld, D., Warshauer, M. E., Sherlock, S., Zauber, A. G., Leder, M., and Payne, R. The epidemiology of testicular cancer in young adults. *Am. J. Epidemiol.*, **112**, 232–246 (1980).

64. Silverberg, S. G. and Makowski, E. L. Endometrial carcinoma in young women taking oral contraceptive agents. *Obstet. Gynecol.*, **46**, 503–506 (1975).

65. Smith, D. C., Prentice, R., Thompson, D. J., and Herrmann, W. L. Association of exogenous estrogen and endometrial carcinoma. *N. Engl. J. Med.*, **293**, 1164–1167 (1975).

66. Smith, O. W. Diethylstilbestrol in the prevention and treatment of complications of pregnancy. *Am. J. Obstet. Gynecol.*, **56**, 821–834 (1948).

67. Smith, O. W. and Smith, G. van S. The influence of diethylstilbestrol on the progress and outcome of pregnancy as based on a comparison of treated with untreated primigravidas. *Am. J. Obstet. Gynecol.*, **58**, 994–1009 (1949).

68. Stadel, B. V., Rubin, G. L., Wingo, P. A., and Schlesselman, J. J. Oral contraceptives and breast cancer in young women (letter). *Lancet*, **i**, 436 (1986).

69. Stadel, B. V., Webster, L. A., Rubin, G. L., Schlesselman, J. J., and Wingo, P. A. Oral contraceptives and breast cancer in young women. *Lancet*, **ii**, 970–973 (1985).

70. Stern, E., Forsythe, A. B., Youkeles, L., and Coffelt, C. F. Steroid contraceptive use and cervical dysplasia: increased risk of progression. *Science*, **196**, 1460–1462 (1977).

71. Swan, S. H. and Brown, W. L. Oral contraceptive use, sexual activity and cervical carcinoma. *Am. J. Obstet. Gynecol.*, **139**, 52–57 (1981).

72. Swan, S. H. and Pettiti, D. B. A review of problems of bias and confounding in epidemiologic studies of cervical neoplasia and oral contraceptive use. *Am. J. Epidemiol.*, **115**, 10–18 (1982).

73. Thomas, D. B. Relationship of oral contraceptives to cervical carcinogenesis. *Obstet. Gynecol.*, **40**, 508–518 (1972).

74. Vessey, M. P., Doll, R., Jones, K., McPherson, K., and Yeates, D. An epidemiological study of oral contraceptives and breast cancer. *Br. Med. J.*, **1**, 1757–1760 (1979).

75. Vessey, M. P., Fairweather, D.V.I., Norman-Smith, B., and Buckley, J. A randomized double-blind controlled trial of the value of stilboestrol therapy in pregnancy: long-term follow-up of mothers and their offspring. *Br. J. Obstet. Gynaecol.*, **90**, 1007–1017 (1983).

76. Vessey, M. P., Lawless, M., McPherson, K., and Yeates, D. Neoplasia of the cervix uteri and contraception—a possible adverse effect of the pill. *Lancet*, **ii**, 930–934 (1983).

77. Vessey, M. P., Lawless, M., McPherson, K., and Yeates, D. Oral contraceptives and cervical cancer. *Lancet*, **ii**, 1358–1359 (1983).

78. Vessey, M. P., McPherson, K., Yeates, D., and Doll, R. Oral contraceptive use and abortion before first term pregnancy in relation to breast cancer risk. *Br. J. Cancer*, **45**, 327–331 (1982).

79. Vihko, R. and Apter, D. Endocrine characteristics of adolescent menstrual cycles: impact of early menarche. *J. Steroid Biochem.*, **20**, 231–234 (1984).

80. Weiss, N. S., and Sayvetz, T. A. Incidence of endometrial cancer in relation to the use of oral contraceptives. *N. Engl. J. Med.*, **302**, 551–554 (1980).

81. Willett, W. C., Bain, C., Hennekens, C. H., Rosner, B., and Speizer, F. E. Oral contraceptives and risk of ovarian cancer. *Cancer*, **48**, 1684–1687 (1981).

82. Worth, A. J. and Boyes, D. A. A case-control study into the possible effects of birth control pills on pre-clinical carcinoma of the cervix. *J. Obstet. Gynecol. Br. Commonwlth.*, **79**, 673–679 (1972).

83. Yager, J. D. and Yager, R. Oral contraceptive steroids as promoters of hepato-carcinogenesis in female Sprague-Dawley rats. *Cancer Res.*, **40**, 3680–3685 (1980).

84. Ziel, H. K. and Finkle, W. D. Increased risk of endometrial carcinoma among users of conjugated estrogens. *N. Engl. J. Med.*, **293**, 1167–1170 (1975).

ADULT T-CELL LEUKEMIA

Suketami Tominaga, Ikuko Kato, and Kazuo Tajima

*Division of Epidemiology, Aichi Cancer Center Research Institute**

In Japan the mortality rate for malignant lymphomas has shown a characteristic geographical distribution, *e.g.*, very high in the southwestern part of the country, especially in the Kyushu district. The survey on adult T-cell leukemia/lymphoma (ATLL), a new disease entity reported by Takatsuki *et al.*, revealed that the high mortality rate for malignant lymphomas in the Kyushu district was attributable to ATLL. As the causal agent, human T-cell leukemia/lymphoma virus type I (HTLV-1), a type of retrovirus, was isolated from T-cell lines derived from ATLL patients, and antibodies to HTLV-1 antigen were detected in sera not only from the patients with ATLL but also from healthy adults in ATLL-endemic areas. In the areas with high incidence rates of ATLL, the positive rate of antibodies to HTLV-1 antigen was also high. From family studies, two main transmission routes of HTLV-1 were suspected, horizontal transmission from carrier-husbands to wives and vertical or horizontal transmission from carrier-mothers to children. As possible risk factors other than HTLV-1, filariasis, undernutrition, thymic function, and genetic factors were discussed in the epidemiological model for ATLL. Future studies must/should clarify the transmission routes of HTLV-1 and promotive factors for ATLL after HTLV-1 infection to prevent this disease.

Adult T-cell leukemia/lymphoma (ATLL), one of the endemic lymphomas, is a new disease entity first described by Takatsuki and his colleagues in 1977 (*18*). Because of the characteristic geographical distribution of this disease, a viral involvement has been suspected in its etiology (*11*). In 1980, a retrovirus (human T-cell leukemia/lymphoma virus type I (HTLV-1) was isolated in the U.S.A. by Poiesz *et al.* in T-cell lines derived from patients with cutaneous T-cell malignancy (*8*). Independent of HTLV-1, adult T-cell leukemia virus (ATLV) was found in T-cell lines derived from ATLL patients in 1981 by Hinuma *et al.* (*2*). Today, these two viruses are regarded to be almost identical (*9, 10*) and to be the main causal agent for ATLL. Moreover, seroepidemiological studies of ATLL and virological and molecular biological studies on HTLV-1 have progressed greatly in recent years. In this paper, we will review the epidemiological approaches to this disease and will discuss an etiological model and future prospects.

Malignant Lymphomas in Japan

The age-adjusted death rate for malignant lymphomas in Japan has always been much lower than in western countries and in the U.S.A. (*11*). However, a marked geographical variation of the mortality within Japan has been observed since 20 years ago.

* Kanokoden 1-1, Tashiro-cho, Chikusa-ku, Nagoya 464, Japan (富永祐民, 加藤育子, 田島和雄).

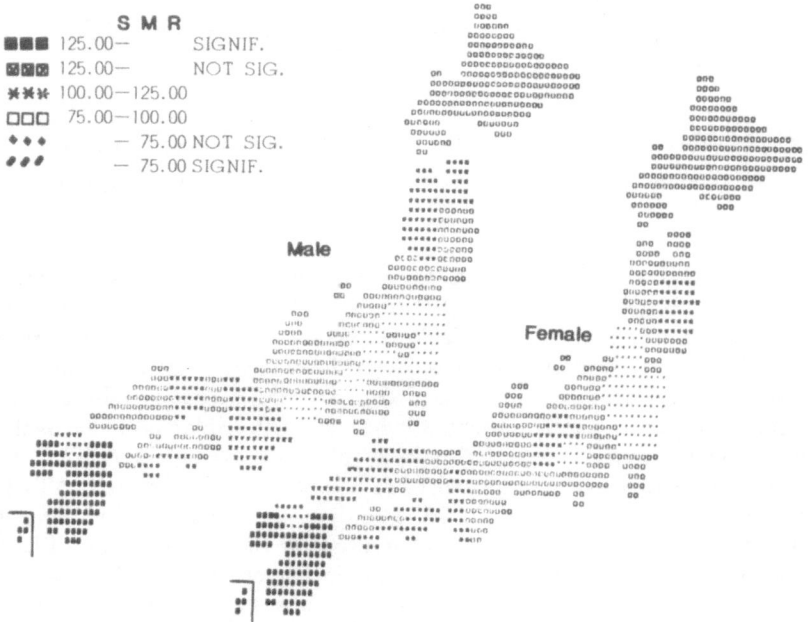

FIG. 1. Maps of geographical comparison of SMR of malignant lymphomas in Japan from 1973 to 1977. Tested at the 5% significance level

Figure 1 shows maps of the standardized mortality ratio (SMR) for malignant lymphomas by prefecture from 1973 to 1977. Several prefectures of the Kyushu district in southwestern Japan show SMRs twice as high as all Japan in both sexes. Moreover, a nationwide study of T- and B-cell lymphomas in Japan suggested that the proportion of T-cell lymphoma among non-Hodgkin lymphoma was very high in the Kyushu district (11, 15).

Epidemiological and Clinico-pathological Features of ATLL

1. Epidemiological features

It has been suggested by clinicians that many cases of ATLL, even if diagnosed in metropolitan areas, had the Kyushu district as place of birth (18). A nationwide survey revealed that the birthplaces of most ATLL patients were clustered in the Kyushu district, especially in rural coastal areas, and coastal areas of southern Shikoku and the Kii Peninsula where the climate is warm and rainy. However, sporadic cases were observed throughout Japan even in mountainous areas (Fig. 2) (16, 17). These findings suggest that the excessive mortality rate for malignant lymphomas in the Kyushu district was due to the high incidence of ATLL. In another part of the world, cases like Japanese ATLL were reportedly found among Caribbean people who might have originated from central Africa (1). Family clustering of ATLL patients and a high frequency of patients family history of malignant lymphomas have also been reported (4).

HTLV-1 detected in T-cell lines derived from ATLL patients is a type of retrovirus sometimes involved in the cause of certain leukemias, lymphomas and sarcomas in various animal species. It was clarified by Hinuma *et al.* that sera from ATL patients regularly reacted in an immunofluorescence test with cytoplasmic antigen of an ATL

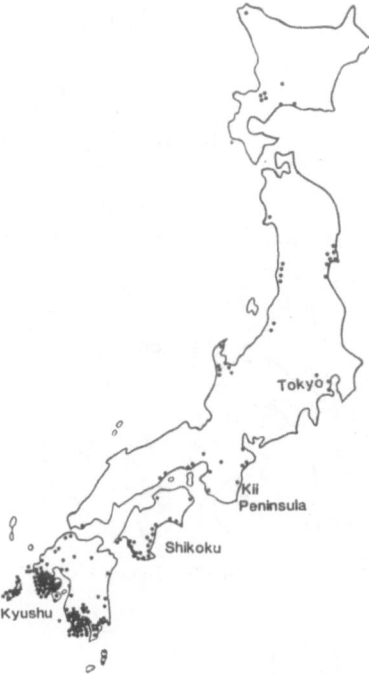

FIG. 2. Distribution of birthplaces of ATLL patients (from the T- and B-cell Malignancy Study Group, 1981) (*16*)

cell line called ATL related antigen (ATLA) (*2*). The integration of the provirus genomes in DNA of leukemia cells from patients with ATLL was also demonstrated (*19*). No oncogenes were detected in the provirus genome, though the complete nucleotide sequence was determined (*10*).

2. Clinico-pathological features

The sex ratio (male/female) is about 1.3, lower than that of other types of lymphomas. The onset is in adulthood, most frequently in the 50s but, ranging from 20s to 80s. The clinical course is mostly acute, although subacute, chronic and smoldering types have also been reported. Leukemic manifestations with or without generalized lymphadenopathy frequently occurs, one of the reasons this disease is called ATLL. Frequent hepatospleno-megaly, hypercalcemia and skin lesions such as erythroderma and nodule formation are observed. Neoplastic cells have peripheral T-cell characteristics (OKT4 positive) and peculiar pleomorphic nuclei. Current anti-leukemic agents are not effective in most cases (*16, 18*).

Epidemiology of HTLV-1

In ATLL-endemic areas, antibodies to ATLA were found not only in sera from ATLL patients but also in those from healthy adults (*2*). The nationwide survey detecting antibodies to ATLA among healthy adults aged 40 years or over revealed that most of the high incidence (6 to 37%) of antibody-positive donors was found in southwestern regions of Japan, corresponding to the ATLL-endemic areas shown in Fig. 3 (*3*).

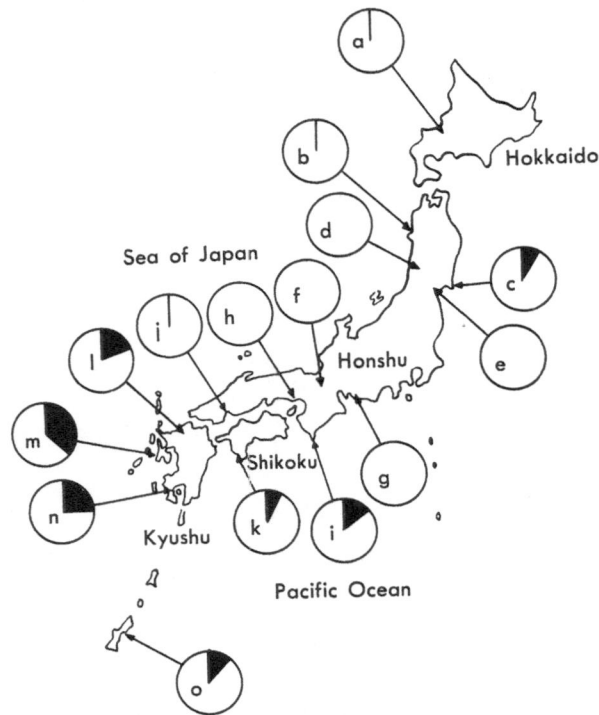

FIG. 3.   Geographical distribution of positive rate(%) of anti-ATLA antibody among healthy adults in Japan (from Hinuma *et al.*, 1982)

The age-specific positive rate of antibodies to ATLA in the endemic areas increased with age, the increase after age 40 being much greater in females than in males. However, the positive rate was very low among children even in the endemic areas (Fig. 4) (*13*). Although sero-conversion against HTLV-1 infection may occur in later life with repeated stimulation by latently infected-HTLV-1 antigen, it is still unknown whether the age distribution of HTLV-1 carriers reflects the age effect and/or a cohort effect.

In an analysis of married couples, more than 80% of wives with a carrier-husband over age 40 were infected with HTLV-1, but only 19% of those were infected with non-carrier-husbands (Table I) (*15*). This suggests that horizontal transmission from carrier-husband to wife, causes an increase in the positive rate of antibodies to ATLA among females in older age groups. Furthermore, HTLV-1-antigens were identified from lymphocytes in the semen of carrier-husbands (*7*). However, as the incidence of ATLL is lower in females than in males in spite of a higher positive rate of antibodies to ATLA among females in older age groups, infection in later life may not lead to the manifestation of ATLL.

In the analyses of the familial infection mode of HTLV-1, almost all children of parents without antibodies to ATLA were also without the antibodies, and about 50% of children older than 20 years from mothers with the antibodies were infected with HTLV-1 (*13*), suggesting vertical or horizontal transmission from mothers to children, though the route of transmission is still unknown. Recently, lymphocytes with HTLV-1 antigen have been identified from breast milk of carrier-mothers (*5*). From these family

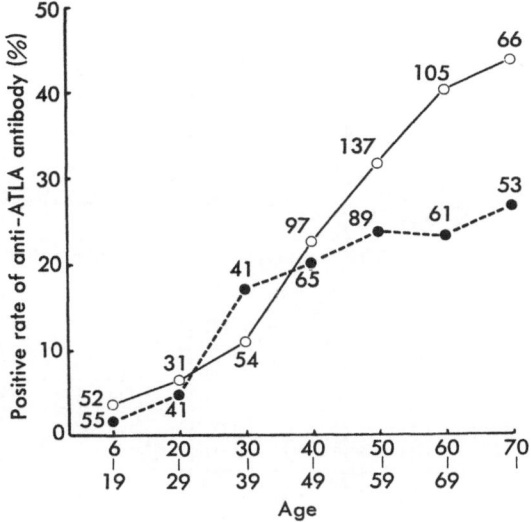

FIG. 4. Age- and sex-specific positive rates of anti-ATLA antibody among 947 persons in the Goto Islands
Figures in graph indicate number of samples. ● males ($n=405$); ○ females ($n=542$).

TABLE I. Distribution of Anti-ATLA Positives among Husbands and Wives According to the Anti-ATLA Positivity of Spouses

Anti-ATLA positivity Positive subjects (+) / Total subjects	Age group of subjects		Total
	40–59	60+	
Wives (+) / Wife with husband (+)	21/27 (78)	11/11 (100)	32/ 38 (84)
Wives (+) / Wife with husband (−)	16/94 (17)	12/51 (24)	28/145 (19)
Husband (+) / Husband with wife (+)	22/32 (69)	13/31 (42)	35/ 63 (56)
Husband (+) / Husband with wife (−)	5/75 (7)	1/54 (2)	6/129 (5)

Figures in parenthesis indicate the positive rate (%) of anti-ATLA antibody in each group.
Data source: Tajima and Hinuma (1985) (15).

studies, very close relation within a family seems to be needed for the transmission of HTLV-1. Other than natural transmission, parenteral infection mainly by whole blood transfusion can be an important route of transmission of the disease.

An Epidemiological Model for ATLL

HTLV-1 virus has been regarded as the most definitive causal agent for ATLL, though some patients with the same clinico-pathological features as ATLL but without evidence of HTLV-1 infection have been observed. Other factors could be related to the development of this disease, however, because ATLL does not develop in most HTLV-1 carriers.

Filariasis was suspected to be involved in part in the etiology of ATLL for the following reasons: the geographical distribution of the prevalent areas of filariasis in the past in Japan resembles those of ATLL; filarial parasites affect the lymphatic vessels and

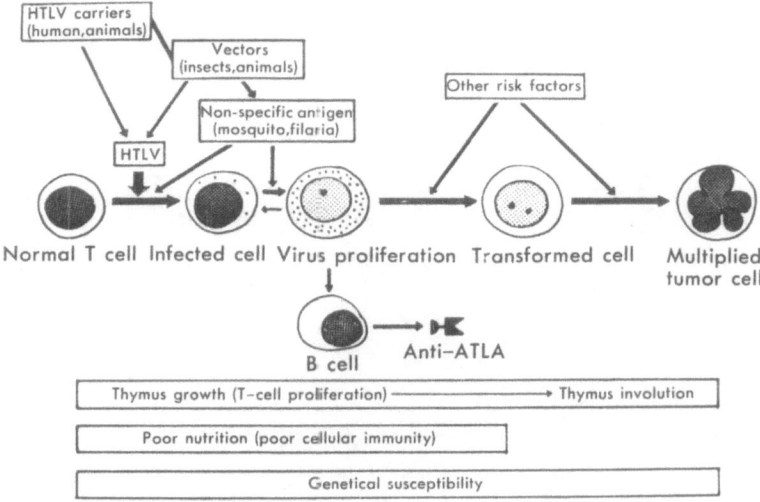

FIG. 4. A model for the epidemiological hypothesis on the action of each risk-factor for ATLL

impair the function of their host's immune system; and the positive rate of antibodies to ATLA was higher among persons with a high antibody titer to filarial antigen than among persons with a low antibody titer to it (*12*, *14*). The existence of certain vectors, such as mosquitoes in filariasis or some kinds of animals, should not be overlooked in consideration of the characteristic climate of the endemic areas.

Genetic factors might influence the course of infection of HTLV-1 and development of ATLL. It has been suggested that poor nutrition in childhood suppresses the growth of the thymic gland and the function of cell-mediated immunity. People of ATLL-endemic areas were undernourished compared with other districts, especially metropolitan areas in the past. The thymic gland, where T-cells divide, differentiate and mature, markedly involuted after 40 years of age when most ATLL patients were diagnosed. Therefore, the lowered function of cell-mediated immunity could be a risk factor for the development of ATLL (*12*). These epidemiological hypotheses are illustrated in Fig. 5.

Future Prospects

There remain several problems to be elucidated in future studies of ATLL. It is of scientific interest to determine the mechanisms of oncogenesis by HTLV-1; it is also anthropologically interesting to search for the origin of this disease. However, the most important point in future studies on ATLL should be its prevention. The prevention of HTLV-1 infection is most essential, so that the routes of infection must be clarified and methods to shut off the suspected routes such as milk and blood transfusion need to be developed, as well as vaccination against HTLV-1. Since an HTLV-1-like virus was detected in several kinds of Old World monkeys including the Japanese monkey (*6*), animal studies will also contribute to the understanding of the route of infection of HTLV-1 and subsequent preventive measures of infection. Elucidation of the natural history of HTLV-1 infection is necessary together with detection of genetic and environmental factors which promote the infection and which are related to the transition from carrier state to preleukemic stage, or from smoldering leukemia to advanced leukemia/ lymphoma. Finally, for ATLL patients, the development of new therapeutic methods is important. Programs against ATLL are expected to be a model in virus-related cancers as well as liver cancer and Burkitt lymphoma.

REFERENCES

1. Blattner, W. A., Kalyanaraman, V. S., Robert-Guroff, M., Lister, T. A., Galton, D.A.G., Sarin, P. S., Crawford, M. H., Catovsky, D., Greaves, M., and Gallo, R. C. The human type-C retrovirus, HTLV, in blacks from the Caribbean region, and relationship to adult T-cell leukemia/lymphoma. *Int. J. Cancer*, **30**, 257–264 (1982).
2. Hinuma, Y., Nagata, K., Hanaoka, M., Nakai, M., Matsumoto, T., Kinoshita, K., Shirakawa, S., and Miyoshi, I. Adult T-cell leukemia: Antigen in an ATL cell line and detection of antibodies to the antigen in human sera. *Proc. Natl. Acad. Sci. U.S.A.*, **78**, 6476–6480 (1981).
3. Hinuma Y., Komoda, H., Chosa, T., Kondo, T., Kohakura, M., Takenaka, T., Kikuchi, M., Ichimaru, M., Yunoki, K., Sato, I., Matsuo, R., Takiuchi, Y., Uchino, H., and Hanaoka, M. Antibodies to adult T-cell leukemia-virus-associated antigen (ATLA) in sera from patients with ATL and controls in Japan: A nationwide sero-epidemiologic study. *Int. J. Cancer*, **29**, 631–635 (1982).
4. Ichimaru, M., Kinoshita, K., Kamihira, S., Yamada, Y., Oyakawa, Y., Amagasaki, T., and Kusano, M. Familial disposition of adult T-cell leukemia and lymphoma. *In* "Adult T cell Leukemia and Related Diseases," eds. M. Hanaoka, K. Takatsuki, and M. Shimoyama, pp. 185–196 (1982). Plenum Press, New York and London.
5. Kinoshita, K., Hino, S., Amagasaki, T., Ikeda, S., Yamada, Y., Suzuyama, J., Momita, S., Toriya, K., Kamihira, S., and Ichimaru, M. Demonstration of adult T-cell leukemia virus antigen in milk from three sero-positive mothers. *Gann*, **75**, 103–105 (1984).
6. Miyoshi, I., Fujishita, M., Taguchi, H., Matsubayashi, K., Miwa, N., and Tanioka, Y. Natural infection in non-human primates with adult T-cell leukemia virus or a closely related agent. *Int. J. Cancer*, **32**, 333–336 (1983).
7. Nakano, S., Ando, Y., Ichijo, M., Moriyama, I., Saito, S., Sugimura, K., and Hinuma, Y. Search for possible route of vertical and horizontal transmission of adult T-cell leukemia virus. *Gann*, **75**, 1044–1045 (1984).
8. Poiesz, B. J., Ruscetti, F. W., Gazdar, A. F., Bunn, P. A., Minna, J. D., and Gallo, R. C. Detection and isolation of type C retrovirus particles from fresh and cultured lymphocytes of a patient with cutaneous T-cell lymphoma. *Proc. Natl. Acad. Sci. U.S.A.*, **77**, 7415–7419 (1980).
9. Popvic, M., Reitz, M. S., Jr., Sarngadharan, M. G., Robert-Guroff, M., Kalyanarman, V. S., Nakao, Y., Miyoshi, I., Minowada, J., Yoshida, M., Ito, Y., and Gallo, R. C. The virus of Japanese adult T-cell leukemia is a member of the human T-cell leukemia virus group. *Nature*, **300**, 63–66 (1982).
10. Seiki, M., Hattori, S., Hirayama, Y., and Yoshida, M. Human adult T-cell leukemia virus: Complete nucleotide sequence of the provirus genome integrated in leukemia cell DNA. *Proc. Natl. Acad. Sci. U.S.A.*, **80**, 3618–3622 (2983).
11. Tajima, K., Tominaga, S., Kuroishi, T., Shimizu, H., and Suchi, T. Geographical features and epidemiological approach to endemic T-cell leukemia/lymphoma in Japan. *Japan. J. Clin. Oncol.*, **9**, 495–504 (1979).
12. Tajima, K., Tominaga, S., Shimizu, H., and Suchi, T. A hypothesis on the etiology of adult T-cell leukemia/lymphoma. *Gann*, **72**, 684–689 (1981).

13. Tajima, K., Tominaga, S., Suchi, T., Kawagoe, T., Komoda, H., Hinuma, Y., Oda, T., and Fujita, K. Epidemiological analysis of the distribution of antibody to adult T-cell leukemia-virus-associated antigen: Possible horizontal trasmission of adult T-cell leukemia *Gann*, **73**, 893–901 (1982).

14. Tajima, K., Fujita, K., Tukidate, S., Oda, T., Tominaga, S., Suchi, T., and Hinuma, Y. Seroepidemiological studies on the effects of filarial parasites on infection of adult T-cell leukemia virus in the Goto Islands, Japan. *Gann*, **74**, 188–191 (1983).

15. Tajima, K. and Hinuma, Y. Epidemiological features of adult T-cell leukemia virus. *In* "Pathological Aspects of Cancer Epidemiology: Immunological Virological Endocrinological and Genetical Factors," eds. G. Mathè and P. Reizenstein, pp. 75–87 (1985). Pergamon Press, Oxford.

16. The T- and B- cell Malignancy Study Group. Statistical analysis of immunologic clinical and histopathologic data on lymphoid malignancies in Japan. *Jpn. J. Clin. Oncol.*, **11**, 15–38 (1981).

17. The T- and B-cell Malignancy Study Group. Statistical analyses of clinico-pathological, virological and epidemiological data on lymphoid malignancies with special reference to adult T-cell leukemia/lymphoma: A report of the second nationwide study of Japan. *Jpn. J. Clin. Oncol.*, **15**, 517–535 (1985).

18. Uchiyama, T., Yodoi, J., Sagawa, K., Takatsuki, K., and Uchino, H. Adult T-cell leukemia: Clinical and hematologic features of 16 cases. *Blood*, **50**, 481–491 (1977).

19. Yoshida, M., Miyoshi, I., and Hinuma, Y. Isolation and characterization of retrovirus from cell lines of human adult T-cell leukemia and its implication in the disease. *Proc. Natl. Acad. Sci. U.S.A.*, **79**, 2031–2035 (1982).

CHEMICAL RISK FACTORS FOR NASOPHARYNGEAL CARCINOMA (NPC)—A REVIEW

J. H-C. Ho

*Department of Radiotherapy and Oncology, Hong Kong Baptist Hospital**

From current epidemiological data, ingestants rather than inhalants are likely to be involved in the aetiology of nasopharyngeal carcinoma in southern Chinese who have the highest incidence of the cancer. Of the ingestants, salted fish fed during early childhood, a traditional food habit of southern Chinese, appears to be a major risk factor. The epidemiological and experimental evidence in support of this hypothesis has been reviewed.

Much epidemiological evidence indicates the importance of environmental risk factors in nasopharyngeal carcinoma (NPC). Mortality from NPC has declined in Chinese Americans of both sexes (10), and American-born, second-generation Chinese have been reported to have a lower risk for NPC than Orient-born first-generation Chinese (24). This could be due to a decline in traditional environmental influence on the risk. Although these studies involved small numbers, deficient census estimates, and possible confounding factors, such as influence on mortality by improvement in therapeutics and possible differences in the composition by dialect community groups and places of origin, the findings are in line with the California data by Zippin et al. (36), Buell (33), and Yu et al. (35), all pointing in the same direction. Furthermore, Buell (4) reported a higher than expected risk for NPC in white males who were born in the Philippines or in China of Caucasian stock with no Mongoloid admixture.

NPC has been known to be prevalent among Singapore Chinese as early as 1912 (30), and probably in Canton, now known as Guangzhou, in 1921 (32). It is, therefore, most likely that, if an environmental risk factor was involved, it is associated with the traditional rather than modern lifestyle of southern Chinese (16), and was one that southern Chinese brought along with them when they migrated to Singapore, Malaysia, and U.S.A. (15) to account for the high risk among the populations of Chinese stock in these countries. The question is whether the major risk factor is an inhalant or ingestant.

Inhalants

In 1924 Dobson (7) postulated that NPC in Chinese was caused by frequent and prolonged exposures to the smoke from burning grass, wood, tobacco, candles, incense (joss sticks), kerosene lamps, and lamps burning peanut oil in poorly ventilated houses. Later, his household smoke hypothesis received support from observations by workers in Kenya (5, 6). The evidence was reviewed by Ho (18, 19) who argued against the hypothesis basing his arguments on the following observations.

---

* Kowloontong, Kowloon, Hong Kong.

a)   A male preponderance in the disease when it is the females who are more exposed to household smoke.

b)   People who live and work in boats and cook in the open in Hong Kong have an NPC incidence rate significantly higher than those who dwell in congested quarters on land (*14, 20*).

c)   Southern Chinese who live in better ventilated dwellings in Singapore and Hong Kong have no less risk of developing NPC than their rural countrymen in China.

d)   Before World War II NPC was rare among Buddhist monks in Hangzhou although they spent much of their time in an incense-laden atmosphere (*31*), but the cancer was not rare in Catholic Macaonese (*19*) and Muslim Malays (*27*), neither of whom burn Chinese incense.

Lin *et al.* (*26*) in a case-control study in Taiwan noted a significant excess of smokers among patients, and that working under poorly ventilated conditions enhanced the risk, as did the use of herbal drugs and nasal balms or oils. In this study the controls were chosen from neighbours of the NPC patients. Unfortunately, the place of origin and the period of stay in the neighbourhood were not matched, and it is well known that Chinese of different places of origin have different risks for the disease. Furthermore, working in a poorly ventilated atmosphere is unlikely to explain the high risk found in people who work and live on boats. The steep rise in the age-specific incidence after 20–24 years of age is also incompatible with an occupational hypothesis (*17, 20*).

Ingestants

Southern Chinese who had settled overseas retained both a high risk of NPC and their food culture and this applies particularly to the consumption of Cantonese salted fish (*19, 20*). Fisherfolks in Hong Kong who have the highest risk for NPC consume salted fish more frequently than land–dwelling Chinese but fewer fresh vegetables and fruit, sources of vitamin C which is known to block nitrosation of amines in the upper gastrointestinal tract (*18*). Many carcinogens, *e.g.*, the nitrosamines, are organotropic when they enter the blood stream after ingestion. Consequently, a cancer developing in a part of the respiratory tract does not necessarily exclude a causal factor derived from ingestants.

To narrow down the enormous number of possible risk factors to be examined the important or critical period, if there is one, of exposure to such factors has first to be identified.

Ho (*18*) compared the male age-specific incidence curves for NPC for Hong Kong Chinese (1965–1969), Singapore Chinese (1950–1961), and for Swedes (1959–1965). In the case of Swedes only transitional cell, squamous, and undifferentiated carcinomas were included. The curves for Chinese in Hong Kong and Singapore showed in common a rapid sustained rise after 20–24 years of age to a peak at 45–54 years, after which the curves begin to decline. This would suggest that the disease in Chinese is unlikely to be due to a continued exposure to an external carcinogen throughout life, as is postulated for most epithelial cancer, *e.g.*, cigarette smoking and bronchial carcinoma of the squamous and small cell type. The curve for Swedes showed, on the other hand, a sustained rise in incidence from 40–44 years of age to 70–74, similar to one encountered in bronchial cancer. The curves for American whites and blacks showed a rise after the third decade of life to a peak at the seventh decade (21). Thus the aetiology of NPC in Swedes and American whites and blacks may differ substantially from that in Chinese. There has been no change in the shape of the age-specific incidence curves for Hong Kong Chinese for three successive five-year periods from 1960 (7), indicating that the environmental determinant, if there is one, was still with the population at least 3 decades ago, if we allow for an average latency period of 20 years or more between initiation of carcinogenesis and clinical diagnosis. By the same reasoning, the steep rise in incidence rates after the age of 20–24 years is an indication that the critical period of exposure to the environmental risk factors is most likely to be in early childhood.

A study of feeding and weaning in Hong Kong Chinese infants by Topley (33) revealed that among traditional foods frequently fed to them in the weaning and post-weaning periods was salted fish added to congee, a rice porridge. A retrospective study of the early environmental backgrounds of young Chinese patients with NPC diagnosed before the age of 25 years found salted fish was the most commonly eaten among the traditional foods fed to them when they were babies (1). As it is impossible for adults to recall their early childhood environments, the results of this study fill an important gap in our knowledge of the most important period of life where the aetiology of NPC is concerned. Twenty-four Chinese NPC patients were interviewed in the study, 22 of them in the presence of their families and 16 in their homes. An interview lasted 2 to 4 hr. It followed a set pattern but was not standardized and did not involve a questionnaire, because it was felt that such less obviously formal interviewing would permit more detailed probing enquiry, especially with regard to follow up of items of interest. A questionnaire covering the same material would be formidably long, daunting the most cooperative of correspondents. Leading questions were scrupulously avoided. Although it is regretted that limited funds did not allow for matched controls to be included in the study, an analysis of results eliminated household inhalants, aerial contaminants, medicines, food therapy, spices, fresh foods, and soya sauce as likely factors in the carcinogenesis. The only foods other than salted fish eaten by all the patients were laap cheung (Cantonese pork sausage), and tau si (a black fermented product made of salted soya bean), but salted fish was most commonly eaten and the only one fed to babies. Furthermore, in childhood they had rarely or never been fed vegetables or fruits, and also most characteristically they had been since childhood sickly, inactive, withdrawn, and choosy about their food. The study concluded that consumption of salted fish and vitamin-C deficiency in early childhood appeared to be important environmental factors.

In Hong Kong a case-control study of the socioeconomic status, past health and food habits of 150 NPC patients and 150 age- and sex-matched controls consisting of patients with other cancers hospitalized in Queen Elizabeth Hospital undertaken by a team of workers from the IARC (11) collaborating with workers in our institute disclosed that salted fish was given to babies just after weaning more often in households with an NPC patient than in control households. A multivariate analysis of the data collected showed that traditional lifestyle and the consumption of salted fish during weaning were independent risk factors for NPC. The other factors that were found to be positively associated with the disease were: belonging to the four lowest occupational classes; practising Buddhism or ancestral worship and having religious altars in the house; and having a history of previous illnesses of the ear or nose after the age of 15 years. The last factor could be related to the beginning of the clinical manifestation of the disease or a tendency to recall symptoms associated with the disease by patients, and is, therefore, of doubtful significance. Factors found to be negatively associated were the eating of bread and tinned food and the use of spices.

In Japan Hirayama (12) studied the correlation between the age-adjusted incidence rate for NPC and the consumption of animal protein, fruits, salted fish as indicated by the ratio of salted fish to the daily intake of raw fish, and the number of Chinese per 100,000 in the population in 9 districts in Japan. He found a negative correlation between NPC incidence and animal protein or fruit consumption, but a relatively high positive correlation (correlation coeficient $r=0.711$) for salted fish consumption, which was higher than that for the proportion of Chinese in the population ($r=0.579$).

In a case-control study carried out in Alaska by Lanier et al. (25) among natives consisting of Eskimos, Aleuts, and Indians, who have a risk for NPC intermediate between the high risk for southern Chinese and the low one for Caucasians, the NPC patients in response to a questionnaire more often reported the use of salted fish in their childhood diet, but the difference was not statistically significant. The Eskimos in Greenland, who have about 30% admixture with Danes (28), also have an intermediate risk for NPC. It would be interesting to carry out a case-control study among them to determine whether they have the same food habits as those in Alaska.

The finding of a high geographic similarity seen in the distribution of *Croton tiglium*, the parent plant for croton oil, as well as other related members of the Euphorbiaceae family, the seeds of which are being used currently as a purgative in southern parts of China, and NPC has led Hirayama and Ito (13) to suspect an aetiological relationship between croton oil and NPC. In their laboratory studies they found that Epstein-Barr virus (EBV)-carrying P3HR-1 and Raji cells showed a dramatic increase in EBV antigens when given a combined treatment with *n*-butyrate and croton oil in nanogram concentrations, and that *Fusobacterium* and other common microbacterial inhabitants of the mouth and nasopharynx of man efficiently produce, in laboratory culture fluids, *n*-butyric acid with EBV-inducer activity. Based on these findings, they hypothesize that NPC is initiated by persisting EBV as an essential basic factor plus the combined action of bacterial fatty acid and traditional intake of promoter substance of plant origin as cofactors, and that the EBV, induced and activated by the mechanisms, initiates the chain of events which ultimately lead to the development of the cancer.

That EBV plays a role as a cofactor in the genesis of NPC has not been established. We still do not know whether DNA of the virus regularly demonstrated in undifferentiated and poorly differentiated NPC cells play a driver's or passenger's role. EBV is an ubiquitous virus and excretion of the virus in the saliva is not confined to southern Chinese. Croton oil bean is undoubtedly being used as a purgative, but the use is not confined to southern parts of China, where NPC is prevalent. Furthermore, because it is a drastic purgative, it is never given to babies or young children. When swallowed it is always quickly washed down with fluids, and its use is very sparing. Consequently, even if an aetiological link between the use of croton oil and NPC exists, it cannot be a strong one.

Armstrong et al. (2) in an epidemiological study of 100 southern Chinese NPC patients and 100 neighbourhood controls in Malaysia found daily consumption of salted fish carried a relative risk (RR) of 17.4 (95% confidence interval=2.7, 111.1) compared with non-consumption. Another study by Yu et al. (34) involving 250 incident cases of southern Chinese patients younger than 35 years of age to ensure a better recall of childhood events and an equal number of friends as controls in Hong Kong showed that the RR for consuming the food at least once a week compared with less than once a month at 10 years of age was 37.7 (95% confidence interval=14.1, 100.4). In this latter study, because the subjects were young many had mothers who could be separately interviewed to check the data obtained from their children. In both studies the cases and controls were sex- and age-matched to within 5 years.

Experimental Evidence in Support of the Salted Fish Hypothesis

Salted fish, uncooked and cooked, has been shown to contain volatile nitrosamines, principally N-nitrosodemethylamine (NDMA) and N-nitrosodiethylamine (NDEA). They are potent procarcinogens in laboratory animals, but their levels were less than 1 μg/kg in most specimens tested and no higher than those encountered in cured meat consumed in Europe (22). It is, however, unique that salted fish is fed to southern Chinese children from infancy, wheras cured meat is consumed by older children and adults among Europeans. Until recently the traditional diet of southern Chinese babies has been peculiarly lacking in variety during weaning, consisting mainly of fresh or salted fish meat added to congee. This lack in variety that might have excluded protective substances, e.g., vitamin-C, in the diet, the frequency of feeding the same carcinogenic agents, and the greater susceptibility of growing tissue in the young may explain the difference in risk. It may also explain Buell's observation (3) that there was a more than expected risk of NPC in pure white males of Caucasian stock born in the Philippines or China, and the development of NPC in three patients of mixed Caucasian and Chinese parentage who were brought up on a predominantly Cantonese type diet (20).

Experiments have shown that Wistar albino (WA) rats fed steamed salted fish would regularly pass urine with mutagenic activity as shown by the Ames test (36) using *Salmonella typhimurium* TA 98 and TA 100 (9). Purchase et al. (29) considered the test to be about 90% accurate in detecting a variety of chemical carcinogens as mutagens. It may, therefore, be presumed that the mutagenic activity in the urine of the experimental rats was derived from the salted fish diet which had caused mutagens, and very probably car cinogens as well, to enter the blood circulation and became excreted by the kidneys into the urine. To see whether such an event occurs also in men, it would not be unethical to apply the test to southern Chinese adults who had eaten much salted fish in the past. So far this has not been done.

Some of the WA rats so fed as a part of their diet for 12–24 months developed invasive carcinomas in their nasal and paranasal regions, whereas none of the control rats fed normal rat chow developed carcinoma (23).

It is difficult to extrapolate animal experimental findings to men, in whom all we can do is to demonstrate what could have occurred and not what did occur. It is possible that men may react likewise when salted fish is consumed, but whether such circulating carcinogens will in due course cause NPC is impossible to say. That such a possibility may occur in certain individuals as a result of combined action with other cofactors is very real in view of the strong epidemiological evidence in support.

It is of special significance that chemical analysis has shown the presence of NDMA and NDEA in the aqueous phase during steaming of salted fish. Since southern Chinese frequently steam their salted fish on top of rice in a cooking utensil with the lid on, some of the aqueous phase containing nitrosamines could as condensate find its way into the

rice and be consumed by someone unknowingly. Chemical carcinogens, including nitrosamines, often find their way into the milk during suckling and they can also pass
through the placenta (8). In designing questionnaires in epidemiological studies these
possiblities should be borne in mind.

Prevention and Outlook

Since there is now evidence to support that salted fish consumption during early
childhood is a major risk factor in southern Chinese, these people should be advised not
to feed their babies and young children this food. Tradition dies hard, but fortunately
hard economics have an even stronger influence. Formerly salted fish was for economic
reasons a very important item of food, especially among the poor. Now not only more
cheap dairy products are available, but also salted fish has become more expensive than
chicken. Consequently, the traditional habit is fast disappearing. The trend began in the
nineteen fifties in Hong Kong. It is tempting to attribute the progressive fall in the annual mortality rates for NPC during 1975–1984 from 15.1 per 100,000 to 12.4 for males
and from 5.6 to 4.0 for females to this food trend.

Acknowledgments
I am grateful to members of the staff of the Medical and Health Department Institute
of Radiology and Oncology for their valuable assistance in my previous epidemiological and
experimental studies on nasopharyngeal carcinoma and to Ms. Grace Ma of the Hong Kong
Baptist Hospital for her secretarial assistance.

REFERENCES

1. Anderson, E. N., Jr., Anderson, M. L., and Ho, J.H.C. Environmental backgrounds of
    young Chinese nasopharyngeal carcinoma patients. *In* "Nasopharyngeal Carcinoma:
    Etiology and Control," eds. G. de-Thé and Y. Ito, IARC Scientific Publications No. 20,
    pp. 231–239 (1978). IARC, Lyon.
2. Armstrong, R. W., Armstrong, M. J., Yu, M. C., and Henderson, B. Salted fish and in-
    halants as risk factors for nasopharyngeal carcinoma. *Cancer Res.*, **43**, 2967–2970 (1983).
3. Buell, P. Nasopharyngeal cancer in Chinese of California. *Br. J. Cancer*, **19**, 459–470
    (1965).
4. Buell, P. Race and place in the etiology of nasopharyngeal cancer: a study based on Cali-
    fornia death certificates. *Int. J. Cancer*, **11**, 268–272 (1973).
5. Clifford, P. Malignant disease of the nasopharynx and paranasal sinuses in Kenya. *In*
    "Cancer of the Nasopharynx, UICC Monograph Series 1," eds. C. S. Muir and K.
    Shanmugaratnam, pp. 82–94 (1967). Munksgaard, Copenhagen.
6. Clifford, P. and Beecher, J. L. Nasopharyngeal cancer in Kenya. Clinical and environmen-
    tal aspects. *Br. J. Cancer*, **18**, 25–43 (1964).
7. Dobson, W. C. Cervical lymphosarcoma. *China Med. J.*, **38**, 786 (1924).
8. Editorial: Transplacental carcinogenesis. *Lancet*, **i**, 1425 (1973).
9. Fong, L.Y.Y., Ho, J.H.C., and Huang, D. P. Preserved foods as possible cancer hazards:
    WA rats fed salted fish have mutagenic urine. *Int. J. Cancer*, **23**, 315–328 (1978).
10. Fraumeni, J. F., Jr. and Mason, T. J. Cancer mortality among Chinese Americans. *J.
    Natl. Cancer Inst.*, **52**, 659–665 (1974).
11. Geser, A., Charney, N., Day, N. E., Ho, H. C., and de-Thé, G. Environmental factors in
    the etiology of nasopharyngeal carcinoma: Report on a case-control study in Hong Kong.

In "Nasopharyngeal Carcinoma: Etiology and Control," eds. G. de-Thé and Y. Ito, IARC Scientific Publications No. 20, pp. 213–229 (1978). IARC, Lyon.

12. Hirayama, T. Descriptive and analytical epidemiology of nasopharyngeal cancer. *In* "Nasopharyngeal Carcinoma: Etiology and Control," eds. G. de-Thé and Y. Ito, IARC Scientific Publications No. 20, pp. 167–189 (1978). IARC, Lyon.

13. Hirayama, T. and Ito, Y. New view of the etiology of nasopharnygeal carcinoma. *Prevent. Med.*, **10**, 614–622 (1981).

14. Ho, H. C. Nasopharnygeal carcinoma in Hong Kong. *In* "Cancer of the Nasopharynx, UICC Monograph Series 1," eds. C. S. Muir and K. Shanmugaratnam, pp. 29–63 (1967). Munksgaard, Copenhagen.

15. Ho, H. C. Epidemiology of nasopharyngeal carcinoma. *J. R. Coll. Surg. Edin.*, **20**, 223–235 (1975).

16. Ho, H. C. Current knowledge of the epidemiology of nasopharyngeal carcinoma—a review. *In* "Oncogenesis and Herpes Virus," eds. P. M. Biggs, G. de-Thé, and L. N. Payne, IARC Scientific Publications No. 2, pp. 357–366 (1972). IARC, Lyon.

17. Ho, H. C. Epidemiology of nasopharyngeal carcinoma. *Gann Monogr. Cancer Res.*, **18**, 49–61 (1976).

18. Ho, J.H.C. Genetic and environmental factors in nasopharyngeal carcinoma. *In* "Recent Advances in Human Tumor Virology and Immunology," eds. W. Nakahara, K. Nishioka, T. Hirayama, and Y. Ito, pp. 275–295 (1971). Japan Sci. Soc. Press ,Tokyo.

19. Ho, J.H.C. Nasopharyngeal carcinoma (NPC). *Adv. Cancer Res.*, **15**, 57–92 (1972).

20. Ho, J.H.C. An epidemiologic and clinical study of nasopharyngeal carcinoma. *Int. J. Rad. Oncol. Biol. Phys.*, **4**, 181–198 (1978).

21. Ho, J.H.C., Chan, C. L., Lau, W. H., Au, G.K.H., and Koo, L. C. Cancer in Hong Kong: Some epidemiological observations. *Natl. Cancer Inst. Monogr.*, **62**, 47–55 (1982).

22. Huang, D. P., Ho, J.H.C., Gough, T. A., and Webb, K. S. Volatile nitrosamines in some traditional Chinese food products. *J. Fd. Safety*, **1**, 1–6 (1977).

23. Huang, D. P., Saw, D., Teoh, T. B., and Ho, J.H.C. Carcinoma of nasal and paranasal regions in rats fed Cantonese salted fish. *In* "Nasopharyngeal Carcinoma: Etiology and Control," eds. G. de-Thé and Y. Ito, IARC Scientific Publications No. 20, pp. 315–328 (1978). IARC, Lyon.

24. King, H. and Haenszel, W. Cancer mortality among foreign and native-born Chinese in the United States. *J. Chronic Dis.*, **26**, 623–646 (1972).

25. Lanier, A., Bender, T., Talbot, M., Wilmeth, S., Tshopp, C., Henle, W., Henle, G., Ritter, D., and Terasaki, P. Nasopharyngeal carcinoma in Alaskan Eskimos, Indians, and Aleuts: a review of cases and study of Epstein-Barr virus, HLA, and environmental risk factors. *Cancer*, **46**, 2100–2106 (1960).

26. Lin, T. M., Chen, K. P., Lin, C. C., Hsu, M. M., Tu, S. M., Chiang, T. C., Jung, P. F., and Hirayama, T. Retrospective study on nasopharyngeal carcinoma. *J. Natl. Cancer Inst.*, **51**, 1403–1408 (1973).

27. Muir, C. S. Nasopharyngeal carcinoma in non-Chinese population. *In* "Oncogenesis and Herpes Virus," eds. P. M. Biggs, G. de-Thé, and L. N. Payne, IARC Scientific Publications No. 2, pp. 367–371 (1972). IARC, Lyon.

28. Nielsen, N. H., Mikkelsen, F., and Hansen, J. P. Nasopharyngeal cancer in Greenland. *Acta Pathol. Microbiol. Scand.*, **85**, 850–858 (1977).

29. Purchase, I.F.H., Longstapf, E., Ashby, J., Styles, J. A., Anderson, D., Lefevre, P. A., and Westwood, F. R. An evaluation of six short-tests for detecting organic chemical carcinogens. *Br. J. Cancer*, **37**, 873–960 (1978).

30. Shanmugaratnam, K. Studies on the etiology of nasopharyngeal carcinoma. *Int. Rev. Exp. Pathol.*, **10**, 361–413 (1971).

31. Sturton, S. D., Wen, H. L., and Sturton, O. G. Etiology of cancer of the naspoharynx. *Cancer*, **19**, 1666–1669 (1966).

32. Todd, P. J. Some practical points in the surgical treatment of cervical tumours. *China Med. J.*, **35**, 21–25 (1921).

33. Topley, M. Cultural and social factors relating to Chinese infant feeding and weaning. *In* "Growing Up in Hong Kong," eds. C. E. Field and F. M. Barber, pp. 56–65 (1973). Hong Kong University Press, Hong Kong.

34. Yu, M. C., Ho, J.H.C., Lai, S. H., and Henderson, B. Cantonese style salted fish as a cause of nasopharyngeal carcinoma: Report of a case-control study in Hong Kong. *Cancer Res.*, **46**, 956–961 (1986).

35. Yu, M. C., Ho, J.H.C., Ross, R. K., and Henderson, B. Nasopharyngeal carcinoma in Chinese salted fish or inhaled smoke? *Prevent. Med.*, **10**, 15–24 (1981).

36. Zippin, C., Tekawa, I. S., Bragg, K. U., Watson, D. A., and Linden, G. Studies on heredity and environment in cancer of the nasopharynx. *J. Natl. Cancer Inst.*, **29**, 483–490 (1962).

OCCUPATIONAL LUNG CANCER IN A TIN MINE IN SOUTH CHINA

Yan Sun

Cancer Institute and Hospital, Chinese Academy of Medical Sciences

Over the past three decades it has been widely recognized that the incidence of lung cancer has been rapidly increasing and is one of the most challenging problems in public health in China. During the past 20 years, an excess of lung cancer has been noticed among workers in a tin mine in South China. The present paper briefly reviews the data of an epidemiological study, mass survey, clinical features, as well as the etiological studies of that occupational lung cancer.

According to a nationwide survey of cancer mortality, lung cancer ranks third in the male population and forth in the female population. A map of the geographic distribution of the mortality rates of lung cancer in different regions shows that they vary widely in China. Several high incidence areas have been found. The mortality of lung cancer in the northeast and some big cities along the coast is much higher than that of other parts. Actually, lung cancer ranks first among common malignancies in Beijing, Shanghai, Tianjin, and some industrial cities. Near the border of South China, in Yunnan province, there are two hot-spots. One of them is a rural lung cancer high incidence area, Xuanwei county, and the other is a tin mine in Gejiu city.

In historical records dating from 2,000 years ago, the Gejiu area was famous for its production of tin. During the mid of 1960s, an excess of lung cancer was noticed among workers in the Yunnan Tin Mine Corporation. Since 1975, the Cancer Institute and Hospital, Chinese Academy of Medical Sciences and the Institute of Health of Chinese Center of Preventive Medicine have been deeply involved in the study of epidemiology, etiology, mass survey, early detection,t reatment, and prevention in that area. A department of oncology in the hospital and an institute were established in Gejiu to carry out clinical and research work on occupational lung cancer.

Epidemiology and Etiology

The average mortality rate of lung cancer in Yunnan province was rather low, 2.60 per 100,000 population, but among workers in the tin mine it was as high as 108.57 per 100,000 during 1973–1975. During recent years, the incidence and mortality of lung cancer have become even higher.

Epidemiologic study shows that during 1954–1983 the incidence of lung cancer was 31.82 to 531.91 (average 308.39) per 100,000, the mortality rate was 20.68 to 517.49 (average 263.29) for workers with a history of mining; that for workers without a history of mining was 4.83 to 39.83 (average 25.48) and 0.00 to 39.83 (average 22.95) per 100,000, respectively (Table I).

---

* Chaoyangqu, Beijing, China.

TABLE I.   Incidence and Mortality from Lung Cancer in Yunnan Tin Mine Corporation, 1954–1983

Year	1954–1959	1960–1964	1965–1969	1970–1974	1975–1979	1980–1983
Miners						
Incidence	31.82	140.16	219.34	390.33	473.12	531.91
Mortality	20.68	98.75	217.61	316.88	358.30	517.49
Non-miners						
Incidence	4.83	11.98	23.83	34.35	32.11	39.83
Mortality	0.00	10.89	23.83	29.14	28.33	39.83

TABLE II.   Relative Risk (RR) of Lung Cancer in Different Occupations

Occupations	Incidence	RR	Mortality	RR
Mining alone	414.08	13.32	359.20	13.48
Melting alone	86.90	2.80	66.80	2.51
Mining+Melting	1,180.30	37.96	729.20	27.38
Others	31.09	1	26.65	1

TABLE III.   Age of Workers Starting to Work in the Mine and the Incidence of Lung Cancer

<15	971.03
15–	171.23
20–	146.31

It is evident that the incidence and mortality of lung cancer among workers have increased markedly over time. In the decades of the sixties, in the Tin Mine Corporation Hospital 8.7% of all deaths were due to this cause. In 1970–1974, the figure became 17.2%, and in 1975–1979 it reached 20.24%. During the past 30 years, 1,448 cases were diagnosed as lung cancer, and 1,253 of them have already died. Among the common malignancies, lung cancer ranks first, and composes 77.86% of all cancer deaths.

The average age of lung cancer patients in the mine is about 55 (19–78), which is 5 years younger than the lung cancer patients in other parts of China. The latent period plus the preclinical stage to the clinical stage is estimated to be about 25–30 years.

The incidence varies with types of employment. Miners and workers with a history of mining have significantly more lung cancer than workers without such a history. Incidence among workers with a history of mining plus melting was as high as 1,180.30 per 100,000. That shows there might be some synergistic carcinogenic factors or promoters in their working environment (Table II).

It can be seen that the younger the age when the workers started mining, the higher the risk of developing lung cancer (Table III). Also, the years employed in mining is an important factor influencing the risk of developing lung cancer (Table IV). From the epidemiologic study, we learned that workers who started to work before the 1940s have a much higher incidence of lung cancer than those who started working after the 1950s; during that time the working conditions improved gradually.

Our preliminary conclusion is that the etiologic factor or factors must exist in the working environment, especially in mining and melting; thus, this is an occupational lung cancer. Yunnan Tin Mine is a multiple metal mine. Several etiologic factors are suspected and studied, principally arsenic, radon, and tobacco smoking. The concentra-

TABLE IV. Years Employed Mining and the Incidence of Lung Cancer

<5	148.9
5–	148.8
10–	282.9
15–	408.6
20–	817.5
25–	1,003.3
30–	1,694.9

TABLE V. Experimental Induction of Lung Cancer in Rats

Group	No. animals	Dys-plasia	Precan-cerous	Lung cancer			Others
				Squamous	Adeno	Mixed	
Control	40	0	0	0	0	0	Lung adenoma 1
As containing ores[a]	112	84	34	13	8	1	Hepatoma 2
Radon inhalation[b]	100	77	11	17	2	3	Lung adenoma 2

[a] 6–10 mg/day×15.
[b] Total dosage 800–3,000 WLM.

TABLE VI. Cumulative Exposure to Arsenic and Mortality from Lung Cancer

Exposure (months)	Mortality of lung cancer		O/E
	Expected	Observed	
<5	2.3454	9	3.84
5–	1.4422	10	6.93
10–	3.3065	28	8.47
30–	2.4318	28	11.51
50–	1.6853	29	17.21
70–	0.9841	26	26.42
90–	0.7908	23	26.08
110–	0.3125	8	25.60
150–	0.1223	4	32.72

TABLE VII. Cumulative Exposure to Radon Daughters and Mortality from Lung Cancer

Dosage exposed (WLM)	Mortality of lung cancer		O/E
	Expected	Observed	
<100	3.6774	12	3.26
100–	3.7475	14	3.74
200–	3.6365	53	14.57
400–	2.3530	51	22.64
600–	0.7769	17	21.98
800–	0.5904	2	20.33
1,000–	0.0938	4	42.46
1,500–	0.0233	2	86.02

tions (mg/m^2) of several metals in the dust powder in the mine are as follows: arsenic 0.0016–0.0147, iron 0.267–0.317, cobalt 0.000026–0.0001, chrome 0.0004–0.0016, cadmium 0.00005–0.00017, nickel 0.00005–0.00038. Over 90% of the dust was less than 10 μm.

In experiments conducted on rats, squamous carcinoma resulted from intra-tracheal infusion of original ores (mainly oxide and sulfate) in 14%, adenocarcinoma in 4.7%, and mixed carcinoma in 1.9% of 212 rats, while none of the 40 rats in the control group, which received normal saline, developed carcinoma (Table V). When two factors were combined, 71.8% of the hamsters developed lung cancer, mainly adenocarcinoma.

Chemical analysis of lung tissue from cancer patients in the mine revealed the arsenic level to be 4 to 100 (average 20.76) times higher than in other persons. Multiple skin keratoses and cancer are also common in the Gejiu area.

The levels of radioactivity from radon and its daughters, the average being 1.1–4.07 units and 0.38–2.38 working level months (WLM) respectively, are also much higher than the normal permissible level in the mine. When the cumulative doses to workers reached 200 WLM, the mortality rates of lung cancer rise 14.57–86.02 times, in proportion to the dosage (Tables VI and VII).

The majority of workers were heavy smokers during their teen years. We compared the incidence of lung cancer among the workers with a history of mining: for smokers it was 525.1, and for non-smokers it was 370.50; for those without a history of mining, it was 59.2 and 0 per 100,000, respectively. But, in 50 patients with short histories of mining, less than 10 years, the majority had smoked for more than 20 years. This means that although smoking does not play an important role in the majority of paitents in that local area, it might be an important factor or co-factor in carcinogenesis in some patients.

Other factors such as nutrition, dietary habits, as well as genetic and immunologic factors are also under investigation.

Clinical Study

Analysis of 916 cases of lung cancer seen at the Department of Oncology revealed that there 874 male (95.4%) and 42 female patients. Among them, 718 (78.4%) were miners 558 (77.7%) had worked underground for more than 10 years, and 712 (99.1%) were smokers. The average patient's age was 55.4 years. Clinically and roentgenologically, 74% of all patients had lung cancer of the central type. Among 403 cases proved by histological examination, there were 269 (66.8%) squamous, 67 (16.6%) small cell, 38 (9.4%) adeno, 11 (2.7%) alveolar, 8 (2%) mixed, 6 large cell, and 6 (1.5%) unclassified carcinomas.

TABLE VIII.   Results of the Mass Survey in Yunnan Tin Mine Corp. (1973–1983)

Years	No. employees entered	No. employees examined	% examined	No. lung cancers	Incidence[a]	No. lung cancer pts. in that year
1973–76	36,574	33,719	92.19	42	124.56	280/4
1977	27,357	21,492	78.51	17	79.10	75
1978	12,748	8,966	70.33	12	133.84	81
1979	7,069	4,634	65.55	12	258.96	77
1980	10,795	6,995	64.80	18	257.33	93
1982	7,450	6,956	93.37	41	589.42	124
1983	8,213	7,644	93.10	42	549.31	98
1984	11,148	10,351	92.53	59	571.98	91[b]

[a] Number of cancer/number examined × 100,000.
[b] Until Nov. 11, 1984.

Since 1974, there were 67 cases of occult carcinoma not detected by chest films, the exfoliative cytology of sputum being positive but routine chest X-ray film negative. Fifty of these have been localized through careful endoscopic, tomographic, and bronchographic examinations. For patients diagnosed in early stages, the results of treatment are rather good.

Mass screening has been carried out every year (Table VIII). Only half of the cancers were detected during the screening, including some early cases and occult cancer.

Some preventive modalities such as retinoic acid and Chinese herbs Sophora subprostrats Chun et T. Chen are being studied and there is some change in the sputum cytology in the treated group as compared with a control group of selected workers with precancerous diseases.

Ongoing Research and Future Plans for Study of Tin Miner's Lung Cancer

In 1984, a research committee was organized for the Tin Miner's lung cancer project and the following research is just getting under way:

1.   Comparison of different mines in China to reveal further the occupational factors in Yunnan Tin Miner's lung cancer;

2.   Histological and electron microscopic scanning studies of lung cancer to observe possible etiologic particles of different metals deposited in the patient's lung tissue;

3.   Case-control study of lung cancer patients to reveal factors influencing carcinogenesis of the lung;

4.   Blood and hair analysis for different metals and nutrients in workers to reveal possible nutritional factors and metals in carcinogenesis;

5.   Experimental study of the induction of lung cancer in animals using related factors or co-factors;

6.   Computerized multiple analysis of related factors in the genesis of lung cancer;

7.   Methods, frequency and efficacy of mass screening for high-risk (male, over 40 years employed in mining over 10 years, smoker) and ultra-high-risk (male, over 45 years, employed in mining or smelting over 20 years, smoker) populations;

8.   Kinetic observation of tumor markers and immunological parameters;

9.   Method to localize the lesion in early stage;

10.   Protocols of multi-modality treatment for different types and stages of lung cancer;

11.   Chemoprevention for the high-risk population.

ETIOLOGIC CLUES FROM CANCER MAPPING IN THE UNITED STATES

Joseph F. Fraumeni, Jr.

*Division of Cancer Etiology, National Cancer Institute**

A series of etiologic clues have been generated from the geographic patterns of cancer at the county level in the United States. This review describes how leads to the determinants of several cancers have been identified through cancer mapping and correlation studies, and it emphasizes their pursuit through case-control studies conducted in high-risk areas of the country.

A landmark achievement of Professor Mitsuo Segi was the development and utilization of mortality and incidence statistics to elucidate the demographic patterns of cancer, thus generating a series of new clues to its etiology. His monographs on cancer occurrence in various countries documented striking international variation for many common cancers. Although some of the global variations may be influenced by a genetic component and by reporting practices in different countries, the major impact of environmental factors was indicated by the patterns of risk among migrant populations, such as the Japanese who moved to Hawaii and California. Stimulated by Professor Segi's observations, Haenszel and Kurihara (18) demonstrated that as migrant groups adopt customs of the new land, their risk of various cancers shifts away from the rate prevailing in the country of origin to approximate that of the host country. The change in incidence for some cancers, notably the colon, was evident within two or three decades of migration, wheras the change for other cancers, notably the breast, required more than one generation. Thus, the international and migrant patterns suggested to many observers that the bulk of human cancer results from environmental influences, including lifestyle practices, and that a large fraction of cancer is potentially preventable.

Cancer Mapping

Although differences in cancer risk within nations have generally been less impressive or informative than international variations, the epidemiology group at the U.S. National Cancer Institute was struck by the fact that many etiologic leads have come from clinical observations of unusual case clusters in small groups of individuals over short periods. It was possible to detect these clusters on clinical grounds because they involved cancers that are ordinarily rare in the general population. We decided to try a systematic approach to evaluate clustering of the more common tumors by examining patterns of cancer mortality at the county level, where the population is small enough to be relatively homogeneous, yet large enough to provide reliable data and stable rates. Our analyses revealed a surprising number and variety of geographic patterns, and some

---

* Bethesda, MD 20892, U.S.A.

cancers displayed so-called "hot spots" that generated not only scientific interest but also public and political concern (7, 17).

Our geographic studies have involved a stepwise approach. First, using mortality data for the 20-year period 1950–1969, age-adjusted rates were calculated by sex and race for 35 cancers in each of the 3,056 counties of the U.S. These were published in a directory of county-by-county rates (23). As might be expected, these tables amounted to a rather unexciting inventory. However, when the rates were plotted in a series of computer-generated maps, the information seemed to come to life and patterns emerged that were sometimes unexpected and provocative. Atlases were published for the white population in 1975 (24) and the non-white population in 1976 (25). For the more common tumors, the maps are now being updated to cover deaths through the 1970s. In addition, an atlas was published for non-neoplastic diseases, with emphasis on conditions that may be etiologically related to cancer (22).

Secondly, the county cancer rates have been correlated with demographic, industrial, and environmental data available at the county level. Despite their limitations, these surveys have helped to refine the etiologic clues produced by the maps and to generate further hypotheses.

Finally, in collaboration with other research groups, we have embarked upon field studies in various parts of the U.S. with unusually high mortality rates. These are mostly case-control studies in which individuals with and without a particular cancer are interviewed for lifetime histories of residence, occupation, smoking, diet, and other suspected risk factors. Comparisons between cases and controls are then made in an attempt to identify the factors responsible for the high cancer rates in certain areas. The approach resembles that taken by Haenszel et al. (19) in case-control studies among migrant and other populations found to have unusual risks.

Lung Cancer

The maps for lung cancer attracted early interest. Among white males, mortality rates were high in New York, New Jersey, and the urban northeast but were even higher in certain seaboard areas of the south. Clusters of elevated rates were seen along the Gulf Coast from Texas to the Florida panhandle, and along the southeast Atlantic coast from Virginia to northern Florida. The excess in urbanized areas of the northeast appeared consistent with patterns of cigarette smoking. However, occupational factors were suspected for the coastal excesses, since the clustering was limited to males, and some correlations were found with industries often seen along the coast, including chemicals, petroleum, paper and pulp mills, and shipbuilding (4). Although only a few areas in the U.S. now have shipyards, it is noteworthy that ship construction and repair was the largest manufacturing industry during World War II, with a peak employment of 1.7 million people in late 1943 (12). Indeed among the 49 counties with large shipyards during the war, there was a consistent pattern of excess mortality rates for respiratory cancer during the period 1950–1969.

The southeast Atlantic coast was selected for three case-control interview studies of lung cancer. In coastal Georgia a significantly increased risk was associated with employment in area shipyards that operated during World War II and were then closed (10). The summary relative-risk estimate was 1.6 after adjusting for smoking, other occupations, and demographic variables. The risk was not limited to any single trade within the industry, such as insulators or pipecoverers who actually handle asbestos. However, there was a synergistic interaction between shipyard employment and tobacco smoking, with the risk for former shipyard workers who smoked heavily being 20 times higher than for nonsmokers who had never been employed in this industry. This is consistent with the multiplicative effect previously observed when asbestos exposures are combined with smoking.

In Tidewater, Virginia, large Navy and private shipyards were present during the war and continue to provide the major industry in the area (11). The relative risk of lung cancer, 1.7, associated with shipbuilding resembled that seen in Georgia, and the increase was primarily among men who began work during the war. In addition, a cluster of mesothelioma was detected among residents in this area, the incidence exceeding the national level by about 4-fold (34). Three-fourths of the cases worked in shipyards, mostly during the war. A high percentage were pipecoverers or pipefitters, but many other trades with presumably lighter exposures to asbestos were reported, suggesting that airborne fibers were not confined to the immediate areas of use. Indeed, among five women identified with mesothelioma in the area, four were wives of shipyard workers, indicating the spread of asbestos beyond the workplace.

In Jacksonville, Florida, which has the highest lung cancer rate of any urban county in the U.S., a strong association was again found with work in shipyards (2). However, an increased risk was seen also among construction workers, particularly those with asbestos exposure, and among workers in the lumber and wood industries, especially those with heavy exposure to wood dusts. Increased risks were also found among workers in the forestry and fishing industries, although the numbers were small. Another high-risk area for lung cancer on the Atlantic coast is Bath, Maine, and a small case-control study has confirmed an increased risk of 1.7 associated with shipbuilding, the major industry in that area since the turn of the century. By combining data from the four studies on the Atlantic coast, synergistic interactions between smoking and shipyard exposures are observed. Case-control studies of lung cancer are now underway in New Jersey, Louisiana, and on the Gulf coast of Texas to clarify the reasons for the high rates in these particular areas. Preliminary analyses of Louisiana data suggest an excess risk among the Cajun population, due at least partly to smoking practices, including the heavy use of hand-rolled cigarettes (28).

In 1969 we reported a cohort study of workers in a copper smelter located in Anaconda, Montana (20). There was an overall 3-fold increased risk of lung cancer, rising to 8-fold among a subgroup of workers most heavily exposed to arsenic trioxide. Thus, on the cancer maps it was not surprising to find a high rate of lung cancer in the county of Montana where the smelter is located, while the state had generally low rates. When we examined the distribution of lung cancer mortality in all U.S. counties with nonferrous primary smelters, we found elevated rates in areas with copper, lead, or zinc smelters which release arsenic during the smelting process, while the rates were not increased in counties with other smelting and refining operations (3). The rates were high in both sexes, suggesting that arsenical emissions from smelter stacks may pose a community risk.

To test this hypothesis a case-control interview study was carried out in the vicinity of a large zinc smelter and steel plant in eastern Pennsylvania (16). Relative risks were determined according to distance of residence from the smelter and the steel plant, and according to residence in areas with high and low levels of various pollutants as measured by soil samples. The risks for lung cancer were elevated among people living near the smelter and in areas with high levels of arsenic and cadmium. These increases in risk were not explained by the effects of smoking or occupational exposure. There was no excess of lung cancer associated with other pollutants or proximity to the steel plant, despite a substantial risk seen among long-term workers in the plant.

Nasal Cancer

Mortality rates for cancers of the nasal cavity and sinuses are about 1/100th of those for lung cancer, with no obvious clustering on the maps for males. For the less common cancers, state economic areas were used for mapping, but this larger unit impairs the sensitivity of the technique to identify clustering of areas with high rates. Since an excess risk of nasal cancer had been reported among furniture makers in England but not in the U.S., we carried out a correlation study among the male population of furniture-industry counties (15). There was an elevated mortality from nasal cancer in these areas, while the rates for most other cancers were at or below expected values, thus indicating the potential for correlation studies to detect occupational clustering not readily seen on the maps. To pursue this lead, we conducted a case-control interview study of nasal cancer in the high-exposure areas of North Carolina and Virginia (13). Employment in the furniture industry was not associated with squamous cell carcinomas, but it increased the risk of adenocarcinoma by 5-fold. In both sexes heavy cigarette smokers showed a 2- to 3-fold excess risk, mainly for squamous cell cancers, the first time that smoking has been linked to cancer of the nasal passages. Among females a 2-fold increased risk was associated with work in the textile industry, which may explain some clustering seen on the nasal cancer maps for females (14).

Bladder Cancer

The distribution of bladder cancer also seemed influenced by occupational exposures, with rates in males being particularly high in New Jersey and other sections of the northeast, in urban areas around the Great Lakes, in southern Louisiana, and in rural areas of New York and northern New England (5). A large case-control study of bladder cancer in several parts of the U.S., undertaken initially to evaluate the possible influence of artificial sweeteners, has been analyzed also for occupational factors, including those operating in high-risk areas. For example, in New Jersey an excess risk of bladder cancer has been identified for a variety of occupational groups associated with chemical and petrochemical exposures (31). In Detroit, an elevated risk of bladder cancer was found among truck drivers, with a significant trend related to increasing duration of employment (32). The relative risk was 5.5 for drivers employed at least 20 years, and 11.9 for drivers operating vehicles with diesel engines. Although the causal nature of this new association is uncertain, other areas participating in the national bladder cancer study have confirmed an excess risk among truck drivers and other groups exposed to motor vehicle exhausts (33).

In females the map for bladder cancer did not show the peculiarities seen in males, except for elevated rates in rural areas of New York and northern New England. Based on preliminary findings from a case-control study in New Hampshire and Vermont, this pattern may result in part from the employment of men and women in the textile and leather industries of this area.

Oral Cancer

One of the most provocative maps was for cancer of the mouth and throat. Among males there were elevated rates in the urban northeast where the levels are relatively high for smoking and alcohol intake, which have synergistic effects on the risk of oral cancer. Among females, however, the rates for oral cancer were highest in rural counties of the south. In a case-control interview study of women in North Carolina, over one-third of the cases were due to the long-standing practice of dipping snuff, that is, placing finely ground powdered tobacco in the mouth between the gum and the cheek (35). The risk of oral cancer associated with snuff among nonsmokers was 4-fold among chronic users, and approached 50-fold for cancers localized to the gum and buccal mucosa, the tissues in direct contact with snuff. The particular ingredient responsible for this risk is uncertain, but high levels of tobacco-specific nitrosamines have been identified in the snuff and saliva of snuff users. This hazard is of special concern in view of the recent upswing in the consumption of smokeless tobacco products in the U.S., the heavy advertising being directed toward young people, and some medical reports even encouraging these products as a substitute for cigarettes.

Esophageal Cancer

Although alcohol potentiates the effects of tobacco smoke on cancers of the esophagus as well as the oral cavity and larynx, it is unclear why the risks for esophageal cancer in the U.S. are so much higher among blacks than whites, especially black males in urban areas. The cancer maps showed that among black males the highest rates in the country occurred in Washington, D. C., exceeding the national level for black males by over 2-fold and for white males by 7-fold. In a case-control study in Washington, D.C., the dominant risk factor among black males was found to be alcohol consumption, which overwhelmed a smaller influence of smoking (30). In addition, an effect was associated with nutritional deficiency, even after adjusting for alcohol intake and socioeconomic status (37). The poor nutrition appeared to encompass a broad dietary deficiency, which could not be narrowed down to any particular food class or micronutrient. Thus, both alcohol consumption and dietary deficiencies appear to contribute to the unusual risk of esophageal cancer in black Americans.

Colorectal Cancer

International correlations and migrant studies have suggested that dietary factors are important in the development of colon and rectal cancers. In the U.S. there is a north/south gradient of colon cancer, with rates in both sexes being 50% lower in the south compared to the northeastern and north central areas of the country (9). It is interesting that lower rates in the south prevail even in areas attracting large numbers of retirees from the north. Is this a reversal of the pattern for colon cancer described among population groups moving from low- to high-risk areas? Preliminary data from a case-control study in Florida retirement communities suggest there is no rapid reduction in risk of colorectal cancer, but the younger the age at migration, the lower the risk (36). It remains to be seen what aspect of the southern environment, lifestyle, or diet may be protective.

Another opportunity for studying colon cancer was provided by an outlier from the usual geographic pattern, namely, a cluster of counties with high rates in a rural agricultural area of eastern Nebraska (29). A case-control interview study revealed that the elevated risk of colon cancer was primarily among persons of Czechoslovakian background, who predominate in the study area. Although our study had limited numbers, the elevated risk among Czechs seemed associated in part with high-fat diets derived from meat and dairy products, with beer drinking, and with familial occurrence of gastrointestinal and certain other cancers. It is noteworthy that recent maps do not show this geographic cluster, since the mortality and incidence rates for colon cancer in this area declined after 1970 to approach the national level, presumably as a consequence of acculturation.

Renal Cancer

Ethnic factors also contribute to the high death rates for kidney cancer in the north central parts of the U.S., as indicated by a case-control study in Minneapolis-St. Paul. For renal adenocarcinoma, which accounts for about 85% of kidney cancer, we found an elevated risk associated with German or Scandinavian background (27). The ethnic associations seemed at least partly explained by dietary factors, as indicated by a high intake of meat and pickled/smoked foods and a relation to obesity, especially in females. In addition, cigarette smokers showed an excess risk of about 60% overall, surpassing 2-fold among heavy smokers. A companion survey of 74 cases of renal pelvis cancers in the area revealed a surprising 6- to 7-fold excess risk among cigarette smokers, reaching 11-fold among heavy smokers, plus increased risks related to certain occupational exposures and to heavy use of phenacetin-containing analgesic drugs (26).

Comment

What have we learned from the U.S. cancer maps? Since Percivall Pott described scrotal cancers among chimney sweeps in 1775, etiologic leads to cancer have come from case clusters occurring in small groups of people. This was the situation with mesothelioma, liver angiosarcomas, and vaginal adenocarcinomas. However, these cancers are quite rare in the general population so that the observation of only a few cases raised suspicion. Clustering of more common tumors is not obvious through clinical experience, but our findings suggest they may be detected by monitoring cancer statistics on a small area scale. Our experience suggests also that county aggregations of cancer may give signals to environmental or lifestyle hazards, although false alarms may sometimes occur as a result of fluctuations in diagnosis, reporting, survival time, and migration. It is noteworthy that the geographic patterns of mortality often run in parallel with incidence data available from the network of cancer registries comprising the Surveillance, Epidemiology and End Results (SEER) program of NCI. For example, the mortality rates for lung cancer have become more prominent in southern areas since 1969 and less evident in the urban north-east, while incidence surveys reveal that Atlanta has shifted from having the lowest to the highest rates in recent data from the SEER program (6).

It is not surprising that the maps are less informative for cancers with favorable survival rates and problems in classification. For endometrial cancer, the mortality patterns are unremarkable, but incidence data have shown elevated rates in the registries on the west coast, including the San Francisco-Oakland area, which can be attributed to regional increases in estrogens prescribed at the time of menopause (1). While mortality rates displayed an overall downward trend, incidence rates rose and then declined when estrogen use was curtailed, a pattern consistent with the observation that estrogen produces mainly localized tumors of the endometrium and acts as a late-stage promoting agent. Although the SEER program covers about 12% of the U.S., the geographic and ethnic patterns of cancer incidence provide information not available from mortality data, and greatly enrich the opportunities for etiologic study.

Although high-risk areas have been the focus of our studies, the maps have also called attention to low-risk populations which provide a complementary strategy for epidemiologic research, as suggested by the comparatively low rates for certain cancers in the south, as well as in certain ethnic and religious groups. Furthermore, the limited amount of geographic variation for certain neoplasms, such as pancreas cancer (8), may itself be a useful pointer.

The cancer maps in the U.S. were soon followed by publication of similar atlases in several European countries, Japan, and most notably China, where remarkable variations occur for several cancer sites (21). Several analytical studies are now underway in high-risk areas of China that may greatly enhance our understanding of cancer etiology and prevention.

The cancer maps from various countries underscore the value of utilizing existing data resources and developing systematic approaches for generating and exploring hypotheses about the causes of cancer and other diseases. Although clinicians and experimentalists will continue to provide crucial leads for epidemiologic testing, it is important that epidemiologists also create new opportunities by strengthening surveillance procedures that may help uncover new health hazards. While it is important to encourage the development and communication of new etiologic leads from a variety of sources, we should strive to ensure that all promising leads are promptly and efficiently tested by analytical studies in the field.

In summary, the clues derived from the U.S. cancer maps have prompted a series of case-control studies that demonstrate the feasibility of this approach in detecting associations with environmental and lifestyle hazards. The evidence to date indicates that some hazards can be identified through the usual observational strategies of epidemiology, but it is likely that others will elude this approach and require multidisciplinary investigations combining the best efforts of epidemiologists and laboratory scientists.

REFERENCES

1. Austin, D. F. and Roe, K. M. The decreasing incidence of endometrial cancer: Public health implications. *Am. J. Public Health*, **72**, 65–68 (1982).
2. Blot, W. J., Davies, J. E., Brown, L. M., Nordwall, C. W., Buiatti, E., Ng, A., and Fraumeni, J. F., Jr. Occupation and the high risk of lung cancer in northeast Florida. *Cancer*, **50**, 364–371 (1982).
3. Blot, W. J. and Fraumeni, J. F., Jr. Arsenical air pollution and lung cancer. *Lancet*, **ii**, 142–144 (1975).
4. Blot, W. J. and Fraumeni, J. F., Jr. Geographic patterns of lung cancer: Industrial correlations. *Am. J. Epidemiol.*, **103**, 539–550 (1976).

5. Blot, W. J. and Fraumeni, J. F., Jr. Geographic patterns of bladder cancer in the United States. *J. Natl. Cancer Inst.*, **61**, 1017–1023 (1978).
6. Blot, W. J. and Fraumeni, J. F., Jr. Changing patterns of lung cancer in the United States. *Am. J. Epidemiol.*, **115**, 664–673 (1982).
7. Blot, W. J. and Fraumeni, J. F., Jr. Geographic epidemiology of cancer in the United States. *In* "Cancer Epidemiology and Prevention," eds. D. Schottenfeld and J. F. Fraumeni, Jr., pp. 179–193 (1982). W. B. Saunders Co., Philadelphia.
8. Blot, W. J., Fraumeni, J. F., Jr., and Stone, B. J. Geographic correlates of pancreas cancer in the United States. *Cancer*, **42**, 373–380 (1978).
9. Blot, W. J., Fraumeni, J. F., Jr., Stone, B. J., and McKay, F. W. Geographic patterns of large bowel cancer in the United States. *J. Natl. Cancer Inst.*, **57**, 1225–1231 (1976).
10. Blot, W. J., Harrington, J. M., Toledo, A., Hoover, R., Heath, C. W., Jr., and Fraumeni, J. F., Jr. Lung cancer after employment in shipyards during World War II. *N. Engl. J. Med.*, **299**, 620–624 (1978).
11. Blot, W. J., Morris, L. E., Stroube, R., Tagnon, I., and Fraumeni, J. F., Jr. Lung and laryngeal cancers in relation to shipyard employment in coastal Virginia. *J. Natl. Cancer Inst.*, **65**, 571–575 (1980).
12. Blot, W. J., Stone, B. J., Fraumeni, J. F., Jr., and Morris, L. E. Cancer mortality in U.S. counties with shipyard industries during World War II. *Environ. Res.*, **18**, 281–290 (1979).
13. Brinton, L. A., Blot, W. J., Becker, J. A., Winn, D. M., Browder, J. P., Farmer, J. C., Jr., and Fraumeni, J. F., Jr. A case-control study of cancers of the nasal cavity and paranasal sinuses. *Am. J. Epidemiol.*, **119**, 896–906 (1984).
14. Brinton, L. A., Blot, W. J., and Fraumeni, J. F., Jr. Nasal cancer in the textile and clothing industries. *Br. J. Ind. Med.*, **42**, 469–474 (1985).
15. Brinton, L. A., Stone, B. J., Blot, W. J., and Fraumeni, J. F., Jr. Nasal cancer in U.S. furniture industry counties. *Lancet*, **ii**, 628 (1976).
16. Brown, L. M., Pottern, L. M., and Blot, W. J. Lung cancer in relation to environmental pollutants emitted from industrial sources. *Environ. Res.*, **34**, 250–261 (1984).
17. Fraumeni, J. F., Jr. The face of cancer in the United States. *Hosp. Practice*, **18**, 81–96 (1983).
18. Haenszel, W. M. and Kurihara, M. Studies of Japanese migrants. I. Mortality from cancer and other diseases among Japanese in the United States. *J. Natl. Cancer Inst.*, **40**, 43–68 (1968).
19. Haenszel, W., Kurihara, M., Segi, M., and Lee, R.K.C. Stomach cancer among Japanese in Hawaii. *J. Natl. Cancer Inst.*, **49**, 969–988 (1972).
20. Lee, A. M. and Fraumeni, J. F., Jr. Arsenic and respiratory cancer in man: An occupational study. *J. Natl. Cancer Inst.*, **42**, 1045–1052 (1969).
21. Li, J. Y., Liu, B. Q., Li, G. Y., Chen, Z. J., Sun, X. D., and Rong, S. D. Atlas of cancer mortality in the People's Republic of China: An aid for cancer control and research. *Int. J. Epidemiol.*, **10**, 127–133 (1981).
22. Mason, T. J., Fraumeni, J. F., Jr., Hoover, R., and Blot, W. J. "An Atlas of Mortality from Selected Diseases," DHEW publ. No. (NIH) 81-2397 (1981). U.S. Government Printing Office, Washington, D. C.
23. Mason, T. J. and McKay, F. W. U. S. Cancer Mortality by County: 1950–1969, DHEW publ. No. (NIH) 74-615 (1974). U. S. Government Printing Office, Washington, D.C.
24. Mason T. J., McKay, F. W., Hoover, R., Blot, W. J., and Fraumeni, J. F., Jr. Atlas of Cancer Mortality for U. S. Counties: 1950–69, DHEW publ. No. (NIH) 75-780 (1975). U. S. Government Printing Office, Washington, D.C.
25. Mason, T. J., McKay, F. W., Hoover, R., Blot, W. J., and Fraumeni, J. F., Jr. Atlas of Cancer Mortality among U.S. Nonwhites: 1950–69, DHEW publ. No. (NIH) 76-1204 (1976). U. S. Government Printing Office, Washington, D.C.

26. McLaughlin, J. K., Blot, W. J., Mandel, J. S., Schuman, L. M., Mehl, E. S., and Fraumeni, J. F., Jr. Etiology of cancer of the renal pelvis. *J. Natl. Cancer Inst.*, **71**, 287–291 (1983).

27. McLaughlin, J. K., Mandel, J. S., Blot, W. J., Schuman, L. M., Mehl, E. S., and Fraumeni, J. F., Jr. A population-based case-control study of renal cell carcinoma. *J. Natl. Cancer Inst.*, **72**, 275–284 (1984).

28. Pickle, L. W., Correa, P., and Fontham, E. Recent case-control studies of lung cancer in the United States. *In* "Lung Cancer: Causes and Prevention," eds. M. Mizell and P. Correa, pp. 101–115 (1984). Verlag Chemie International, Inc., Deerfield Beach.

29. Pickle, L. W., Greene, M. H., Ziegler, R. G., Toledo, A., Hoover, R., Lynch, H. T., and Fraumeni, J. F., Jr. Colorectal cancer in rural Nebraska. *Cancer Res.*, **44**, 363–369 (1984).

30. Pottern, L. M., Morris, L. E., Blot, W. J., Ziegler, R. G., and Fraumeni, J. F., Jr. Esophageal cancer among black men in Washington, D. C. I. Alcohol, tobacco, and other risk factors. *J. Natl. Cancer Inst.*, **67**, 777–783 (1981).

31. Schoenberg, J. B., Stemhagen, A., Mogielnicki, A. P., Altman, R., Abe, T., and Mason, T. J. Case-control study of bladder cancer in New Jersey. I. Occupational exposures in white males. *J. Natl. Cancer Inst.*, **72**, 973–981 (1984).

32. Silverman, D. T., Hoover, R. N., Albert, S., and Graff, K. M. Occupation and cancer of the lower urinary tract in Detroit. *J. Natl. Cancer Inst.*, **70**, 237–245 (1983).

33. Silverman, D. T., Hoover, R. N., Mason, T. J., and Swanson, G. M. Motor exhaust-related occupations and bladder cancer. *Cancer Res.*, **46**, 2113–2116 (1986).

34. Tagnon, I., Blot, W. J., Stroube, R. B., Day, N. E., Morris, L. E., Peace, B. B., and Fraumeni, J. F., Jr. Mesothelioma associated with the shipbuilding industry in coastal Virginia. *Cancer Res.*, **40**, 3875–3879 (1980).

35. Winn, D. M., Blot, W. J., Shy, C. M., Pickle, L. W., Toledo, A., and Fraumeni, J. F., Jr. Snuff dipping and oral cancer among women in the southern United States. *N. Engl. J. Med.*, **304**, 745–749 (1981).

36. Ziegler, R. G., Devesa, S. S., and Fraumeni, J. F., Jr. Epidemiologic patterns of colorectal cancer. *In* "Important Advances in Oncology 1986," eds. V. T. DeVita, Jr., S. Hellman, and A. S. Rosenberg, pp. 209–232 (1986). J. B. Lippincott, Philadelphia.

37. Ziegler, R. G., Morris, L. E., Blot, W. J., Pottern, L. M., Hoover, R., and Fraumeni, J. F., Jr. Esophageal cancer among black men in Washington, D. C. II. Role of nutrition. *J. Natl. Cancer Inst.*, **67**, 1199–1206 (1981).

INTERNATIONAL
COMPARATIVE STUDY

Gann Monograph on Cancer Research 33, 1987

COMPARATIVE EPIDEMIOLOGY OF CANCER IN THE UNITED STATES AND JAPAN: PREVENTIVE IMPLICATIONS

Ernst L. Wynder[*1] and Tomohiko Hiyama[*2]

American Health Foundation[*1] *and Department of Field Research, Center for Adult Disease*[*2]

In accordance with changes in lifestyle factors, mortality rates for selected cancer sites have changed in both the United States and Japan. In line with increased dietary fat intake in Japan, breast and colon cancer mortality rates have steadily increased. Rising lung cancer mortality rates in both countries appear to reflect increasing levels of tobacco consumption. In the subgroup of younger U.S. white males, however, recent reduction in *per capita* tar consumption appears to be reducing lung cancer risk.

Recent epidemiological studies have provided accumulating evidence of an association between lifestyle-related factors and cancer incidence. Examination of the time changes in incidence/mortality rates and lifestyle factors may contribute to the identification of the decisive variables affecting their association. The comparable quality of national vital statistics records maintained by the U.S. and Japan allows comparison of trends in lifestyle and cancer occurrence which may provide valuable clues on cancer etiology.

Comparison of Dietary Factors and Diet-related Cancer Rates

Japanese dietary intake patterns have changed rapidly during the past 30 years toward an increasingly "westernized" diet characterized by high fat and low carbohydrate levels (Table I: *11, 12, 25–27*). In the early 1950s, Japanese daily *per capita* nutritional intake was 1,900 calories. This level has since increased to 2,900 calories per day in the late 1970s, but remains only four-fifths the U.S. level. The Japanese increase in calorie intake has been due primarily to increased fat intake, which during a 25–30 year period has risen from 10–20 to 82 g *per capita* per day. The direction of the time trend in daily cereal consumption has been quite the opposite, decreasing during the same time period from 422 to 316 g *per capita*.

Accordingly, the proportion of daily calorie intake attributable to fat increased in Japan from 9% in 1955 to 24% in 1980 (*18*). This is, of course, still lower than the U.S. level, which has remained relatively constant during a 25–30 year period at about 40% (*34*).

In line with increased fat intake in the Japanese diet, the incidence of cancers thought to be associated with fat intake, *i.e.*, cancer of the breast, colon, and prostate, has also

---

[*1] New York, New York 10017, U.S.A.

[*2] Nakamichi 1-3-3, Higashinari-ku, Osaka 537, Japan (日山與彦).

TABLE I.   Changes in Per Day *Per Capita* Consumption of Selected
Nutrients in the U.S. and Japan

Period	Calories		Cereals (g)		Fat (g)		Protein (g)	
	U.S.	Japan	U.S.	Japan	U.S.	Japan	U.S.	Japan
1948–1950	3,180	1,900	210	—	138.6	10.6	89.2	49.4
1951–1953	3,130	1,930	201	—	136.2	21.4	89.8	60.6
1955–1959	3,156	2,214	186	422	149.2	26.1	99.2	68.5
1960–1964	3,160	2,350	182	410	150.9	37.0	99.5	72.3
1965–1969	3,232	2,432	178	380	158.0	50.6	102.0	76.4
1970–1974	3,223	2,555	174	346	165.8	64.8	104.1	80.9
1975–1977	3,537	2,847	176	331	163.8	72.3	106.2	86.5
1978–1980	3,632	2,916	176	316	169.2	81.6	106.7	93.4

— data not available.   Sources: FAO (*11, 12*) and OECD (*25–27*).

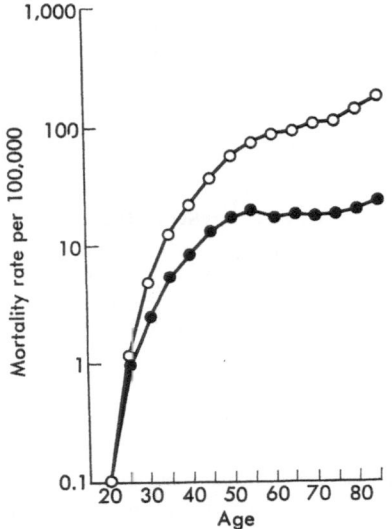

FIG. 1.   Age-specific mortality rate of breast cancer in the U.S. and Japan in 1980
O U.S. white women; ● Japanese women.

risen in Japan (*21*). Age-adjusted breast cancer mortality has increased among Japanese females, climbing to 5.4 per 100,000 in 1980. This rate, however, is still considerably lower than that in U.S. white females whose rate was 21.9 in 1980. The difference in mortality between the two populations applies principally to the rates among older women (Fig. 1; *16, 22*). However, as a result of prominent increases in mortality among the older age groups in Japan (Fig. 2; *16, 22, 35*), the pattern of age-specific mortality began to change in the direction of that observed in epidemic populations.

Since breast cancer is hormone-dependent, alterations in hormone metabolism caused by dietary fat may mediate breast cancer development. In regard to premenopausal women, total plasma estrogen levels in healthy Caucasian and Japanese women and in breast cancer patients are comparable (*14*). Plasma estrogens rise in postmenopausal women mainly by aromatization of androstenedione to estrone and testosterone to estradiol

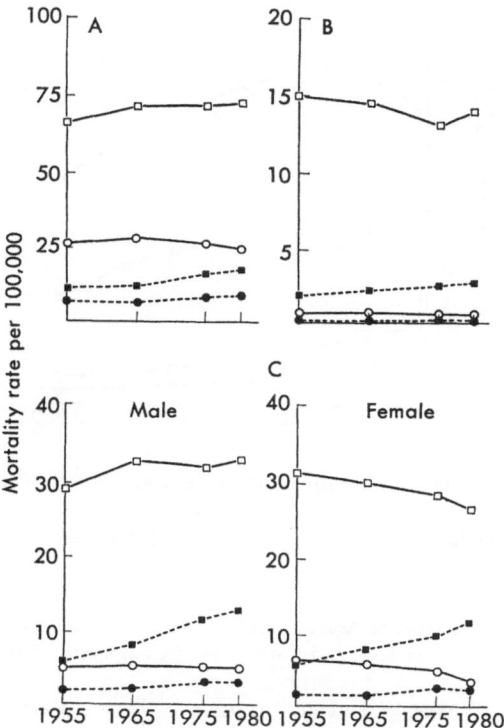

Fig. 2. Age-specific mortality rates for selected cancer sites for U.S white and Japanese, 1955–1980
A: breast. B: prostate. C: colon. ○ U.S. white (35–49); □ U.S. white (50–64); ● Japanese (35–49); ■ Japanese (50–64).

(7). Plasma testosterone levels are lower among premenopausal Japanese women than Caucasian women, although a westernized diet has been shown to increase testosterone levels in Japanese women (13). Consistent with these data is a study showing that a vegetarian diet fed to U.S. men decreased their plasma estradiol levels (30).

In experimental studies, Tannenbaum found that high-fat diets enhanced both chemically induced and spontaneous mammary cancer in rodents (31). Carroll and co-workers shed light on another key aspect of the fat effect, namely, that the type of fat was equally as important as the amount of fat consumed (4). Recently, Cohen and Thompson reported that an oil rich in monoenoic fatty acid, namely, olive oil, does not promote mammary tumor development (5). It is possible, therefore, that the moderate increase in the breast cancer mortality rate among U.S. postmenopausal white females (8) may relate to the disproportionate increase in polyunsaturated fat intake seen in that group (2). The decrease in mortality among premenopausal U.S. white females may reflect a protective effect of early pregnancy only on the mothers of the postwar "baby boom" (1). The hormonal mechanisms affecting breast cancer are complex, with prostaglandin likely to play a role as well (19). Their synthesis, which is derivatives of leinoic, also appears to be affected by dietary fat (17).

The colon cancer mortality rate also increased in Japan, particularly among older age groups (Fig. 2). Along with the increase in mortality rates, the shift in anatomical

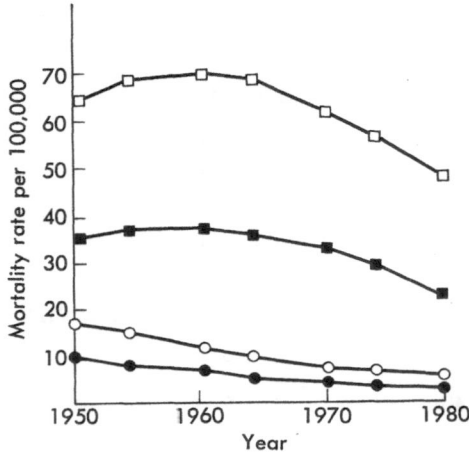

FIG. 3.   Age-adjusted mortality rates for gastric cancer for U.S. white and Japanese, 1950–1980
○ U.S. white, male;   ● U.S. white, female;   □ Japanese, male;   ■ Japanese, female.

TABLE II.   Estimated Strengths of Association between Diet-related Factors Associated with Gastric Cancer Risk and Categories of Comparative Studies

Dietary factors	Time-trend	Inter-country	Intra-country	North/south gradient	Migra-tion	Case/control	Experi-mental
Carbohydrate	++	+++	+	+	++	+++	++
Nitrate/nitrite	++	++	++	+	+	+++	++
Salt (salted/pickled foods)	++	++	++	—	++	+++	+++
Vegetables	++	++	++	+++	+	+++	Not tested
Fruits	+	++	+	+++	+	++	Not tested
Vitamin C	+	+	+	+++	+	+	++
Vitamin A	+	+	++	+++	+	+++	++
Refrigeration	++	—	—	—	—	—	Not tested

Estimated strength of association: +++ strong;   ++ moderate;   + weak/none;   — no evidence.

distribution of colon cancer in Japan has changed toward that of a high-risk population: left-side colon cancer has become the most common subsite; the ratio of cecum-ascending to sigmoid colon cancer incidence fell from 1.4 in 1959–1964 to 0.7 in 1973–1977 for males, and from 2.0 to 1.0 for females in Miyagi, Japan. In the U.S. state of Connecticut, on the other hand, these rates were 0.6 and 0.8 for males and 0.9 and 0.8 for females during the same period (6, 10, 36).

Animal experimental studies have suggested that colon tumor promotion results through a mechanism involving increased colonic bile acid content (23, 28). Dietary fat affects endogenous cholesterol biosynthesis, which in turn leads to increased bile acid biosynthesis. In humans, a significant increase in the excretion of total bile acid was found among U.S. males and females compared with Japanese (29). Dietary fiber, which is said to reduce colon cancer risk by increasing stool bulk, resulting in a dilution of tumorigenic compounds and bile acid concentration (3), is higher in Japan (20 g per day vs. 15 g in the U.S.).

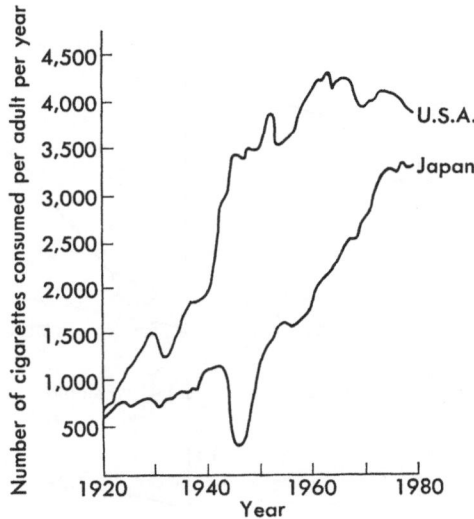

FIG. 4. Number of cigarettes consumed per adult per year in the U.S. and Japan, 1920–1979

Age-adjusted gastric cancer mortality has been decreasing since as early as the 1920s in the U.S., reaching levels of 5.5 per 100,000 white males and 2.6 per 100,000 white females. In Japan, it had been increasing until the late 1950s, at which point the direction of the time trend inverted. It was 47.9 per 100,000 males and 23.8 per 100,000 females in 1980, still considerably higher than among U.S. whites (Fig. 3; *16, 21, 22*). This declining gastric cancer mortality may be primarily due to the decrease in intestinal type gastric cancer, which is linked with environmental factors, undoubtedly dietary factors. Several etiological hypotheses for gastric cancer risk are proposed, although no single etiologic factor has yet been confirmed (Table II).

Comparisons of Tobacco Consumption and Tobacco-related Cancer

In the U.S., *per capita* cigarette consumption has climbed steadily over a three-decade period, reaching its peak in 1963 before beginning a sudden decline (Fig. 4; *20, 33*). This decrease has been primarily due to the decrease in the percentage of smokers among adult males. The proportion of smokers fell from 52% to 38% between 1965 and 1980 (*33*). For adult females, the percentage of smokers was relatively constant from the mid-1960s to the mid-1970s—34% in 1965, 33% in 1976—and appeared to begin decreasing thereafter, reaching 30% in 1980. After the appearance of the first scientific publications suggesting an association between smoking and lung cancer (*38*), the tar and nicotine content of U.S. cigarettes decreased from 37 mg and 2.7 mg, respectively, in 1955 to 14 mg and 1 mg, respectively, in 1980 (*24*). Filter-tipped cigarettes were introduced in the U.S. in the 1950s, and by 1982 reached a market share of 93%.

These changes in tobacco consumption led to a decrease in estimated tar consumption per adult male, this effect first appearing in the decline in lung cancer mortality among young males (Fig. 5; *16, 22, 35*), an effect seen more markedly in Great Britain where a rise in the incidence of lung cancer occurred earlier than in the U.S. (*9*). The

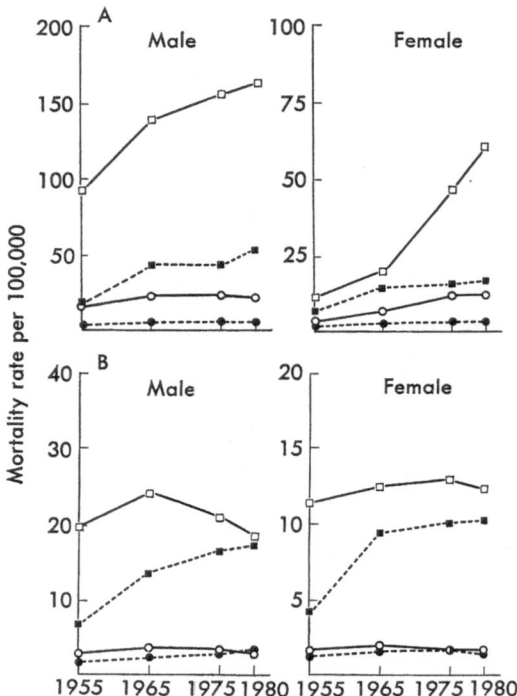

FIG. 5. Age-specific mortality rates for selected cancer sites for U.S. whites and
Japanese, 1955–1980
A: lung. B: pancreas. ○ U.S. white (35–49); □ U.S. white (50–64); ● Japanese
(35–49); ■ Japanese (50–64).

age-specific mortality rates among males aged 30–49 years began to decline in the late
1970s. The decrease in mortality rates has not yet been observed among females in any
age group, although it is encouraging to note that in the 30–39 year-old age group it was
leveling off as of the late 1970s. This plateau may be due in part to the availability and
increasing popularity of low-tar cigarettes, judging from the relatively stable percentage
of smokers among women.

In Japan, *per capita* cigarette consumption has been increasing steadily since the
early 1950s (Fig. 4), accompanied by a concurrent increase in lung cancer mortality.
The finding of a plateau of age-specific lung cancer mortality among older age groups
during the period 1965–1975 may reflect the decline in cigarette consumption during
World War II. Age-adjusted lung cancer mortality will continue to climb among Japanese
males as a result of the constantly high percentage of smokers (75–80%; *32*) and increasing *per capita* cigarette consumption. The percentage of smokers, however, began to
decline in the late 1970s (*32*). Further observations will be necessary to track this trend.

The pancreatic cancer mortality rate increased markedly in Japan in younger as well
as older age groups (Fig. 5). On the other hand, age-specific mortality for 35–49 and 50–
64 year-olds began to decline among U.S. whites in the early 1970s for males, and in the
late 1970s for females, the difference in mortality rates almost disappearing by 1980.
Red meat consumption, which Hirayama reported to be related to pancreatic cancer
(*15*), has been increasing rapidly in Japan (*11*, *12*, *25–27*), although its level is still only

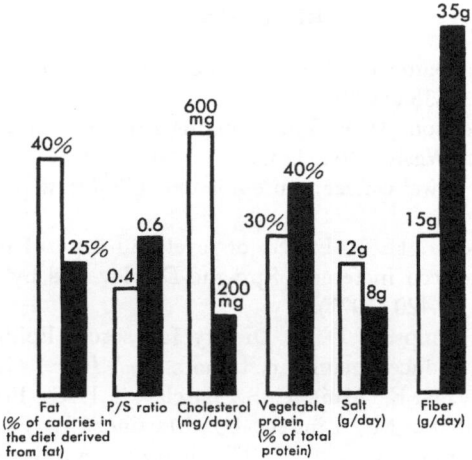

FIG. 6. American Health Foundation Food Plan
□ typical American diet; ■ American Health Foundation Recommended diet.

half that of the U.S. The relatively constant, or even increased, U.S. level cannot account for the decrease in pancreatic cancer mortality observed in the U.S. The increase in mortality of pancreatic cancer in Japan deserves more attention since it may harbor new clues to identify risk factors in addition to cigarette smoking and high-fat diet.

It is clear that many chronic diseases are related to lifestyle and are therefore avoidable, as is observed in the lung cancer mortality rates among young U.S. white males, and the dramatic decline in gastric cancer mortality seen throughout the world. In the area of product modification, we recommend that manufacturers reduce average cigarette tar yield to 10 mg. The idea, of course, is to move toward a non-smoking society. Anti-smoking education campaigns in the U.S. are significantly more advanced than in Japan, and undoubtedly responsible for a decline in the number of smokers and an increase in the number of individuals who have quit smoking. We suggest that the Japanese authorities implement some of the American anti-smoking strategies. Regarding changes in dietary habits, in our American Health Foundation Food Plan, we encourage lower intake of fat and salt, and increased intake of fiber (Fig. 6).

We strongly believe that school health education is a most important component of any long-term health strategy relating to the improvement of health habits, and we therefore developed the "Know Your Body" school health education program the basic purpose of which is to promote among school children an attitude of greater responsibility toward their own personal health (37).

It is our hope that in the next 10 years the occurrence of those cancers known to relate to environmental causes will decline through an improvement in those lifestyle factors that are subject to personal control.

Acknowledgments

This research was supported by National Cancer Institute Program Project Grant No. CA32617 and Center Grant No. CA17613, and American Health Cancer Society Special Institutional Grant SIG-8. The authors thank Mr. Monte Hewson for assistance in manuscript preparation.

REFERENCES

1. Blot, W. J. Changing patterns of breast cancer among American women, 1980. *Am. J. Public Health*, **70**, 823–835 (1980).
2. Brewster, L. and Jacobson, M. F. The changing American diet (1978). Center for Science in the Public Interest, Washington, D.C.
3. Burkitt, D. P. Large bowel cancer: An epidemiologic jigsaw puzzle. *J. Natl. Cancer Inst.*, **54**, 3–6 (1975).
4. Carroll, K.K. and Khor, H. T. Effects of level and type of dietary fat on incidence of mammary tumors induced in female Sprague-Dawley rats by 7, 12-dimethyl-benz(a)anthracene. *Lipids*, **6**, 415–420 (1971).
5. Cohen, L. A. and Thompson, D. O. Dietary fat, serum lipids and the development of N-nitrosomethylurea-induced mammary tumors. *Fed. Proc.*, **43**, 614 (1984).
6. De Jong, U. W., Day, N. E., Muir, C. S., Barclay, T.H.C., Bras, G., Foster, F. H., Jussawalla, D. J., Kurihara, M., Linden, G., Martinez, I., Payne, P. M., Pedersen, E., Ringertz, N., and Shanmugaratnam, T. The distribution of cancer within the large bowel. *Int. J. Cancer*, **10**, 463–477 (1972).
7. Deslypere, J. P., Verdonck, L., and Vernmeulen A. Fat tissue: A steroid reservoir and site of steroid metabolism. *J. Clin. Endocr. Metab.*, **61**, 564–570 (1983).
8. Devesa, S. S., Pollack, E. S., and Young, J. L. Assessing the validity of observed cancer incidence trends. *Am. J. Epidemiol.*, **119**, 274–291, (1984).
9. Doll, R. and Peto, R. The causes of cancer. *J. Natl. Cancer Inst.*, **66**, 1191–1308 (1981).
10. Eisenberg, H. Cancer in Connecticut: Incidence and rates, 1935–1962 (1966). Connecticut State Dept. of Health, Hartford.
11. Food and Agriculture Organization of the United Nations. Production Yearbook, 1955 (1955). United Nations, Rome.
12. Food and Agriculture Organization of the United Nations. Production Yearbook, 1981 (1982). United Nations, Rome.
13. Hill, P., Garbaczewski, L., Kasumi, F., Kuno, K., Helman, P., and Wynder E. L. Breast cancer: Diet and hormone metabolism. *In* "Banbury Report 8: Hormones and Breast Cancer," eds. M. C. Pike, P. K. Siiteri, and C. W. Welsch, pp. 257–277 (1981). Cold Spring Harbor Laboratory, Cold Spring Harbor.
14. Hill, P. and Wynder, E. L. Unpublished manuscript.
15. Hirayama, T. A large-scale cohort study on relationship between diet and selected cancers of digestive organs. *In* "Banbury Report 7: Gastrointestinal Cancer Endogenous Factors," eds. W. R. Bruce, P. Correa, and M. Lipkin, pp. 409–429 (1981). Cold Spring Harbor Laboratory, Cold Spring Harbor.
16. Horm, J. Personal communication.
17. Horrobin, D. F. The regulation of prostaglandin biosyntheses by the manipulation of essential fatty acid metabolism. *Rev. Drug Met. Drug Interact.*, **4**, 339–383 (1983).
18. Japanese Ministry of Health and Welfare, Bureau of Public Health. Kokumin-Eiyo-No Genjo (Current Status of National Nutrition) 1980 (1981). Japanese Ministry of Health and Welfare, Tokyo.
19. Karmali, P. A. Review: Prostaglandins and cancer. *Prostaglandins Med.*, **5**, 11–28 (1980).
20. Kristein, M. K. Forty years of U.S. cigarette smoking and heart disease and cancer mortality rates. *J. Chron. Dis.*, **37**, 317–323 (1984).
21. Kurihara, M., Aoki, K., and Tomonaga, S. "Cancer Mortality Statistics in the World" (1985). The University of Nagoya Press, Nagoya.
22. Ministry of Health and Welfare of Japan. Vital Statistics, 1980 (1982). Ministry of Health and Welfare, Tokyo.
23. Narisawa, T., Magadia, N. E., Weisburger, J. H., and Wynder, E. L. Promoting effect of

bile acids on colon carcinogenesis after intrarectal instillation of N-methyl-N'-nitro-N-nitrosoguanidine in rats. *J. Natl. Cancer Inst.*, **53**, 1093–1097 (1974).

24. Office on Smoking and Health. The Health Consequences of Smoking: Cardiovascular Disease (1984). U. S. Dept. of Health and Human Services, Rockwell, Md.
25. Organization for Economic Cooperation and Development. Food Consumption Statistics. 1955–1973 (1975). Organization for Economic Cooperation and Development, Paris.
26. Organization for Economic Cooperation and Development. Food Consumption Statistics, 1970–1975 (1978). Organization for Economic Cooperation and Development, Paris.
27. Organization for Economic Cooperation and Development. Food Consumption Statistics, 1973–1982 (1985). Organization for Economic Cooperation and Development, Paris.
28. Reddy, B. S., Watanabe, K., and Weisburger, J. H. Effect of high-fat diet on colon carcinogenesis in F-344 rats treated with 1,2-dimethylhydrazine, methylazoxymethanol acetate or methylnitrosourea. *Cancer Res.*, **37**, 4156–4159 (1977).
29. Reddy, B. S. and Wynder, E. L. Large bowel carcinogenesis: Fecal constituents of populations with diverse incidence rates of colon cancer. *J. Natl. Cancer Inst.*, **50**, 1437–1442 (1973).
30. Rosenthal, M. B., Barnard, R. J., Rose, D. P., Inkeles, S., Hall, J., and Pritikin, N. Effects of a high complex carbohydrate, low fat, low cholesterol diet on levels of serum lipids and estradiol. *Am. J. Med.*, **78**, 23–27 (1985).
31. Tannenbaum, A. The genesis and growth of tumors. III. Effects of a high fat diet. *Cancer Res.*, **2**, 468–475 (1942).
32. The Japan Tobacco and Salt Public Monopoly Corporation. The Annual Statistical Report, 1982 (1982). The Japan Tobacco and Salt Public Monopoly Corporation, Tokyo (in Japanese).
33. Tominaga, S. Smoking in Japan. *In* "The UICC Smoking Control Workshop, Nagoya," eds. S. Tominaga and K. Aoki, pp. 27–35 (1982). The University of Nagoya Press, Nagoya.
34. U. S. Bureau of Census. Statistical Abstract of the United States, 1983 (1984). U. S. Government Printing Office, Washington, D.C.
35. Young, J. L., Percy, C. L., and Asire, A. J. Surveillance, Epidemiology and End Results: Incidence and Mortality Data, 1973–1977 (1981). NIH Publication No. 81-2330. U. S. Department of Health and Human Services, Bethesda, Md.
36. Waterhouse, J., Muir, C., Correa, P., and Powell, J. "Cancer Incidence in Five Continents," Vol. III (1976). IARC, Lyon.
37. Williams, C. L., Arnold C. B., and Wynder, E. L. Primary prevention of chronic disease beginning in childhood; The "Know Your Body" program: Design of study. *Prev. Med.*, **6**, 344–357 (1977).
38. Wynder, E. L. and Graham, E. A. Tobacco smoking as a possible etiologic factor in bronchiogenic carcinoma: A study of six hundred and eighty-four proved cases. *JAMA*, **143**, 329–336 (1950).

U.S.-JAPAN COOPERATIVE CANCER RESEARCH PROGRAM REPORT OF A WORKSHOP ON ADULT-TYPE CANCER UNDER AGE 30

Robert W. MILLER[1] and Haruo SUGANO,[2]

Clinical Epidemiology Branch, National Cancer Institute[1] and Cancer Institute[2]

Many binational differences in cancer occurrence under age 30 were identified from review of data presented at this U.S.-Japan workshop. Etiologic influences may be more readily detected when cancers occur much earlier in life than usual. The number of cases of stomach cancer, about 550 annually, allows for sizable multi-hospital studies. Within-country differences in occurrence, as for Kaposi's sarcoma in San Francisco, noted in the Surveillance, Epidemiology and End Results (SEER) data, illustrate that in this age-group etiologically significant clusters can be detected. A seemingly high rate of vaginal cancer in the U.S., 1973–1982, may be due to maternal use of diethylstilbestrol during pregnancy. One might look, through case-control studies, for transplacental carcinogens in the etiology of cancers at 15–29 years of age. The deficiency of Wilms' tumor and of congenital aniridia with the tumor in Japan suggests that the segment of chromosome 11 with the genes for these disorders is less mutable than in people elsewhere.

Professor Mitsuo Segi foresaw the importance of international comparisons in cancer research, and created the first data resource for this purpose. He also saw the benefits in binational collaborative research, and realized them in the case-control studies of migrants from Japan to Hawaii as compared with Japanese who did not migrate. In this work he teamed up with Mr. William Haenszel of the National Cancer Institute in Bethesda. In a sense this was a forerunner of the U.S.-Japan Cooperative Cancer Research Program, which was initiated in 1974. The Program has been highly productive through its workshops, exchange of scientists and the exchange of resources. The differences in cancer occurrence in the two countries provide the stimulus for new ideas, as illustrated by one such workshop reported here.

New understanding of the etiology and pathogenesis of cancer may come from studying its occurrence at unlikely ages or anatomic sites. With this in mind, a workshop on adult-type cancer in persons under 30 years of age was held in Tokyo on March 11–13, 1985, under the sponsorship of the U.S.-Japan Cooperative Cancer Research Program.

For the U.S. good estimates of the national incidence of cancer by site and histologic type are available through the Surveillance, Epidemiology and End Results (SEER) Program of the National Cancer Institute. About 10% of the U.S. population

---

[1] Bethesda, Maryland 20892, U.S.A.

[2] 1-37-1 Kami-Ikebukuro, Toshima-ku, Tokyo 170, Japan (菅野晴夫).

is covered by the registry, and more than 95% of diagnoses have been histologically studied. Young (Bethesda) had prepared detailed tables to show these data by age, sex, and certain subsites for whites, blacks and Japanese-Americans, 1973–1982.

Japanese national data are available through death-certificate diagnoses, which in every country are of variable accuracy and completeness. They are population-based, however, and are representative of the cancer experience according to current practice as it relates to making diagnoses and coding them on death certificates. Comparisons between mortality and morbidity will, of course, be better for cancers that are quickly fatal than for those with long survival. In this report, the data are given as numbers of cases rather than rates to bring to mind the opportunities for studies of case-series. Data from the Nagasaki Tumor Registry, presented by Hoel, Mabuchi and Davis (Hiroshima), and Ikeda (Nagasaki), will be used to supplement observations concerning individual cancer sites. These data are not yet population-based, and have other problems in ascertainment. Some data were also presented from the Hiroshima Tumor Tissue Registry, and from a variety of special registries; *e.g.*, the All-Japan Children's Cancer Registry, the Autopsy Annuals in Japan, and the Bone Tumor Registry in Japan.

A substantial number of findings deserve additional study, especially certain marked differences in the occurrence of specific cancers in the two countries and unexpected clusters within countries.

Oral Cancers

Tongue

Cancer of the tongue caused 102 deaths (9/year) under 30 in Japan, and 46 new cases annually in the U.S. Because xeroderma pigmentosum (XP), a genetic disorder, predisposes to cancer of the tip of the tongue in young people (*11*), the location of the neoplasm is of interest, and was readily ascertained in the SEER Program. The tip was the most frequently affected location. Of the 31 cases in which the location was specified, 16 were at the tip and another five were in the anterior two-thirds. Examination of other clinical data should show if any of these patients had XP.

Gastrointestinal Cancers

1. Esophagus

It is surprising that any cancers of the esophagus were reported in the two series, but three deaths occurred annually in Japan, and an estimated five new cases were reported annually in the U.S. Again a genetic disorder may be involved, for tylosis predisposes to esophageal cancer (*2*).

2. Stomach cancer

The well-known high rate of stomach cancer in Japan was also found among young adults. The SEER Program showed that 50 new cases per year occurred among U.S. whites as compared with about 550 deaths per year under age 30 in Japan. Correa (New Orleans) noted that in Japan diffuse carcinoma predominates in the young, as contrasted with the intestinal type later in life. The diffuse type was thought to vary little in frequency with age, sex, race, migration or geography, but the frequency is clearly higher in young Japanese than in young people in Western countries. This finding indicates a need to reevaluate the conventional wisdom concerning the stability of rates for the diffuse form of gastric cancer, and to study its origins in young Japanese.

The female predominance is of interest: 3,472 females *vs.* 2,483 males in the Japanese death-certificate series. By contrast, the SEER data showed a male predominance: 33 to 17.

Correa suggested a multi-center study in Japan to accumulate a substantial number of cases, with pedigrees noted and a search made for genetic markers, such as blood type for persons with diffuse *vs.* intestinal types of stomach cancer. The role of genetics seems to be stronger than that of the environment. The high mortality rates indicate that specimens and information can be rapidly accumulated in Japan.

3. Colon cancer

Stemmermann (Honolulu) reported that among records for Japanese-Americans seen at Kuakini Hospital, he found seven with colon cancer under 30, one with multiple polyposis, two in single polyps, and the other four had rapidly fatal disease. The Hiroshima Tumor Tissue Registry, 1973–1982, accessioned 33 cases of colon cancer under age 30. One patient had polyposis coli and three had cancers that arose from isolated polyps. In the summary of data from the Autopsy Annuals in Japan, 1974–1982, 64 males and 47 females under 30 were diagnosed as having cancer of the colon or rectum. The distribution of these cases by histologic subtypes and anatomic sites could be compared with those of the Stemmermann's small case-series.

Utsunomiya (Tokyo) presented data from the Japanese Polyposis Registry System. The frequency of multiple polyposis is about the same in Japan as in England, one in 22,000 births. Of 185 Japanese patients with polyposis coli diagnosed under 30 years, 57 had cancer of the colon. Colon cancer is usually mucinous when the onset is early in life (*1*). This was in accord with observations at Kuakini Hospital, but in Hiroshima only one of 33 cases under age 30 was specified as mucinous.

Stemmermann and Utsunomiya concluded that there was no evidence of a strong genetic influence on colon cancer under age 30. The SEER cases, however, might be studied for a family history of colon cancer; *i.e.*, familial colon cancer without polyposis. There are about 277 new cases of colon cancer per year under 30 in U.S. whites.

4. Pancreatic cancer

Cancer of the pancreas caused an average of 33 deaths per year under age 30 in Japan, and the number of new cases annually among U.S. whites was about the same. Study of case-series in each country, might reveal clues to etiology or mechanisms that have eluded detection in the many large studies of older persons with this cancer.

5. Liver cancer

Hepatoblastoma is a neoplasm of children with a peak soon after birth. Hepatocellular carcinoma, the adult form of liver cancer, has been the subject of several U.S.-Japan workshops, and was not dealt with at this one.

Cancer of the gallbladder late in life is substantially more common in Japan than in the U.S. The numbers under 30 years were low in both countries, but the 11 deaths annually in Japan were about the same as the annual number of new cases among U.S. whites.

Respiratory System

1. Maxillary sinuses

The high rate of maxillary sinus cancer in Japan is well known there. An excess under 30 years of age is suggested by the mortality data, 17 deaths per year, which is about the same as the number of new cases annually among U.S. whites.

2. Lungs and bronchi

Japan averages 66 deaths a year from cancer of the lung and bronchus under age 30, as compared with 135 new cases annually among U.S. whites according to the SEER data. However, carcinoid was the diagnosis in 39 females and 21 males. Study of the series of 60 carcinoids would be of interest, perhaps in conjunction with carcinoids of the appendix, which clustered in Seattle (due to selective reporting?).

Cancers of the lungs and bronchi other than carcinoids in U.S. whites affected 35 females and 40 males. Virtually all were said to be primary in bronchopulmonary tissue. The lack of a sex difference in the U.S. is of interest. The histories of cases in this series may be informative. For example, information might be obtained to determine if the affected people were smokers who had been exposed in schoolrooms to the fallout from asbestos-sprayed ceilings. In this connection it is interesting to note that among the 75 bronchopulmonary cancer cases, seven males and no females had oat cell tumors, 12 (both sexes) had squamous cell cancer, 18 had adenocarcinoma, and 38 had other types, The family histories might reveal a propensity toward certain of the cell types.

Bone Cancer

The SEER data showed osteosarcoma and Ewing's sarcoma to be equally frequent in males (153 *vs.* 156 cases) but there was a deficiency of Ewing's tumor in females (138 *vs.* 81). Miller (Bethesda) had examined these data by skeletal site affected, and found that Ewing's sarcoma occurred especially in the axial skeleton and legs, wheras osteosarcoma occurred primarily in the long bones, particularly of the legs. Namba (Hiroshima) believed the anatomic distribution reflected the marrow orgins of Ewing's sarcoma as contrasted with the origins of osteosarcoma at centers of bone growth.

Data from the Bone Tumor Registry in Japan, 1972–1982, presented by Furuya (Tokyo) showed a marked deficiency in Ewing's sarcoma relative to osteosarcoma as compared with SEER data:

Bone cancer	U.S. whites		Japan	
	M	F	M	F
Osteosarcoma	153	138	629	413
Ewing's sarcoma	156	81	84	68
OS/ES	1.0	1.7	7.5	6.1

A marked deficiency of Ewing's sarcoma in U.S. blacks has previously been recognized (*13*). The deficiency persists despite the long presence of blacks in the U.S. Presumably U.S. whites and blacks have similar childhood exposures, but blacks are rarely affected by Ewing's sarcoma, as if they are genetically resistant.

1. Soft-tissue sarcomas

Differences in criteria for classifying subtypes of soft-tissue cancers make it difficult to compare the two sets of data. One finding of possible interest concerns 63 persons with nerve sheath tumors under 30 years of age registered in the SEER Program. It would be interesting to determine how many were isolated findings or part of multiple neurofibromatosis.

2. Skin

Skin cancer is rare under 30 years of age, except in the genetic disorder, XP. Takebe (Kyoto) reported that in a series of 184 Japanese patients with XP 98 have developed skin cancer. Susceptibility is due to a defect in repair in DNA after exposure to ultraviolet light. The greater the reduction in unscheduled DNA synthesis (UDS), the more severe are the symptoms in XP. In Japan the distribution of cases according to the seven genetic complementation groups and the variant group is different from those in the U.S., Europe, and Egypt, where XP is especially prevalent. Of 56 XP families in Japan, 48 are in complementation A or the variant group. Elsewhere there is heavier representation from groups C and D, and much less from the variant group. The average age for the onset of skin cancer in group A and those with less than 5% UDS was 9.4 years. The closer the UDS level was to normal, the older was the age at onset of skin cancer.

To date, complementation group F (four families) has been found only in Japan. In Korea the distribution by complementation groups appears to be different from that in Japan, but to date only four cases have been studied. The incidence of XP in Japan is estimated to be one in 100,000 which is higher than in other countries.

Takebe said that Bloom's syndrome, a genetic disorder primarily of Ashkenazic Jews, has been found in nine Japanese. Two have developed cancer, including one with lung carcinoma at 39 years. A special Bloom's syndrome registry developed by German (3) consists of 100 patients, 25 of whom have developed cancer (leukemia, lymphoma, and carcinomas), usually under 30 years of age. These syndromes illustrate how genetic factors can play a role in the development of adult-type cancers at much earlier ages than usual. One might look for formes frustes of genetic disorders in persons with early onset of adult-type cancer.

3. Melanoma

Melanoma is apparently much less frequent in Japanese than in U.S. whites. The influence of ultraviolet light in its induction is blocked by skin pigmentation. The SEER data show that in the decade studied, 681 males and 1,047 females had melanomas. The well characterized sex difference in anatomic distribution was found: less involvement of the face and scalp of females, but much more on the extremities than in males.

Kasuga (Tokyo) reported that the Annual of Pathological Autopsy Cases in Japan (APAC), 1958–1982, described 69 melanomas under 30 years of age, and 29 from surgical cases seen at the Cancer Institute in Tokyo, 1947–1981. Of particular interest was the finding that 16 of the 69 cases from APAC were of the leptomeninges, a seemingly high frequency.

The peak was at about 20 years of age. Under 30 years of age, 23.2% of melanomas were of the meninges, as compared with 2.0% of melanomas in persons 30 years of age or older. It would be important to confirm this observation from other data, if possible, and to determine if involvement of the meninges was familial or associated with other disorders in the patient or family. Melanomas of the mucosa were said to be more frequent in Japan than in Western countries.

Genital Cancers

1. Prostate

Cancer early in life coded to the prostate is likely to be rhabdomyosarcoma. The SEER data show eight cases at 15–29 years of age, and five at less than this age. The cell-types would be of interest. In Japan there were 56 deaths from cancer of the prostate, 46 of them at 15–29 years of age.

2. Testis

The peak in testicular cancer among U.S. whites rises sharply from 15–19 years (221 cases) to 25–29 years (801 cases). The total under 30 years of age was 1,721. Therapy to date was been very effective, far more so than in Japan, where there was an average of 75 deaths a year. If there is indeed a much greater frequency of testicular cancer in the U.S. than in Japan, the difference may be similar to that between whites and blacks in the U.S. blacks have essentially no peak in the frequency of testicular cancer, and are thus apparently resistant to all the main types: seminoma, embryonal carcinoma, and teratoma.

Japanese and U.S. whites show a small peak in embryonal carcinoma at 0–4 years, but blacks do not. One wonders why both groups have peaks soon after birth, but only U.S. whites have a second peak in young adulthood.

3. Ovary

The most interesting feature from the data available was a seemingly high frequency of benign teratomas in Nagasaki Prefecture as indicated by the Tumor Tissue Registry. In 1979, the most recent year for which an annual tabulation had been made, there were 51 cases. Coverage has improved over time since 1972, so the number of cases ascertained has been increasing. The data available show the peak age at diagnosis to be 20–29. Familial cases are thought to be rare. In Willis' series of 50, six were bilateral (16). One thousand cases or more should be available for study through the Tissue Registries in Nagasaki and Hiroshima. Through such study, risk factors (personal, familial or community) and other characteristics of these tumors may be identified.

Tokuoka (Hiroshima) reported that among women of all ages, 194 ovarian cancers had been ascertained in the extended Life-Span Study sample of the Radiation Effects Research Foundation (RERF). A statistically significant linear increase was observed with increasing radiation dose, but only in 1965–1980, the last half of the study-interval. The risk was greatest for females under 20 at the time of the bomb. The minimum latent period was 15–20 years.

A series of 106 benign ovarian tumors ascertained at autopsy also revealed a statistically significant increase in tumors as the radiation dose increased. No particular cell type was associated with radiation exposure with respect either to benign or malignant tumors of the ovary.

4. Germ cell tumors

The SEER data were readily tabulated. The three histologic types (germinoma, teratoma and embryonal carcinoma) were about equal in frequency. The gonads were, of course, the most frequently affected organ, with a great male preponderance, 1,548 *vs.* 212 per year among U.S. whites. The two most frequently affected non-gonadal sites also showed a great male preponderance: mediastinum 54 *vs.* 7, and pineal 30 *vs.* 5.

Mori (Tokyo) discussed pineal tumors in Japan. Pineocytoma is rare except in infants. The distribution of 131 cases by cell type was:

	Number	%
Germinoma	76	58
Teratoma, benign	19	14
Teratoma, malignant	11	8
Others	25	19
Total	131	99

The peak was at 10–14 years in males, and the sex-ratio, males/females, was 4:1. Koide, in a review of the Autopsy Annuals in Japan found 3,382 brain tumors in a decade, 214 (6.3%) of which were in the pineal (*10*). In another series at Tokyo University, Hasegawa and Mori found 24 (17.5%) pineal tumors among 137 brain tumors (*4*). Other studies indicate that pineal tumors are about 12 times more common in Japan than elsewhere, and the elevation appears to continue after migration to Hawaii. If so, the excess would be attributable to genetic predisposition. In Japan, a case-control study with special attention to the family history might be of interest. Mori said he had observed two patients with pineal tumors and maldevelopment of both eyes.

Pierce (Denver) summarized experimental studies in which embryonal carcinoma cells or other cancer cells were injected into blastocysts of the mouse. With regard to peculiarities in the occurrence of sex-cell cancers in the human, he said explanations are not available from animal experimentation. We do not know why the rates for choriocarcinoma are so high in Southeast Asia. The neoplasm has not been induced in mice, and the only animal in which it or a similar tumor has been described is the armadillo.

We do not know why whites have a towering peak in the frequency of testicular cancer in adolescence and young adulthood, whereas non-whites do not. Pierce said that in the mouse, testicular cancer is induced experimentally by a gene.

Germ cell tumors of all three main types in the SEER Program were about ten times more frequent in males than females at each of the main anatomic sites. Why? Pierce replied that no explanation was available from experimental studies in which the sex ratio cannot be altered, regardless of cell type.

Developmental biology lacks good probes and good ways to "get into" the embryo. The malignant cell and its phenotypic imprint are now being incorporated into normal development, and the fate of the malignant cell can be followed. Pierce was sure that studies of the blastocyst will reveal how primary embryonic induction works. It is generally believed that embryonic induction is non-specific, but by working with known quantities of inductors, and taking into account possible changes in receptors compounded by the necessity of cell contact, Pierce thought the problem could be solved.

5. Breast

The well-known lower rate for breast cancer in Japan than among U.S. women applies, as expected, to women under 30 years of age. Among U.S. white women in this age-group an estimated 679 new cases of breast cancer develop, and among Japanese about 35 deaths occur annually. Notably, 14 white women in SEER were 15–19 years of age at diagnosis, and in Japan, five deaths from breast cancer were coded as being 10–14 years and three as 15–19 years. Further investigation of these cases would reveal if these tumors were typical breast cancers, and they may be of etiologic interest—with regard to the family history, for example.

Specimens of breast cancer from the Tumor Tissue Registries in Hiroshima and Nagasaki, along with others from biopsies and autopsies at hospitals in the area were reviewed by a panel of six experts, three each from the U.S. and Japan. Tokuoka (Hiroshima) stated that among the 300 specimens, no difference by subtype was found in radiation-induced cancers as compared with those in unexposed women. A strong dose-response relationship was observed among each of the 10-year age cohorts exposed at 10–39 years of age, but there was no excess breast cancer among women who were 40–49 years old at the time of the bomb (ATB). Beyond age 50, the dose-response effect was again seen. Recently, when females exposed before 10 years of age reached the usual age for development of breast cancer, they exhibited an excess in frequency that, in time, may exceed that for older age groups ATB. The frequency of bilateral cases seemed to increased with increasing dose.

In response to the question, do oral contraceptives increase the frequency of breast cancer, the U.S. side learned that less than 5% of Japanese women use these drugs. They are available only on a physician's prescription, a circumstance which discourages their use.

Sakamoto and Sugano (Tokyo) reported that at the Cancer Institute Hospital in Tokyo, they had studied 63 cases of breast cancer in women 20–29 years of age in 1946–1980. The distribution by subtypes was different than in older groups. The younger women had the highest percentage of papillotubular neoplasms, and the lowest percentage of the scirrhous type. Medullary tubular lesions had a constant rate at all ages. Ten-year survival was less good under 30 years of age. Risk factors for breast cancer were not more frequent in this age group; i.e., family history of the neoplasm, bilaterality or the presence of fibrocystic disease.

6. Uterine cervix

Because of ealier sexual activity in the U.S., the rates of cancer of the uterine cervix are likely to rise earlier in life and be higher there than in Japan. Among white women under 30 in the U.S., the SEER program revealed 792 new cases annually. Mortality rates have been declining, however, because of earlier detection through use of the Pap smear and prompt treatment. In the U.S., according to Kessler (Baltimore), an increase in the incidence of in situ cancer of the cervix has been accompanied by a decrease in that for invasive carcinoma.

He said that the youngest age at onset of uterine cervical cancer is in the teens among U.S. blacks and in the early twenties among whites. The SEER Program, however, ascertained four cases annually among whites 10–14 years of age and 18 cases at 15–19 years. Marriage to a man whose previous wife had this cancer increases the risk 2.5-fold for the new wife, he said.

Present knowledge about viruses in the etiology of cervical cancer indicates that either herpes type I or II may be involved. The evidence for a role of human papilloma virus is still weak. Types 6 and 11 have been found in cervical cancer.

7. Vagina

The SEER Program listed 48 women with vaginal carcinoma. The years covered, 1973–1982, followed the discovery in 1971 (5) that maternal use of diethylstilbestrol (DES) during pregnancy caused about 1 in 1,000 daughters to develop clear cell adeno-carcinoma of the vagina or cervix at 8–29 years. The 42 cases at 15–29 years of age registered by the SEER Program may well be of this type, which was previously very rare so early in life. This suggests that early onset of other adult-type tumors may be due to transplacental carcinogenesis.

8. Vulva

The SEER Program listed 32 women under 30 years with cancer of the vulva. All of them were 15–29 years of age. A case-control study might reveal risk factors more easily than studies of larger samples of affected older women, whose longer life-histories may make etiologic influences less discernable.

9. Choriocarcinoma

In the SEER Program carcinoma of the placenta was observed in 78 white women under age 30. Except for one diagnosed at 10–14 years, all occurred at 15–29 years. The high frequency of choriocarcinoma among women in China and neighboring countries is well known. A high proportion are cured by chemotherapy, even when metastases are extensive. The frequency of hydatidiform moles, a precursor, is 1 in 1,200 births in the U.S., 1 in 300 in Japan and 1 in 100 in Southeast Asia. The Trophoblastic Disease Registry in Japan in 1974–1979 listed 10,989 hydatidiform moles, 516 invasive moles and 330 choriocarcinomas.

Moles increase in frequency with advancing maternal age. The effect of migration to the U.S. was not clear with respect to the frequency of hydatidiform moles among Japanese or people from Southeast Asia.

Because most complete moles arise from duplication of a haploid sperm in a functionally empty ovum, malignant transformation is thought to result from homozygosity of a recessive mutant gene. Normally a gene controls cell growth, but upon mutation it can no longer do so, and malignant growth may occur (8).

10. Urinary bladder

Cancer of the urinary bladder affects 134 U.S. white males and 60 white females under age 30 annually according to SEER data. All but 9 were 10 years of age or older. The cell type was not available at the time of the meeting, but case-series previously reported indicate that virtually all who were over 10 years of age had transitional cell carcinoma. Cohen (Omaha) stated that these studies had shown no clustering of cases, excess of familial occurrence, or relation to known (or suspected) carcinogens that affect the bladder (cigarette smoking, occupational exposure, analgesic abuse or cyclophosphamide therapy).

Cohen stated that the histology is the same in both countries. Transitional cell carcinoma may be: a) papillary, 75–90% of all bladder cancer, which is usually non-invasive and recurs frequently—50% of patients have a recurrence in one year, and 90% in 5 years; or b) non-papillary, which has bizarre cells in high-grade lesions—treatable but often invasive before diagnosis, so the 5-year survival rate is low.

Bladder carcinoma under age 30, according to previous studies, is almost limited to males, but the SEER data indicate that in U.S. whites the sex ratio, 2.5 : 1, is similar to that observed in older age-groups. Promoters, such as saccharine or caffeine, prenatally should have little effect because the cell proliferation they can cause is likely to have no effect on cells that are already proliferating at maximal speed in the fetus. Instead, one should look for prenatal influences among exposures such as cigarette smoke, that interact with DNA. Because maternal use of cigarettes during pregnancy causes low birth weight for gestational age, the birth weights of young adults with transitional cell carcinoma of the bladder would be of interest. The SEER cases might, through a case-control study, be so evaluated.

Hematopoietic System

Differences between the U.S. and Japan in the frequencies of cancers of the blood-forming organs have been evaluated by several recent workshops under the binational Cooperative Cancer Research Program (7). The focus has been on a reciprocal relationship between certain lymphoreticular neoplasms (low frequency in Japan) and certain autoimmune diseases (high frequency in Japan).

The neoplasms are nodular lymphoma; Hodgkin's disease under age 30; acute lymphocytic leukemia in children, which did not develop a peak in frequency at 4 years of age until two decades after the peak developed in the U.S.; and chronic lymphocytic leukemia in adults. The autoimmune diseases known to be more frequent in Japan than in the U.S. include systemic lupus erythematosus (SLE), Hashimoto's thyroiditis, and Takayasu's aortitis. Presumably lymphocyte function is different in Japanese than in U.S. whites. In effect, the Japanese have greater protection against the lymphomas, and increased susceptibility to the autoimmune diseases. A similar excess of SLE has been found in Hawaii among all Asians (9, 15). Namba (Hiroshima) described how he used the Tumor Tissue Registry to detect the low frequency of nodular lymphoma. Similar review by Namba of specimens on file in Honolulu was encouraged, comparing whites with the several Asian groups there. The histologic study, as Sugano put it, would then be made "by the same eyes."

The SEER data revealed six cases of multiple myeloma under age 30. The youngest was a boy 9 years of age, whose diagnosis was confirmed by electrophoretic studies and bone marrow study. In Japan 56 deaths under 30, 1968–1978, were ascribed to multiple myeloma, the diagnosis of which is notoriously variable in its accuracy.

The SEER data also revealed 12 cases of Kaposi's sarcoma, nine of them in single males living in San Francisco. The diagnoses were made in 1981–1982, and illustrate that luck is needed in establishing registries for detecting geographically localized clusters. It also exemplifies how a small excess of a rare cancer in a registry can be etiologically important.

Thyroid Cancer

The SEER data showed that thyroid cancer was the diagnosis among whites for 300 males and 1,275 females under 30. The sex ratio was thus 1 : 4.25, similar to that in Japan. A. Sakamoto (Tokyo) had studied cases from the Thyroid Cancer Registry in Japan, which had accessioned 6,012 cases, 1977–1982, 736 of which were under 30 years of age. This resource, previously unknown to the U.S. participants, may afford the opportunity to use record-linkage to find persons in the fixed study-samples of RERF who developed thyroid cancer after they migrated from Hiroshima or Nagasaki.

In another series studied by Sakamoto, among 56 cases under age 30 seen at the Cancer Institute Hospital in Tokyo, 10 (18%) had chronic thyroiditis. This seems to be an important subset from which further understanding of the relationship between the two diseases can be explored.

The Japanese have a great excess of latent carcinomas of the thyroid incidentally discovered at autopsy. There is no age gradient. Stemmermann pointed out that some of the latent lesions were partially or totally sclerosed, suggesting that they arose (and were frozen in place) long ago.

Children's Cancer

Kobayashi (Tokyo) presented data from the All-Japan Children's Cancer Registry, 1969–1982, an extension of data previously published by Hirayama (6). These data have long indicated a deficiency in the frequency of Wilm's tumor (WT) as measured against that for neuroblastoma (Nb). In the SEER Program the ratio, Nb/WT was 441/319= 1.38. In Japan it was 1,691/800=2.11. Wilms' tumor has a relatively constant occurrence throughout the world, although an excess among blacks in the Philadelphia area has recently been reported (12). The question, then, is whether in Japan the rate of Nb is high or that for WT is low. The rates are not available as yet.

Retinoblastoma (Rb) appears to be much more common in Japan than in the U.S. The relative frequencies of Nb, Rb, and WT in each country are:

	SEER	Japan
Nb	49.6%	46.5%
Rb	14.5	31.5
WT	35.9	22.0
	100.0	100.0

Rb varies markedly in frequency geographically. The rates are very high in India and Pakistan. Neuroblastoma varies in the other direction: it is virtually absent in Central Africa (3). In Japan there appears to be an excess of Rb and a deficiency of WT.

Kobayashi said (personal communication) that congenital aniridia with Wilms' tumor occurred only half as often in the Japanese series as in Western countries. Among the 800 patients with WT only 4 or 5 instead of 10 had aniridia. The eye defect is due to partial deletion of the short arm of chromosome 11. Retinoblastoma occurs in a syndrome due to partial deletion of the long arm of chromosome 13. Variation in rates for these cancers may be due to differences in an inherent capacity to maintain chromosomal integrity. Such differences have been reported by Mitelman (14) with regard to chromosomes associated with certain other cancers.

REFERENCES

1. Cain, A. S. and Longino, L. A. Carcinoma of the colon in children. *J. Pediat. Surg.*, **5**, 527–532 (1970).
2. Day, N. E. and Munoz, N. Esophagus. *In* "Cancer Epidemiology and Prevention," eds.

      D. Schottenfeld and J. F. Fraumeni, Jr., pp. 612–613 (1982). W. B. Saunders Co., Phila-
      delphia.
   3. German, J., Bloom, D., and Passarge, E. Bloom's syndrome. VII. Progress report for
      1978. *Clin. Genet.*, **15**, 361–367 (1978).
   4. Hasegawa, A. and Mori, W. Pituitary-adrenal axis in pinealoma. *Acta. Pathol. Japon.*, **32**,
      925–931 (1982).
   5. Herbst, A. L., Ulfelder, H., and Poskanzer, D. C. Adenocarcinoma of the vagina. Associa-
      tion of maternal stilbestrol therapy with tumor appearance in young women. *N. Engl. J.
      Med.*, **284**, 878–881 (1971).
   6. Hirayama, T. Descriptive and analytical epidemiology of childhood malignancy in Japan.
      In "Recent Advances in Managements of Children with Cancer," ed. N. Kobayashi,
      pp. 17–43 (1980). Children's Cancer Association of Japan, Tokyo.
   7. Kadin, M. E., Berard, C. W., Nanba, K., and Wakasa, H. Lymphoproliferative diseases
      in Japan and western countries. *Hum. Pathol.*, **14**, 745–772 (1983).
   8. Kajii, T., Kurashige, H., Ohama, K., and Uchino, F. XY and XX complete moles: Clini-
      cal and morphologic correlations. *Am. J. Obstet. Gynecol.*, **150**, 57–64 (1984).
   9. Kaslow, R. A., High rate of death caused by systemic lupus erythematosus among U. S.
      residents of Asian descent. *Arthritis Rheum.*, **25**, 414–418 (1982).
  10. Koide, O., Watanabe, Y., and Sato, K. A pathological survey of intracranial germinoma
      and pinealoma in Japan. *Cancer*, **45**, 2119–2130 (1980).
  11. Kraemer, K. H., Lee, M. M., and Scotto, J. DNA protects against cutaneous and internal
      neoplasia: Evidence from xeroderma pigmentosum. *Carcinogenesis*, **5**, 511–514 (1984).
  12. Kramer, S., Meadows, A. T., Jarrett, P., and Evans, A. E. The incidence of childhood
      cancer: Experience of a decade in a population-based registry. *J. Natl. Cancer Inst.*, **70**,
      49–55 (1983).
  13. Miller, R. W. Ethnic differences in cancer occurrence: Genetic and environmental differ-
      ences with particular reference to neuroblastoma. *Progr. Cancer Res. Ther.*, **3**, 1–17 (1977).
  14. Mitelman, F. and Levan, G. Clustering of aberrations to specific chromosomes in human
      neoplasms. III. Incidence and geographic distribution of chromosome aberrations in 856
      cases. *Hereditas*, **89**, 207–232 (1979).
  15. Serdula, M. K. and Rhoads, G. G. Frequency of systemic lupus erythematosus in different
      ethnic groups in Hawaii. *Arthritis Rheum.*, **22**, 328–333 (1979).
  16. Willis, R. A. "Pathology of Tumors," p. 947 (1960). Butterworths, New York.

REARRANGING SEGI'S CANCER MORTALITY STATISTICS BY FACTOR AND CLUSTER ANALYSIS

Pelayo CORREA, Diego ZAVALA, and Frank GROVES

Department of Pathology, Louisiana State University Medical Center*

Factor and cluster analyses were applied to age-standardized mortality rates for 1978, previously published by Segi for 46 countries. Seven distinct cancer profiles are described and illustrated. Speculations are offered concerning etiologic factors probably related to such profiles as: affluence, meat-related and milk-related high fat diets, alcohol, tannins, and different types of tobacco exposure. These analyses emphasize the usefulness of Segi's pioneer work in the field of cancer etiology.

One of Professor Mitsuo Segi's important scientific contributions was the computation of international mortality statistics. He applied the age-specific rates of each country to a hypothetical population structure by combining the populations of the countries whose data were being analyzed (*9*). This population model was later "rounded" to provide us with the "world" population model, widely used and adopted by "Cancer Incidence in Five Continents" (*3*). Segi's publications have been of great value in etiologic research and provided information on the countries ranked by their level of risk for each specific cancer site.

Segi's data can be of further help in etiologic analysis if data reduction techniques, such as factor and cluster analysis (*2*), are used. This contribution intends to demonstrate the utility of this approach.

Data Reduction and Analysis

This study is based on age-adjusted death rates (AADR) for 1978, of 11 cancer sites in males and 2 in females, of the 34 countries. For most cancer sites common to both sexes, there is a high correlation between male and female mortality rates. Thus, the inferences from correlations obtained from male AADRs and female AADRs would not differ greatly from those correlations obtained using AADR for one sex only.

In the absence of raw data to calculate a pooled AADR for all countries, an arithmetic mean for each of the 13 selected tumor sites was computed for 46 countries in 1978. This average was used as a denominator to obtain standardized rate ratios (SRR). A profile of the log of the SRR was plotted for each country; 12 countries were excluded from further analysis because their mortality rates for virtually all neoplasms fell far below the average which suggests a serious under-registration bias. The countries excluded are Bulgaria, the Dominican Republic, Ecuador, Egypt, Fiji, Greece, Guatemala, Mauritius, Nicaragua, Romania, Thailand, and Yugoslavia.

---

* New Orleans, Louisiana 70112, U.S.A.

TABLE I. Product Moment Correlation Coefficient

		1	2	3	4	5	6
1	Oral cavity and pharynx	1.0	0.68	0.60	0.05	0.23	−0.25
2	Esophagus		1.0	0.53	0.03	0.10	−0.11
3	Larynx			1.0	−0.01	0.08	−0.17
4	Colon				1.0	0.57	0.79
5	Rectum					1.0	0.36
6	Breast						1.0
7	Lung						
8	Skin						
9	Prostate						
10	Leukemia						
11	Lymphoma						
12	Stomach						
13	Cervix						

Cancer of the uterus and bone cancer were excluded from the analysis. Mortality statistics for cancer of the uterus are hindered by mis-classification with respect to corpus and other unspecified parts of the uterus. The epidemiology of bone cancer is confounded by its being represented by a single code which groups together very different cell types, presumably having different etiologies, and by the failure to distinguish between primary and metastatic tumors.

As a first step of the analysis, SRR were recalculated after the above exclusions, and a Pearson's product-moment correlation coefficient matrix was obtained. This correlation matrix was used in a principal-factor analysis with varimax rotation (12). In "Principal Factor Analysis," intercountry mortality variations for several tumor sites are summarized in terms of linear combinations of a smaller number of distinct and meaningful factors. Each factor can be thought of as a common underlying "dimension of variability" in the data. More specifically, with factor analysis one can identify and quantify that part of the total international variation in cancer mortality that is shared by a group of sites. The common factor analytic model assumes that the variance in each site-specific AADR consists of common variance and unique variance. Common variance is that part of the variation of the AADR for a given cancer site which is in common or shared with the variation in AADR for one or more cancer sites. Unique variance is that part of the variation in AADR for a given cancer site which is specific to that cancer site alone.

The second step of the analysis was to assemble the countries into distinct groups by applying "cluster analysis" to the factor scores for each country which were calculated in the first step. A cluster is a group of countries with common cancer mortality patterns manifested in similar scores on the two factors previously derived, suggesting possible common etiological characteristics. The countries within each set have similar mortality profiles for cancers of the various sites, while the average profile for each group is substantially different from the profiles for the other group of countries.

Cancer Profiles ("Factors") and Clusters

The product-moment correlation matrix of the 13 SRR is shown in Table I. Cancers of the oropharynx, larynx, and esophagus were strongly correlated. Likewise, the

Matrix 13 Tumor Sites in 34 Countries, 1978

7	8	9	10	11	12	13
0.17	−0.27	−0.23	−0.22	−0.36	−0.14	−0.06
0.17	−0.37	−0.19	−0.48	−0.41	0.09	0.02
0.05	−0.29	0.11	−0.11	−0.47	0.00	−0.21
0.55	0.41	0.44	0.42	0.51	−0.62	−0.49
0.57	0.07	0.25	0.04	0.14	−0.16	−0.18
0.56	0.35	0.47	0.43	0.65	−0.60	−0.34
1.0	0.02	0.17	0.12	0.33	−0.35	−0.29
	1.0	0.39	0.40	0.56	−0.42	−0.10
		1.0	0.36	0.49	−0.44	−0.19
			1.0	0.58	−0.38	−0.36
				1.0	−0.65	−0.40
					1.0	0.50
						1.0

SRR of the rectum, breast, lung, skin, prostate, leukemia, lymphoma were positively correlated with colon mortality index. Stomach and cervix showed positive correlation with each other but a negative correlation with colon, breast, lung, skin, prostate, leukemia, and lymphoma.

These three apparent groups of correlated site-specific rates are summarized quite well by just two independent factors. In this study, a cancer site is considered to be significantly related to a factor if the loading for that site on that factor is at least 0.50. The elements of the two factors obtained are listed below:

Factor	Cancer-sites
1	High: colon, rectum, lung, breast, prostate, and lymphoma
	Low: cervix and stomach
2	High: oral cavity/pharynx, larynx, and esophagus

Skin cancer and leukemia, although apparently belonging to the first group, are weakly correlated with both factors as reflected by the low (less than 0.50) absolute value of their factor loadings.

Countries with similar site-specific cancer mortality patterns were identified by cluster analysis; the six clusters of countries obtained are listed in Table II with their corresponding factor scores as well as the average scores for each cluster. France was not grouped into any cluster and is listed as the seventh cluster. Figure 1 shows the profiles of the resulting clusters.

The 13 countries in the first cluster are characterized by high Factor 1 scores, with moderate but consistently negative scores on Factor 2. This cluster includes most of the Anglo-Saxon, industrialized countries of Western and Central Europe, North America, and Oceania. They also have low mortality levels for those cancer sites defined by Factor 2.

Nine countries scored low (below −0.50) on Factor 1, which corresponds to patterns of high stomach and cervical cancer, common in developing countries. In keeping with this pattern, Chile, Costa Rica, and Venezuela are ranked lowest on Factor 1. Japan ranks low in this factor as well, and this is clearly attributable to high stomach cancer mortality in this country. Other countries scoring in the bottom nine for Factor 1 are Hong Kong, Singapore, Poland, Portugal, and Spain.

The second cluster groups Argentina and Cuba with the Mediterranean countries

TABLE II. Results of Cluster Analysis—List of Countries as Selected in Seven Clusters

	Factor 1	Factor 2		Factor 1	Factor 2
Cluster 1			Cluster 3		
Average	0.71	−0.34	Average	0.08	−1.23
Australia	0.70	−0.84	Finland	−0.21	−1.00
Austria	0.31	0.11	Iceland	−0.31	−1.34
Canada	0.97	−0.53	Israel	0.56	−1.53
Denmark	0.66	−0.57	Norway	0.13	−1.09
England and Wales	0.53	−0.20	Sweden	0.24	−1.20
Germany, F. R.	0.31	−0.24			
Ireland	0.97	0.05	Cluster 4		
Netherlands	0.64	−0.61	Average	−2.11	−0.37
New Zealand	1.02	−0.62	Chile	−2.10	−0.09
Northern Ireland	0.63	−0.26	Costa Rica	−2.37	−0.87
Scotland	0.96	−0.09	Japan	−2.03	−0.08
Switzerland	0.58	−0.04	Venezuela	−1.95	−0.59
United States	1.01	−0.67			
			Cluster 5		
			Average	0.74	1.25
Cluster 2			Luxembourg	0.88	1.16
Average	−0.35	0.42	Uruguay	0.59	1.33
Argentina	−0.23	0.59			
Cuba	−0.26	0.16	Cluster 6		
Hungary	0.45	0.40	Average	−0.63	2.13
Italy	0.25	0.44	Hong Kong	−0.57	2.31
Poland	−1.17	0.22	Singapore	−0.69	1.95
Portugal	−0.71	0.56			
Spain	−0.76	0.60	Cluster 7		
			France	0.97	2.33

of Portugal, Spain, and Italy; Hungary and Poland are also included. This cluster is characterized by moderate negative scores for Factor 1 and moderate positive scores for Factor 2. The only tumor site for which these countries display a pronounced excess of mortality is larynx.

In Cluster 3, Israel is grouped with the Scandinavian countries of Finland, Iceland, Norway, and Sweden. Their scores for Factor 2 are quite low, with scores being near zero on Factor 1. These countries have high indexed mortality rates for skin, prostate, and lymphoma, similar to the countries in Cluster 1, but lower levels of mortality for colon, lung, and breast cancer. The five countries scoring lowest on Factor 2 are Finland, Norway, Sweden, Iceland, and Israel.

Cluster 4 identifies three Latin American countries with extremely low Factor 1 scores, reflected in high stomach and cervical cancer rates and unusually low rates for lymphoma, leukemia, prostate, breast, colon, rectum, and lung. Japan is included here as well. These countries contrast well with countries in the first cluster defined above.

The fifth cluster includes two countries, Luxembourg, and Uruguay. They have relatively high positive scores on Factor 1 and high positive scores on Factor 2.

Singapore and Hong Kong were retained as the sixth cluster with very high Factor 2 scores (oral cavity/pharynx, larynx, and esophagus) and negative but moderate scores for Factor 1.

Finally, France has an extremely high score on Factor 2 and a relatively high score

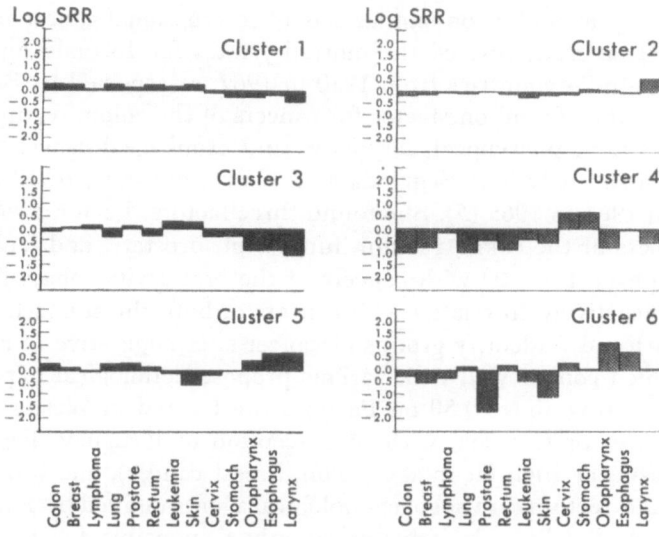

FIG. 1. Cancer profiles identified by cluster analysis

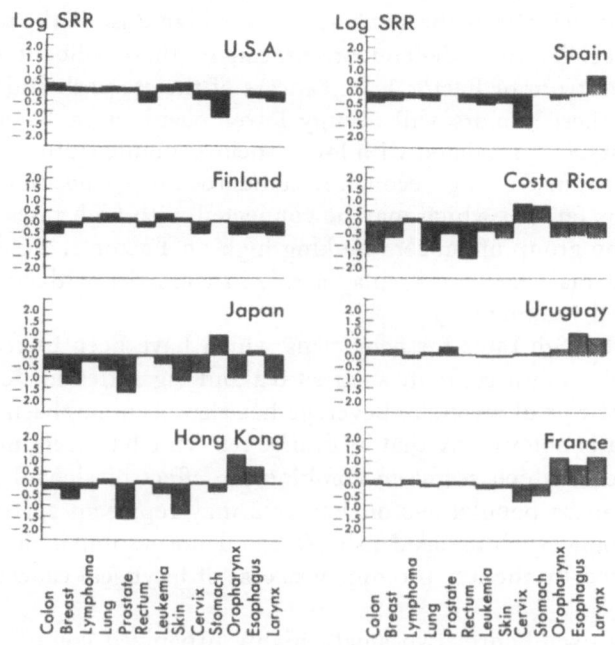

FIG. 2. Cancer profiles for selected countries

on Factor 1. These scores are reflected in a pronounced excess in mortality from cancers of esophagus, mouth, pharynx, and larynx, with a deficit for cervix and stomach.

Interpretation

Our results based on Segi's data for 1978 agree reasonably well with the findings in previous factor-analytic studies on similar sets of international cancer mortality rates in previous years. Yanai *et al.* studied the mortality rates for 13 male tumor sites and 14 female tumor sites in 24 countries from 1950 to 1967, as reported by Segi (*15*). In both males and females, they found one factor for cancers of the colon, rectum, and lung, and another factor for oral, pharyngeal, laryngeal, and esophageal cancer mortality. M. A. Howell applied factor analysis to Segi's data for cancer mortality of 10 male tumor sites in 41 countries in 1964 to 1965 (*5*). She found three factors. Factor 1 was positively correlated with cancers of the colon, rectum, lung, skin, prostate, and leukemia. A second factor linked esophageal cancer with cancers of the oral cavity, pharynx, and larynx. A third factor was negatively correlated with cancers of both the stomach and larynx.

Our Factors 1 and 2 identify groups of cancer sites suggestive of common etiological exposures, which concur well with various proposed etiological hypotheses. Most of the 15 countries scoring above 0.50 on Factor 1 are located in Western or Central Europe, North America or Oceania, with the exception of Uruguay. High cigarette consumption (lung cancer), high fat intake (colon, breast cancer), and low fiber diets (cancer of the colon and rectum) are suspect etiological agents defined by Factor 1. Economic affluence underlines the lifestyle items apparently responsible for Factor 1. Although smoking is prevalent throughout the world, the countries where smoking-related cancers display higher rates combine an early start of the habit (around World War I) and an economic affluence which allows the smokers to use a high dose of the product. Similarly, high fat diets, especially meat-dependent, prevail in these affluent countries. At the lower end of the spectrum of Factor 1 are cancers of the stomach and cervix. Countries with high rates of these tumors will occupy lower positions in Factor 1 rankings. In general, these tumors are associated with lower socioeconomic status. Japan is an exception in this regard because of high economic standard, but its position can be explained on the basis of a low fat diet which may be connected with high rates for gastric cancer and low rates for the group of cancers ranking high on Factor 1. Besides low economic status, the so-called male factor may play a role in countries with high cervical cancer rates, low in Factor 1 ranking (*11*).

Factor 2 reflects high rates for neoplasms which have been linked with the use of substances of a high tannin content, such as tea and cigarettes made of black tobacco (*1, 7, 8, 10, 14*). The role of alcoholic beverage has also been emphasized for these sites, and in this regard it is noteworthy that in France red wine has been implicated in larynx and esophagus cancer, which seems to combine the effect of alcohol and tannins. The high ranking of Chinese populations on Factor 2 may represent specific causes of nasopharyngeal carcinoma, such as aged fish (*16*), and not so much the effect of alcohol. This is also suggested by the less prominent excess of laryngeal cancer in these populations.

Uruguay and Luxembourg, two small, highly urbanized countries, also rank high in Factor 2 scores. Countries with moderate scores on Factors 1 and 2 include the Mediterranean countries of Portugal, Spain, and Italy. Hungary and Argentina are also in this group. It is noteworthy that in these countries there has been a high consumption of red wine and black tobacco.

High laryngeal cancer mortality in the Mediterranean countries as well as in Argentina and Cuba has been noted before. The important contrast in these countries, however, is that while in Argentina and Cuba both lung and larynx cancer mortality are high, in the Mediterranean countries oral and esophageal rather than lung cancer mortality match the high larynx cancer mortality, These differences may indicate differences in the use of black tobacco and the types of alcoholic beverages.

Figure 1 depicts the average cancer mortality profile for all countries belonging to each cluster. Figure 2 gives individual examples of countries representing each cluster. The United States represents the typical rates of Cluster 1. The only exception is rectal cancer, which may be artifactual and related to differences in coding tumors of the recto-sigmoid to rectum in some countries and to colon in others. In few words, this cluster represents affluent societies with high tobacco use and high fat diet. Cluster 2, well represented by Spain, represents the larynx cluster, probably related to black tobacco and alcohol consumption. Cluster 3, represented by Finland, is similar to Cluster 1 except that the high fat diet depends more on milk than on meat. Cluster 4 may indicate low fat and low exposure to tobacco in previous decades, represented by Costa Rica with high gastric and high cervical cancer rates and by Japan where the only apparent present-day cancer epidemic is that of gastric cancer. Cluster 5, represented by Uruguay, depicts the least favorable situation with fat-related, smoking-related, tannin-related, and alcohol-related cancer epidemics. Cluster 6 apparently characterizes some Chinese populations whose cancer epidemics are limited to the nasopharynx and esophagus. The last cluster, exclusively represented by France, has a profile similar to that of Uruguay except that it seems to have brought under control the cervical and gastric cancer epidemics.

Acknowledgment

This work was supported by Grant No. P01-CA-28842 from the National Cancer Institute, National Institutes of Health.

REFERENCES

1. Cook-Mozaffari, T. J., Azordegan, F., Day, N. E., Ressicaud, A., Sabai, C., and Aramesh, B. Oesophageal cancer studies in the Caspian Littoral of Iran: results of a case-control study. *Br. J. Cancer*, **39**, 293–309 (1979).
2. Dillon, W. R. and Goldstein, M. "Multivariate Analysis. Methods and Applications." J. Wiley and Sons, New York (1984).
3. Doll, R. Comparison between registries. Age-standardized rates. *In* "Cancer Incidence in Five Continents," eds. J. H. Waterhouse, C. Muir, P. Correa, and J. Powell, pp. 453–459 (1976). IARC Lyon, France.
4. Dunham, L. and Bailar, J. World maps of cancer mortality rates and frequency ratios. *J. Natl. Cancer Inst.*, **14**, 155–203 (1968).
5. Howell, M. A. Factor analysis of international mortality data and per capita food consumption. *Br. J. Cancer*, **29**, 328–336 (1974).
6. Joly, G. Dark tobacco and lung in Cuba. *J. Natl. Cancer Inst.*, **70**, 1033–1039 (1983).
7. Morton, J. F. Tentative correlations of plant usage and esophageal cancer zones. *Economic Botany*, **24**, 217–226 (1970).
8. Segi, M. Tea-gruel as a possible factor for cancer of the esophagus. *Gann*, **66**, 199–202 (1975).
9. Segi, M. "Age-adjusted Death Rates for Cancer for Selected Sites (A-classification) in 46 Countries in 1978," (1984). Segi Institute of Cancer Epidemiology, Nagoya, Japan.
10. Simarak, S., de Jong, U.W., Breslow, N., and Dahl, C. J. Cancer of the oral cavity, pharynx, larynx and lung in North Thailand: case-control study and analysis of cigar smoke. *Br. J. Cancer*, **36**, 130–139 (1977).

11. Skegg, D. C., Corwin, P. A., Paul, C., and Doll, R. Importance of the male factor in cancer of the cervix. *Lancet*, **ii**, 581–583 (1982).

12. "Statistical Analysis System, User's Guide: Statistics," First edition (1982). SAS Institute Inc., Cary, North Carolina.

13. Tuyns, A. and Audigier, J. Double wave cohort increase for oesophageal and laryngeal cancer in France—relation to reduced alcohol consumption during the Second World War. *Digestion*, **14**, 197–208 (1976).

14. Vassalo, A., Correa, P., DeStefani, E., Cendan, M., Zavala, D., Chen, V., Carzoglio, J., and Deneo-Pellegrini, H. Esophageal cancer in Uruguay: a case-control study. *J. Natl. Cancer Inst.*, **75**, 1005–1009 (1985).

15. Yanai, H., Inaba, Y., Takagi, H., and Yamamoto, S. Multivariate analysis of cancer mortality for selected sites in 24 countries. *Environ. Health Perspect.*, **32**, 83–101 (1979).

16. Yu, M. C., Ho, J.H.C., Shiu-Hung, L., and Henderson, B. E. Cantonese-style salted fish as a cause of nasopharyngeal carcinoma: report of a case-control study in Hong Kong, *Cancer Res.*, **46**, 956–961 (1986).

AUTHOR INDEX

SUBJECT INDEX